GMO FREE
Child

A Parent's Guide to Dietary Cleanup of Genetically Modified Organisms

INKWATER
PRESS

PORTLAND · OREGON
INKWATERPRESS.COM

BY APRIL SCOTT, HHC

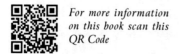

*For more information
on this book scan this
QR Code*

Publisher: Inkwater Press | www.inkwaterpress.com

ISBN-13 978-1-62901-395-4 | ISBN-10 1-62901-395-1

Printed in the U.S.A.

1 3 5 7 9 10 8 6 4 2

Dedications

This book is dedicated to my lovely daughters, my magnificent grandchildren and to all children suffering the ill-effects of the SAD GMO Diet. May all parents revolt on your behalf. And to my wonderful husband and great love, I could not have done this without you!

Much love,
April Scott
The Cleanfood Advocate

For my dad, David H. Saragosa:

The Seven Deadly Sins are:

Wealth without Work
Pleasure without conscience
Knowledge without character
Business without morality
Science without humanity
Worship without sacrifice
Politics without principle

- Mahatma Gandhi

Acknowledgments

I have deep gratitude for the contributions of the following individuals to this book and their valiant efforts to stop this Public Health Emergency.

Jeffrey Smith
Dr. Thierry Vrain
Dr. Nancy Swanson
Dr. Stephanie Seneff
Dr. Les Berenson
Diana Reeves
Amber King

Table of Contents

Introduction

Our Story

I was a single mom working 10-hour days most of which were spent in high gear. Regrettably, I paid little attention to the quality of food I fed my family. I had little interest in cooking and quick meals were simply a means to stop the rumbling tummies and get on with the day. I went about my business totally oblivious to the concept of buyer beware or the nutritional needs of little bodies. outside the misfortunes of the USDA Food Pyramid.

I was raised with a special love and patriotism for my country, "land of the free, home of the brave." I trusted that our government had our best interest at heart. At the same time, I was also taught to be suspicious of the political rhetoric, behind the facade of the "American Dream." Being a child of the 70s, I wanted to believe the best about everyone, including the leaders of *our great country tis of thee.* I know it sounds naive looking back; I should have taken more stock in my mother's examples, cooking from scratch, growing a garden, using herbs and such. We rarely ate at restaurants; however, that was typical before the "microwave processed food revolution." Sure we had mac and cheese, helpers of hamburger and even McDonalds, but an explosion of nutritionally deficient, processed foods began to saturate the US market in the 80s, tagging along the GMO "Green Revolution" of the 90s. Now mind you, that decade, I earned a bachelor's degree in criminology with a minor in broadcast media and began working for a major news station as a talk show producer. I didn't have my head in the sand, or so I thought.

It still took me until the Spring of 2008 to catch on to the changes that had occurred when I happened upon the documentary film *The Future of Food,* by Deborah Koons Garcia; that hit me with a bombshell of shock and disbelief. [1] How did I have no idea that an estimated 75-80 percent of our food supply had been genetically rearranged? [1] Why hadn't I been told? Why hadn't I voted on it? How could this have happened? Had I been asleep for the past decade? This whole revelation threw me into a whirlwind of panic, anxiety and a deep depression. To top it off, the time-line nearly clashed with the discovery that my youngest child had developed more than 62 food and environmental allergies; it was the perfect storm. So, you can only imagine my dismay as I riffled diligently through my cabinets and fridge, only to find a myriad of questionable GMO options that filled my grocery cart just the day before.

Devastated, I slumped to the floor in tears, infuriated at the circumstances and feeling hopeless against the mountains of madness I had just discovered. I was furious at our gatekeepers for letting this happen. I, like so many parents, thought the FDA and USDA had our back. I trusted them. Didn't they have families of their own to feed?

After pausing for a total breakdown, I pulled up my big girl panties, trashed hundreds of dollars in food-like products and headed for the natural food store for my GMO-Free education. In blind confusion, I spent more on food that day than I usually did in a whole month, justifying the necessary expenses for the safe-guard of my daughter's health.

Thankfully, now I'm able to arm you with the knowledge and experience I've gained, along with time/money saving tips, and tools to empower you and help you stay the course with your GMO-Free child.

Prior to these disturbing revelations about the food changes, my daughter had been suffering from allergies, chronic headaches, severe nasal congestion (since infancy), dark circles under her eyes (most days), learning and extreme behavioral challenges, along with a myriad of seemingly disconnected symptoms, which I now believe may be related to Autism Spectrum Disorder (ASD), though I've yet to have that confirmed.

The more I found out the more adamant I became that I wasn't going to take any chances with Rya's fragile health following these damages, I believe for the most part, were caused by my uneducated, GMO-glyphosate laden pregnancy and subsequent exposures to the Standard American Diet (SAD), along with other unknown environmental risk factors. I was floored by the (industry independent) GMO feeding studies on animals showing a variety of concerning outcomes and health conditions like chronic digestive and immune system malfunction, allergies, liver damage, tumors and even cancer. All of my light bulbs blew up at once. As we'll discuss later, there have been more than a few highly competent scientists whose GMO research has led to some very unexpected results. Some of these surprising outcomes have thoroughly crushed their careers after the researchers went public with their safety concerns. See Chapter 2 "Independent Science."

So what if I was chained to a rock and hard place. I wasn't going to compromise my child's wellbeing any further for a few lousy dollars. Realistically though, it was a whole different story; in the beginning, I barely surpassed income for the Food Stamp limit. I didn't make enough money as an administrative assistant for the state. There wasn't any wiggle room in my strict budget to allow for such luxuries like clean organic, allergy-free specialty foods, or so I thought. Sometimes I couldn't even afford socks without holes for that matter. Regardless of my tight budget, I resolved that I would live in my car before I would submit to the notion of feeding my child a mishmash of genetically altered *Frankenfoods*, when the feeding studies showed such concerning health effects. Meanwhile, I introduced my new nemesis to everyone I knew. I lodged lengthy complaints to anyone who would listen, many of which are still considered instrumental in state government and public health. Nobody listened; they said things like, "It's just a conspiracy theory" or worse, "We're all going to die from something anyway."

I felt alone and abandoned in hell by people I trusted and whose intelligence I admired. They thought I had lost my marbles, brainwashed by some food conspiracy cult that kidnapped me over the weekend. Nobody understood what I was going through. Besides, they shoot the messenger - don't they?

I began publishing cheeky online articles after a friend introduced me to the editors of *Salem-News.com*. Tim and Bonnie King host a group of former journalists gone rouge. These edgy, online truthtellers cross the lines of traditional journalism with hundreds of thousands of international readers a month, scouring their pages for the real-raw story behind the big-media facade. The editors welcomed my so-called "conspiracy" and no-nonsense critical approach to the government collusion surrounding our contaminated food supply. They allowed me, in article after article, to blaze out criticisms of the FDA, USDA, EPA and Monsanto free of censorship. That was just the beginning.

Back to School

I knew if I was going to be able to feed my kid with 62 food allergies and successfully navigate the detriments of the Standard American Diet (SAD), I had better re-learn everything, so I went back to school. While still working those 10-hour shifts I spent nights, weekends and even lunch hours studying to become a holistic health and nutrition coach. I earned my certification from the Institute for Integrative Nutrition (IIN) and the American Association of Drugless Practitioners (AADP). Of course, IIN challenged everything I thought I knew about food, health and nutrition. It was money very well spent. I discovered a new route to wellbeing, avoiding the paths and pitfalls of self-destruction using whole food and plant-based options, rather than pharmaceutical means. If we are to heal ourselves and our broken medical system, then we must free ourselves of the mindset that there is a pill for every ill.

I have seen considerable, amazing improvements in the people around me and in my daughter's health, behavior and cognitive abilities, since our *cleanfood* commitment began. I will share some testimonials in Chapter 5. It does take some time, consistency and dedication to experience the full effects of this lifestyle! You'll probably begin feeling better and seeing a significant difference in your child in the first week or so; and that will indeed keep you engaged for the long haul.

Although navigating the GMO food supply (without labels) has some steep learning curves, there are many great options for you to discover. And I'm going to lend you my daily mantra. Be sure to memorize it and repeat it often. You will indeed need it. Ready, here it goes – *It's a process, not an event!* This handy little statement will keep you sane; it will help you maintain your motherly (or fatherly) composure, regardless of the circumstances before you. It is relevant to everything you're about to learn, so every time you say it, let it remind you of your commitment and most of all that you are doing your best to navigate a difficult situation. It takes time to establish a new way of living for you and your GMO-Free child. Please be patient with yourself and them.

Once you begin the process it will build energy rather quickly. Please remember I'm here to support and guide you with my extensive knowledge and experience navigating this GMO mine-field as a broke single mom. I'm optimistic that the momentum of the GMO-Free movement, as well as product labeling trends, will continue to expand our market options as producers respond to those who vote with their dollars.

Unfortunately many children and adults appear to be suffering countless ill effects from long-term consumption of GMO foods. Of course we can't be completely certain without a good labeling and tracking system in place, because let's face it, if *you can't track it, you can't control it*. We don't know for sure which foods contain GMO ingredients, and which do not, without labeling. Therefore producers cannot be implicated in the cause and effect relationships between their products and the symptoms in your child, if any, do indeed exist. It is no secret that a record number of our children are experiencing a myriad of serious health effects, and disorders never seen before in such gigantic proportions, since GMOs began infiltrating our food supply in 1996.

Robyn O'Brien is an author, public speaker and mother of four. She launched the AllergyKids Foundation after her youngest had a severe allergic reaction to unknown GMO ingredients in her breakfast [2]. Robyn is dedicated to educating parents about recent changes in our food supply and the striking increases in the rate of allergies, asthma, ADHD and autism in the last two decades, since they introduced GMOs to the public market. Following this contamination we have seen a:

- 400% increase in allergies
- 300% increase in asthma
- 400% increase in ADHD
- 1,500 to 6,000% increase in Autism-Spectrum Disorders (ASD). [2]

I will introduce you to several more unsung heroes of the GMO-Free movement in the coming chapters, including medical doctors, scientists and parents who are saying enough is enough.

You will read the lab results in animal feeding studies that are running parallel to our current childhood epidemics. So far scientists say there have not been any "official" human GMO feeding studies behind laboratory doors.

Our children are acting as the lab rats of this experiment and they are suffering like never before. Under these horrific circumstances, we must look at every possible causation factor, honing in on what has changed for our children over the course of the past 20 years. What is causing such high levels of illness amongst our youngest, most vulnerable citizens? After you read this book I think perhaps you will have an answer to that.

You will get to know parents, like yourself, that are struggling to manage the health of their children within the confines of the GMO food box. I know that you will become inspired to make lasting changes that will help you raise a happy, healthy GMO-Free child.

The GMO Rubik's Cube

I recall a wise scientist, Michael Antoniou, raving about the recently discovered "health risks of genetically modified foods and glyphosate-based herbicides." He says scientists didn't understand the outcomes of genetic transfer in the early days of genetic engineering. They thought they could just move around a few genes, and they would function independently, without any consideration for how they perform as a whole organism? *Bravo scientists*, I smugly thought to myself. That epiphany took hold of me immediately, when I figured out that they were redesigning the very structure of our genetic core and the keys to life on this planet. It was obvious from the start that this would cause an environmental catastrophe that this world has never seen, along with an enormous assault on public health and the human rights of every individual. This indiscriminate attack was generated behind closed doors, and carried out with machine gun tactics, against an unsuspecting public with our most vulnerable citizens in the line of fire.

Over the course of two decades, this war on our children has delivered widespread surges in childhood epidemics and disorders, becoming the very epitome of evidentiary proof of a full-blown public health emergency, as our children are chained to the front lines of battle as the barometers of a revolution. The toll is high and I'm not willing to pay it. I promise that I will not stand by silently and let them experiment on your child, much less my own. That is the reason I am here including you in this very important discussion. You don't know, what you don't know. I come to you with a mother bear perspective, as a criminologist, writer, researcher, holistic health coach and small farmer.

It is my humble opinion, along with over 800 independent scientists and those *Millions Against Monsanto,* that the mix-and-match process of gene recoding and the crossing of kingdom barriers is inherently foolish. It raised all my red flags from the get-go. I don't think you need to be a brilliant scientist at all to see the pitfalls of their destructive plan. I took biology in high school and again in college. I have a bachelor's degree in criminology with a minor in broadcast media. I produced four talk radio shows a day, before there was even an internet and also worked as a copywriter for a major news station in Portland, Oregon. Think of me as a trained pit bull that likes to dig, and this situation has reeked like rotten meat since I got my first sniff in 2008. As you can imagine, I'm quite skilled at sorting out the BS from the evidentiary proof to come to a logical, common sense conclusion. For example, you can't put the genetic code to life on a Rubik's Cube, (metaphor alert), without a clear expectation of severe health and ecological consequences that are inevitable from such an undertaking.

I'm sure you played with a Rubik's Cube as a child or, at least, you observed others within the throws of the conundrum. What happened? Within minutes it was an array of assorted colors for which there was no turning back. You could spend days trying to get one side all green again, and then you had five more sides to contend with and so you gave up. Few folks had the wherewithal or attention span to complete the puzzle.

Now imagine that Rubik's Cube and replace the colors with separate genes (keys to life) from different species of plants, animals, bacteria and viruses. Now, randomly twist and turn that cube, add generous helpings of glyphosate, antibiotics, and various chemical fertilizers and then feed it to your child. This process is creating a synthetic mish-mash of genes and new life forms this world has never seen. For example, ever see a pig with a cowhide? Monsanto has done it. There is no telling how many combinations of new organisms and mutated life forms will result affecting the entire food chain, our planet and our children's children, for all generations to come. This asinine experiment is changing the very core of our existence, and it is our job as parents to do everything we can to shield our children from the repercussions; and teach them how to feed themselves into adulthood and beyond within this hostile food environment.

I recall an article in the *New England Journal of Medicine*, "A Potential Decline in Life Expectancy in the United States in the 21st Century," reporting that the health of our children is diminishing so fast that the life expectancy of this generation's children is expected to be shorter than their parents. That is largely due to significant spikes in childhood obesity rates, heart disease and Type 2 diabetes in our nation's children. [1]

I'm not here to be a fear monger but simply a messenger with the candid truth that will no longer sit by quietly, letting your child become a barometer in the GMO food experiment, without your knowledge and consent! Atrocities are being perpetuated upon our children through the food they need to survive. They are all of our children and we are all responsible for what is taking place here. If we don't speak up and resist the pretty packages and plastic lies, we will all be in this sinking boat together.

You, like many parents, might find yourself witness to dramatic changes in the health, behavior and mental capabilities of your child within days and weeks of going GMO-Free.

If your child is suffering like mine was, quite possibly, you will begin to recognize your real child behind the myriad of unexplainable symptoms.

Don't forget we are available on our private *Facebook* page with updated information, support and answers when you need them. Perhaps you have a favorite recipe that you want to convert? Let us help. Come visit: *facebook.com/groups/1589064821351920/*

CHAPTER 1

Why GMO?

"Monsanto should not have to vouchsafe the safety of biotech food.... Our interest is in selling as much of it as possible. Assuring its safety is the FDA's job."

> —Phil Angell, Director of Corporate Communications, Monsanto, quoted in *New York Times Magazine*, October 25, 1998.

"Ultimately, it is the food producer who is responsible for assuring safety."

> — FDA, "Statement of Policy: Foods Derived from New Plant Varieties" (GMO Policy), *Federal Register*, Vol. 57, No. 104 (1992), p. 22991

What are Genetically Modified Organisms?

Foods derived from genetically modified organisms (GMO or GM) are also referred to as transgenic or simply genetically engineered (GE). The terms are used interchangeably throughout science and this text. [1, 2]

In simplified terms, the process of genetic engineering can be described as a synthetic re-configuration of the genetic material or DNA (deoxyribonucleic acid) from a variety of non-related plants and animals that normally wouldn't mix.

Genes are selected, cloned and driven into the cellular structure of the host plant, using an invasive gene gun technique to penetrate the plant's natural barriers. A second approach uses a soil bacteria called Agrobacterium that causes tumors in plants, or galls in trees. This allows the new genes to transfer themselves into the host's DNA. [3, 4] Genes taken from the cauliflower mosaic virus (CaMV), used as a promoter, will allow this new combination to take hold and multiply within the plant's cells.

Of course, there are other approaches to hacking our genetic codes and new ones are most certainly on the horizon. The bottom line is that this mixing and matching of our genetic data has many scientists pointing to one concerning aspect of this development, and that is the perception of control over the inherent features and traits of plants and animals. [3, 4, 5] This perception of control over genetic factors, and nature, is simply an illusionary concept.

In June 2015, I was thrilled to interview consumer advocate and GMO-Free world champion, Jeffrey Smith, a best-selling author and award winning producer of the book and film *Genetic Roulette: The Gamble of Our Lives.* This movie is a mind-blowing exposé, revealing the inside-scoop behind big biotech food and the real science that has been ignored. Since its 2012 release, *Genetic Roulette* has continued to capture the attention of international audiences and governments alike, while prompting a passionate storm of controversy and activism for the state of our food supply and environmental health.

As a major critic of GMO technology, he explains it like this:

> Scientists take genes from one species like bacteria or viruses and make millions of copies and put it into a gene gun and shoot it to implant millions of cells, using the bacteria to infect the cells; then they clone the cells into plants. Following that process our farmers spray Roundup herbicide on those crops that are designed to withstand the toxic chemical without dying.

Types of GMOs

The documentary film *Bought* defines three categories of GMOs:

1. <u>Bt toxins</u>: engineered into corn, soy and cotton plants. They are specifically designed to produce the toxin within the plant itself. The toxins work because they burst the stomachs of insects that come into contact. The corn is registered with the EPA as a pesticide. [6]

2. <u>Roundup Ready</u>: plants that are re-engineered to survive large amounts of pesticide applications without dying. The US sprays around 5 billion pounds of Roundup on crops each year. This method kills everything but the plant. About 68 percent of GM crops are herbicide tolerant. [6]

3. GMOs that don't use pesticides at all are those that have been created with special genetic traits using promoter genes to wake up latent genes that have been suppressed. [6]

In coming chapters, we'll discuss concerns around potential consequences of waking up latent genes, for example, cancer in our populations.

Who is Monsanto?

Although Monsanto is not the only biotech company genetically remastering our planet, they are the largest company with many pharmaceutical and agricultural subsidiaries under their corporate umbrella. [7]

Monsanto started in 1901 as a chemical company. They currently are the largest seed developer in the world. Prior to genetically engineered crops, their first product on the market was one called saccharine, which is a main ingredient in the sugar alternative Sweet'N Low. Monsanto's past also embraces some of the world's most controversial developments like agent orange, DDT, aspartame, dioxins, sulphuric acid, Astroturf, polychlorinated biphenyls (PCBs) which are used in the development of plastic and other chemical compounds, synthetic fabrics, pesticides, herbicides like Roundup, rBGH (recombinant Bovine Growth Hormone) and much, much more. In addition, they were heavily involved in uranium research for the Manhattan Project. [7] Knowing this I was curious about what Monsanto had to say for themselves. So I checked out their website boasting the following:

> Our Human Rights Policy is guided by the Universal Declaration on Human Rights, which provides the most widely recognized definition of human rights... Whereas recognition of the inherent dignity and of the equal and inalienable rights of all members of the human family is the foundation of freedom, justice and peace in the world; Whereas disregard and contempt for human rights have resulted in barbarous acts which have outraged the conscience of mankind, and the advent of a world in which human beings shall enjoy freedom of speech and belief and freedom from fear and want has been proclaimed as the highest aspiration of the common people; Whereas it is essential, if man is not to be compelled to have recourse, as a last resort, to rebellion against tyranny and oppression, that human rights should be protected by the rule of law... [8]

Stay tuned to see if this mission rings true throughout the state of their business affairs.

Why Did They Develop GMOs?

GMO products are sold with the following benefit claims:

- Resistant to weeds, pests and other diseases
- Larger yields
- Less pesticide use
- Better texture, flavor and nutrition
- Longer shelf life
- Sustainable practices [9]

A Patent on Life

The "genetic revolution" gave Monsanto a patent on life. This controversial move eliminated government restrictions on the patenting of living organisms. Food crops and other products of nature were excluded from patenting for over 200 years, because of moral grounds. In the 1930s this restriction was slightly amended, as they allowed plant breeders to begin patenting their work, although the patent did not extend to the plants or seeds after the first generation seedlings. [10]

Everything changed after 1978, when microbiologist and engineer for General Electric, Ananda Mohan Chakrabarty, submitted a patent request for an oil-eating microorganism. The patent office turned him down flat, but General Electric and Chakrabarty took the matter all the way to the Supreme Court. The judges overruled the patent office decision in Chakrabarty's favor. This world changing decision opened the floodgates for Monsanto's gene revolution. [10]

He Who Controls the Food...

The concept behind the patenting of seeds was, from the beginning, an attempt to capitalize on nature itself. It's speculated that Monsanto has claim to everything that contains their genetically engineered organisms, whether that be seeds, plants, animals or perhaps even people. This gives corporations the power to own and control life. [10]

In the documentary film *The Future of Food* we see Monsanto buying up major seed companies, left and right, during the 90s'. Basically the pesticide industry spent 8 million dollars buying up seed companies. Taking advantage of new patent laws, these industries began patenting traditional seeds that had not been patented before. They even went into the seed banks that were established to protect biodiversity, got samples of unpatented varieties from vaults, and applied for patents on them. As long as they were there first they got the patent. [10]

Monsanto owns over 11,000 patents in the US and worldwide. With that, the company is able to create the one seed that will replace all the others, and since they own all the others, they conveniently control production and distribution. [10]

Henry Kissinger said it best, *"Control oil and you control nations; control food and you control the people."*

GMO vs. Traditional Crossbreeding

"Genetic engineering is to traditional Crossbreeding, what the nuclear bomb was to the sword."

Andrew Kimbrell, Center for Food Safety

Farmers have been crossbreeding plants for generations and the word in the field is that genetic modification techniques are no different. That could not be further from the truth. Nature designed it so that traditional gardeners were able to cultivate new varieties of crops, through years of selective breeding, by cross-pollinating two different but related plants, thus taking six to ten generations to develop. Eventually they could create a new type of plant that was more suited to their soil or climate, as well as more disease and insect resistant. [11]

Later on, hybrid plants were able to do this within one generation as discovered by Charles Darwin and his associate Gregor Mendel, a scientist and Roman Catholic monk. They were able to take two different plants and crossbreed them to create traits in their crops that were more desirable for growers. This gave growers more control and the selective methods were termed, F1 hybrids. [11, 12] This brought us canola, sweet corn, cantaloupes, seedless watermelons, tangelos and clementine oranges. [12]

As it turns out, the big hybrid disappointment for farmers was, and still is, the poor outcomes in the second generation planting of those novel types. Often those hybrid seeds won't regenerate correctly, if at all. When they do, they are often deformed or lack the qualities they were bred for originally. [13]

Rebsie Fairholm is the "the daughter of the soil." She calls hybrid "the one-hit wonder," indicating that hybrids cause some frustration for many gardeners in their seed saving efforts. She notes they are often a crap-shoot when you want to maintain those special varieties without going back to the seed producers who are making a racket on sales. [13]

It is estimated that 70 percent of food grown worldwide is from backyards and small farms. Farmers never had to buy seeds before. Poor rural villages, around the world, have survived for thousands of years because of their traditional plant breeding and seed saving techniques passed on from generation to generation, village to village, hand to land. [14.15]

In the documentary film *One Man, One Cow, One Planet* it is calculated that some of these biotech seeds cost Indian farmers nearly 400 percent more than conventional seeds, and farmers complain that their yields are often about 30 percent less. Indian dealers get huge commissions for GM related product sales, although a 2006 report said 60 percent of Indian farmers using GMO seeds could not recoup their investment, let alone feed their families. [14]

Poor farmers who never even had to buy seeds, now have to also purchase fertilizer and chemicals. Plus the seeds often need more water to thrive than traditional crops do. This keeps the farmers in a cycle of debt perpetually having to buy new seeds and chemicals every year. [11, 14, 15]

Indian and Latin American farmers have been left with no choice but to sell their farms and migrate to bustling cities to look for work. Many farmers don't leave their land; instead they choose suicide as an escape route from the financial burden and the shame of not being able to feed their families. [11, 15, 16, 17]

Control of our seeds, and thus our food, was intentionally taken from the soil of our farmers and put into the hands of a few multinational corporations that do not have our best interest at heart. As a result, the world has lost about 75 percent of our crop biodiversity. [11] As opposed to traditional and natural breeding techniques, genetic engineering methods bore us a whole different animal. This technology crisscrosses biological kingdoms through gene splicing techniques, penetrating foreign DNA from different classes of plants and animals into the cells of unrelated species. [18] Although this new food often looks, smell and in some cases, tastes the same as its historical counterparts, you can be certain that what you are eating today is not the same as Grandma used to make.

Crossing Kingdoms

GMO crops are the result of crossing multiple kingdoms and classes of species whose natural barriers would never intersect without artificial means. [18] As noted earlier, this "Rubik's Cube" type method mixes genetic codes (keys to life) from different species of plants, animals, bacteria and viruses. Essentially, they randomly twist and turn this theoretical cube adding generous helpings of glyphosate, antibiotics and various chemical fertilizers. [18] This technology creates a synthetic mish-mash of genes and mutated life forms this world has never seen. For example, the new GMO salmon has genetic material from an eel-sort of fish and a Pacific Chinook salmon that produces growth hormones, causing it to grow twice as big as your wild salmon.

In my 2010 article "Speak Now or Forever Hold Your Fish" I encouraged consumers to participate in the public comment period by writing the FDA Veterinary Medicine Advisory Committee, which presides over these matters. [19]

And in the film *Genetic Roulette*, Smith reveals that labs are now mixing pig and cow genes so that pigs will grow cowhides! Furthermore, spider genes are being inserted into goats, so they can milk them and get spider web proteins to make bulletproof vests. Human genes, Smith says, are also being mixed up with corn genes to make spermicides. [20]

Why Poison?

The Encyclopedia Britannica says, "In regard to poisoning, chemicals can be divided into three broad groups: agricultural and industrial chemicals, drugs and health care products, and biological poisons—i.e., plant and animal sources." [21] Most agricultural chemicals are pesticides which include other categories like insecticides, herbicides, fungicides, fumigants, and also rodenticides. [21]

The first pesticides were mostly made from arsenic and hydrogen cyanide. Farmers abandoned these early versions because they were seen as ineffective and/or too toxic for frequent use. Then came the second generation of pesticides that included synthetic organic compounds, synthetic, meaning manmade and organic, containing carbon, but we won't confuse that with organic farming. We'll get to that later. [22]

Silent Spring & DDT

The first synthetic pesticides were chlorinated hydrocarbons (or organochlorine) called dichlorodiphenyltrichloroethane or better known as DDT. An Austrian chemist named Othmar Zeidler first developed the compound in 1874, although he didn't recognize that it could be used as an insecticide. [23]

In the mid-1930s a Swiss chemist named Paul Muller began to search for an effective insecticide whose potent toxicity would be fatal enough to kill the "maximum number" of insects, but that wouldn't be too toxic to plants or warm-blooded animals. The chemical also needed to be non-water soluble, so he could be sure that it would stay in the environment for long periods of time and not get washed away (off). DDT fit the bill perfectly (or so it was thought) and it was cheap to make. A few years later the Swiss government put it into circulation. Following their footsteps the United States Department of Agriculture (USDA) wasn't far behind. Then the infamous Monsanto Corporation took over production in 1944 developing the chemical themselves. [23]

Outspoken environmental champion Rachel Carson shocked the world when she released an international best-selling book called *Silent Spring* in 1962, revealing the toxic effects of DDT on the health of humans, wildlife and our environment. Her publication caused widespread public concern and controversy, and it also led to the development of the US Environmental Protection Agency (EPA) which was created to protect human and environmental health as the guardians of our land, air and water. Where are those assurances now? [24]

The *New York Times* says *Silent Spring* sold more than two million copies, and it made a powerful case for the idea that if humankind poisoned nature, nature would in turn poison humankind. "Our heedless and destructive acts enter into the vast cycles of the earth and in time return to bring hazard to ourselves," Carson told a subcommittee. [25] As a result, in 1972, EPA outright banned DDT citing toxic effects on wildlife, the environment and probable health risks. For example, it impairs reproduction in animals and possibly humans.

Studies have continued to focus on DDT, finding that the chemical accumulates in fatty tissue and causes live tumors in animals. DDT is classified as a probable human carcinogen by the US and other international authorities. [26]

Roundup Ready

Not far behind the DDT debacle, a Swiss chemist named Henri Martin worked feverishly to develop a charming little molecule called glyphosate in the 50s. By 1964, Stauffer Chemicals had swooped in and applied for patent on it as a chelating agent, seeing that it would easily bind to metals. In the early days it was used to clean industrial pipes, until it was discovered that the chemical kills plants by inhibiting some of their key processes. [27]

Monsanto was still reeling from the whole DDT humiliation when they got their hands on the patent for glyphosate in 1969; they were able to pull it off as an active ingredient in their herbicide Roundup. Quickly, they shoved it onto the market for starry-eyed consumers as a biodegradable, non-toxic and broad-spectrum herbicide, gaining top world markets in the 1980s. [28]

During our interview Jeffrey Smith said,

> the drive to genetically engineered crops was largely set up around the glyphosate patent by Monsanto. They created Roundup Ready crops that were allowed to be

sprayed with glyphosate-based herbicides like Roundup. Glyphosate products have extended their dominance in the weed killer market making Roundup the most popular herbicide...the genetic engineering process affords patents to the producers and gives them unprecedented control of the entire food supply and in some cases the chemicals that are associated with it.

Why Bt Corn?

Jeffrey Smith is admired by millions for his diligence, passion and the raw courage he shows carrying forth the message no one really wants to hear. During our interview I asked him to clue me in a little more about Bt corn and its significance to our food supply:

Bt stands for Bacillus Thuringiensis which is soil bacteria. It's known that certain varieties produce toxins that kill insects by breaking holes in their stomachs. It was used as a spray by gathering up the spores in the bacteria putting them into an aerosol form and spraying it on crops during times of high infestation. It kills the insects and then washes off and biodegrades rather quickly. The engineers have taken the bacterium, made changes in the genetic structure and inserted it into corn and cotton varieties, so that the plants do the killing, producing toxins thousands of times the concentration of the spray form. It's designed to be more toxic than the spray, and unlike the spray it doesn't wash off or biodegrade.

Agent Orange and 2,4-D (incl. 2,4-D update)

The interview circled around to the topic of Agent Orange used during the Vietnam War to kill vegetation so troops could make their way through dense jungle foliage, and it made the enemy troops visible. Curious as to how it is related to our food, I invited Jeffrey Smith to tell me about (what was) the newly approved 2,4-D pesticide, Enlist Duo, and its relationship to what we eat:

Historically, Agent Orange had two different toxins in it and half of it was 2,4-D which is being evaluated now by the WHO, and according to science I've read, has as much or probably more evidence of being a carcinogen than glyphosate which was declared a human carcinogen. The process that created 2,4-D can create dioxins, and dioxins have a high relation to cancer and birth defects... companies claim they now have cleaner ways to produce 2,4-D; 2,4-D is also sold out of China, and their 2,4-D has been tested recently with high levels of dioxins. So the "Agent Orange" crops, or so they are called, will likely result in a highly toxic 2,4-D, as well as dioxins being used at much higher levels. 2,4-D can vaporize, leave one field and travel to another field; causing crop damage and possible health problems. They're very hard to control and the expectation is that these "Agent Orange" crops will increase its usage by as much as 20 fold or more.

Important update: Following this discussion, EPA reversed its decision in November 2015 revoking the approval for Enlist Duo, the 2, 4-D pesticide for agricultural use. [29]

Although 2,4-D is not allowed on food crops being grown in the US, at the moment, are we importing foods likely contaminated (accidently on purpose) with this chemical?

In *One Man, One Cow, One Planet*, Director Thomas Burstyn offers an undercover glimpse into the Indian biotech business, where 2,4-D is being sold and marketed everywhere as a your common herbicidal solution for the everyday farmer [14].

GMO Government Collusion

Let me begin by stating, I do not write this book with any political agenda outside of the health and safety of our children and the food they eat. Regardless of left and right perspectives, there are many on both sides of the political trumpet, supporting and opposing the GMO feeding experiment. Let's examine the political strategies that led us here.

GMO food policies have been par for the course over the last four administrations. Monsanto's influence *has* been steadfast across party lines, regardless of whether our president was a Republican or Democrat. [20]

One of the government's biggest roles is supposed to be the protection and safeguarding of our food supply and consumer products. Instead, Monsanto has been given free access to do what they want, with not only our food supply but also the genetic heritage of life itself, with a total renovation of our plant and animal species without our knowledge or consent.

The FDA says they weren't aware of any information or safety concerns around the consumption of genetically engineered foods when they went to market in 1996. Then a 1998 lawsuit opened up a big can of GMO worms as 44,000 internal memos started flowing into public hands, directly contradicting FDA's safety claims. The lawsuit was initiated by a public interest attorney named Steven M. Druker, asserting that the FDA was lying from the beginning with an illusion of regulation surrounding GMO foods. Druker appears with Smith in *Genetic Roulette,* exposing the deceit, after reviewing all 44,000 documents containing numerous examples of blatant misrepresentation and falsehoods surrounding the safety and policies of GMO foods, particularly around the claims of "overwhelming consensus" among their staff members and scientists, when actually the opposite was true. [20]

Smith points out, "The overwhelming consensus among the scientists working at the FDA was not only that GMOs were different, but that they were dangerous...they could lead to allergies toxins, new diseases and nutritional problems," which, he says, *is* according to FDA's own accounts. Why did they ignore their own scientists? Smith wants to know. [20]

George H.W Bush is in the "De-reg Business"

In the documentary film *The World According to Monsanto* we see a

1987 news clip of then Vice President George Bush Sr. on a field trip to the Monsanto plant. It looks like he's splicing a few genes in the lab when Monsanto executives complain about difficulties getting around health and environmental regulations with their new Roundup Ready soy; Bush advises them, "Call me, we're in the de-reg business, maybe we can help." And help he did. [20,30]

By 1992, Bush was well established in his presidency with Monsanto's agenda not far behind. Then Vice President Dan Quayle announced, as part of the Regulatory Relief Initiative, there would be no regulatory oversight the of new genetically modified foods, outside standard regulation received by conventional food crops. He said the American biotechnology industry would reap huge profits, *"as long as we resist the spread of unnecessary regulations."*

FDA scientists reportedly were outraged, pointing out significant issues with the lack of testing and serious health effects reported in the animal feeding studies. Those objections were ignored. [3] Bush hired Michael Taylor, Monsanto's former attorney, creating a position for him in the FDA as deputy commissioner of policy. GMO food received a quick, free-market pass and the FDA gave it a rating of "Generally Recognized as Safe" (GRAS) and deemed it substantially equivalent to other foods. [3] In order to be granted patents (on life) for GMOs they had to prove their biotech product was significantly different from nature's versions, while also claiming they were the same as conventional food sources. Monsanto bought the best of both worlds, so the 1992 federal policy was finalized that eventually sent GMOs to your kitchen table [20].

Free Trade & the Clinton GMO Love Affair

The Clinton family, including Bill Clinton, is said to have "dined regularly on organic foods including wagyu (highest quality beef) and grass-fed beef." [31] They also, reportedly, ate quite a bit from their own organic White House garden. Walter Scheib was the White House Executive Chef until 2005. He said, "all produce was grown without the use of fertilizers and pesticides."

Meanwhile, Clinton appointed former Monsanto attorney,

Michael Taylor to head the FDA where he approved the highly controversial rBGH (GMO) chemical for use in milk-producing cows for the rest of us. [31, 32] At least one financial report shows the Clinton Foundation received donations from Monsanto averaging between $501,250 and $1 million. It's likely, this wasn't a onetime deal. [33]

Bill Clinton opened the floodgates when he signed the North American Free Trade Agreement (NAFTA) in 1993, which was a trade pact between the United States, Canada, and Mexico that eliminated nearly all the tariffs and trade restrictions between the three nations. [34] Little did we know that this would establish the open door trade policy on forth-coming GMO products three years down the line. Later NAFTA dramatically increased US exports of GMO corn to Mexico (unlabeled) threatening contamination of its ancient maize varieties, while wreaking havoc on the corn crops of traditional Mexican farmers.[35]

According to a report from the Institute for Policy Studies (IPS), the 1996 Farm Bill created another big change in policy for American farmers. That legislation was said to have set in motion an unspoken policy of "get big or get out" where farmers were expected to significantly increase production for export markets, including those to Mexico. The report says, almost immediately, the commodities market dropped out sharply, prompting Congress to issue emergency payments to farmers which later are integrated into what became the farm subsidies program. IPS statistics show that in 2007, small family farms made up only about one-third of total producers. That led to a shift where a handful of large corporations were controlling production making it more difficult for smaller farmers to get fair market prices for their commodities. [36]

With NAFTA and the new World Trade Organization (WTO) opening up global exports, corporations were able to grow larger while consolidating across the U.S. and the world. American jobs were shipped overseas despite the promises of increased employment opportunities. Clinton negotiated 300 trade agreements with other countries during his presidency, including those with China. [36] Clinton's free trade agreements imposed a pivotal lock on the American economy, shipping our jobs overseas and limiting access to genuine "Made in the USA" products while increasing GMO exports.

Currently, we are seeing a significant upsurge in countries banning imports of our GMO food commodities. By October 2015, more than 38 countries banned the cultivation of GMOs within their borders. [37]

The *Examiner* says Clinton passed The Food Quality Protection Act in 1996 changing the Food, Drug, and Cosmetic Act. This eliminated the Delaney clause with its strict requirements relating to pesticide contamination in our food. This replacement allowed pesticide residues in the food supply, whether they were carcinogenic or not, as long as, "ill effects occur only after some critical level of exposure is reached." [38]

Why don't they consider the potential health risks of accumulated exposure since contact rarely happens in single doses?

Clinton moved further up his GMO agenda with free trade and even hired a former Monsanto corporate lobbyist to represent American consumers on a transatlantic committee that was set up to avoid a trade war over genetically engineered foods, says the *San Francisco Chronicle* report. The *Chronicle* describes friction between the US and Europe because of disagreements over food issues that had "torpedoed," they say, during the 1999 World Trade Organization (WTO) talks in Seattle which, *"threatened to erupt into a transatlantic trade war."* The committee was established as a final attempt to settle their differences; so leaders created the 20-person Biotechnology Consultative Forum to work out a compromise. A letter was sent out advising members to "suggest a compromise on labeling, safety testing, and other regulatory issues."

Consumer and environmental groups were furious at the State Department after they were invited to represent opponents of bioengineered foods, and then instead, the key post was given to Carol Tucker Foreman, although she had lobbied for Monsanto's rBGH drug policy and was, apparently, not so opposed to the GMO agenda. [39]

George W. Bush

"Laura Bush was 'adamant' about organics," says Walter Scheib, former White House Chef, according to a *New York Times* article. He says Laura Bush, "insisted that fresh, organic foods be served in the White House," although she didn't talk about it outside the house much. The article clearly asserts, "Bush matched Clinton's zeal for propping up industrial farming but also tried to weaken organic standards." [40]

Bush appointed Attorney General John Ashcroft who reports receiving $10,000 from Monsanto during the congressional elections. The donation was more than any congressional candidate had gotten before. The *Guardian* says that Ashcroft worked to promote GMO crops in developing countries and helped to persuade Europe to accept them.

Moreover, Bush also hired a lawyer named Tommy Thompson, the former governor of Wisconsin, as Secretary of Health and Human Services. Thompson was a vocal GM supporter, who also accepted campaign funds from Monsanto. He even set up a biotech growing zone while working with 13 other state governors to launch a campaign promoting GMOs. The *Guardian* says that the efforts were funded, in part, by Monsanto.

The article also details Bush's appointment of Ann Veneman as the new Secretary of Agriculture. Previously, she was on the board of directors for Calgene, before it was a Monsanto company. She played a key role in world trade negotiations favoring US exports of GMO crops to developing countries. [41]

Donald Rumsfeld served three terms in Congress and was the Secretary of Defense under President Ford and then again under President Bush. He served as the president and CEO of Searle Pharmaceuticals, and apparently made $12 million on its sale to Monsanto. [42] The USDA issued new legal guidance in 2004, under Bush, to allow use of antibiotics in organic dairy cows, along with synthetic pesticides on organic farms. Also the scope was narrowed for federal organic certifications related to crops and livestock. This meant that national organic standards would "exclude fish, nutritional supplements, pet food, fertilizers, cosmetics, and personal-care products."[43]

The Organic Consumer's Association (OCA) reports that Bush signed a 2007 proposal allowing 38 new non-organic ingredients in products with the USDA Organic seal, even though more than 10,000 e-mails and letters were received from consumers and farmers adamantly opposing the measure. Bush's USDA suddenly ended a government program testing pesticide levels in produce and field crops claiming the program cost was too high. [44]

Organic farmers were deeply concerned that the USDA was pushing to rewrite the organic standards without any input from the organic community, consumers or even the National Organic Standards Board. [45]

The Bush Administration furthered the GMO agenda and Clinton's free trade agreements, locking the perpetual shackles of America's economy and health to the biotech food chain.

Hope and Change

In 2008, with a new president and a new agenda, those fighting against Monsanto looked to President Obama for the "transparency, hope and change," he had promised them. Obama supporters waited in vain for him to label GMOs, as he slipped from the icy promises of the campaign trail. Initially, the first lady, unlike her predecessors, was open with the public about her new-found preference for organic foods. Michelle Obama told *The New Yorker,*

> in my household, over the last year we have just shifted to organic … And the fruit-juice-box thing, and we think— we *think*—that's juice. And you start reading the labels and you realize there's high-fructose corn syrup in every- thing we're eating. [sic] Every jelly, every juice. Everything that's in a bottle or a package is like poison in a way that most people don't even know. [46]

Following the election, the Center for Food Safety (CFS)

requested an official reassessment of the GMO policy, *"in light of the change in administration."* What happened?

Obama sent a clear message right off, appointing long-time GMO supporter Tom Vilsack for USDA Secretary. In 2009, Vilsack filed a response in California District Court on behalf of Obama, addressing the CFS request, verifying that the official stance on GMOs had not changed with the new administration. [47] Despite over 250,000 letters opposing it, President Obama signed the Monsanto Protection Act (Farmer's Assurance Provision) into law, as part of an appropriations bill in 2013, allowing genetically modified seeds to be planted even if a federal court ordered them to stop. "Blatantly unethical, and possibly unenforceable, the Act ignores the fact that Monsanto has already been above the law for decades," notes Aviva Shen Editor of *Think Progress*. [48,49] Environmentalists and consumer groups were relieved when it expired that same year. [50]

The *Huffington Post* reports on the expiration saying Oregon Senator Jeff Merkley worked with legislative leaders to ensure the Farmer Assurance Provision rider expired before it could be extended. Merkley applauded those who helped him to avert the extension:

> This is a victory for all those who think special interests shouldn't get special deals. This secret rider, which was slipped into a must-pass spending bill earlier this year, instructed the Secretary of Agriculture to allow GMO crops to be cultivated and sold even when our courts had found they posed a potential risk to farmers of nearby crops, the environment, and human health. I applaud the hundreds of Americans who have worked hard to end this diabolical provision. [50]

This wasn't the first time biotech special interests were put above the law. In 2010, a federal court ordered the planting of genetically altered sugar beets be halted pending the outcome of an environmental study. The USDA overrode the judge's decision and deregulated the crop anyway, claiming the setback would cause a sugar shortage. [51]

The Monsanto Protection Act was repackaged and it reappeared as part of the Safe and Accurate Food Labeling Act Of 2015 or H.R. 1599, and CFS reported that it was worse than ever. Representative Mike Pompeo drafted different versions of the bill, which was dubbed the "Denying Americans the Right to Know Act," or the DARK Act, by those who opposed it, because it voided states' rights allowing them to mandate GMO labeling. [52. 53, 54]

By May 2016, over 70 labeling bills were introduced in more than 30 states, with H.R. 1599 on their heels, threatening to overturn voter-approved laws passed in Vermont, Connecticut, and Maine, along with any future labeling laws. [55]

In July 2015, this dangerous legislation was approved by the House, moving forward in a must-pass federal spending bill. Surprisingly, in December, they announced that H.R. 1599 would not be part of the bill after all. "We are very pleased that Congress has apparently decided not to undermine Americans' right to know about the food they purchase and feed their families," said Andrew Kimbrell, Executive Director of Center for Food Safety:

> Adding a rider to the budget bill that would nullify state laws requiring labeling and even forbidden [sic] federal agencies from mandating labeling would have been profoundly undemocratic and nothing short of legislative malfeasance. We will remain vigilant over the coming days and into the next legislative session to ensure our right to know is protected. [56]

In 2016, Congress caved to industry pressure passing the long dreaded legislation to the detriment and dismay of US citizens.

What is TPP?

The Trans-Pacific Partnership (TPP) and the Transatlantic Trade and Investment Partnership (TTIP) are enormous international trade deals designed and packaged for and by corporations, while heavily endorsed by lawmakers directly supporting the biotech food monopoly. [57]

The Trans-Pacific Partnership trade deal is being fast-tracked, in secret, through Congress. It's even been called the DARK Act on steroids. Similarly, the agreement, cloaked in secrecy, looks to restrict GMO labeling around the world making it illegal. [58]

A *New York Times* editorial says,

> National security secrecy may be appropriate to protect us from our enemies; it should not be used to protect our politicians from us....for an administration that paints itself as dedicated to transparency and public input, the insistence on extensive secrecy in trade is disappointing and disingenuous. [58]

The *International Business Times* reports that the deal has been negotiated in secret with 11 other countries that represent 40 percent of our U.S imports. [59]

2016—New President, New Agenda?

In 2016, Hillary Clinton forges yet another path to the White House. She's a political tigress, a mother and woman many regard for her feminist take-charge attitude, but what does Hillary Clinton really represent, better yet, whom?

A *Washington Times* article points to a speech given at a biotech conference in San Diego where she openly supported GMOs, while advising biotech executives to consider an image makeover because, "Genetically modified sounds Frankensteinish—drought-resistant sounds like something you'd want....be more careful, so you don't raise that red flag immediately." [60]

Monsanto and Dow Chemical publicly support the Clinton Foundation with sizable donations. In addition, Clinton has made it no secret that she endorses the Feed the Future Global Initiative, designed to promote GMO technology to vulnerable populations around the world. On the other hand, we find that Hillary's personal eating habits contradict her open devotion to *Frankenfood*. Her former White House Chef Walter Scheib, reported that he was obligated to serve foods from local growers and suppliers, while prioritizing GMO-Free/organic for the Clintons. This has been the standard trend of our first families who continue to demand wholesome pesticide and GMO-Free foods, while promoting genetically engineered foods to a public that doesn't want them. [60]

Hillary used to work for the Rose Law Firm representing Monsanto and other agribusinesses as well as Tyson and the Wal-Mart Corporation.

During the 2008 election season, Good Morning America's "Brian Ross Investigates" shows footage of Hillary Clinton on the Wal-Mart Board of Directors. She held this position for six years (1986-92) during times the corporation fought hard to keep out the advancing unions. [61]

As the young First Lady of Arkansas, Hillary proudly promoted the "Buy American" program in 1991 to support American jobs. The video shows her at the podium surrounded by red, white and blue signs saying "USA PROUD" as Hillary boasts, "One reason we want to buy America is because we love America." [61]

Ross reported the story for NBC News in 2008:

> Walmart continued to get most of its products overseas, during its 'Buy American' program and some of the foreign made clothing was later found to be sold under 'Made in America' signs in Walmart stores, all at a time while Hillary Clinton served on the Walmart board. [61]

Harvard Law says an estimated 200 children, some 11 years old and even younger, were discovered sewing clothing for Hanes, Wal-Mart, J.C. Penney and Puma at the Harvest Rich factory in Bangladesh. They say the children disclosed that they were routinely being slapped and beaten, sometimes even falling down from exhaustion, being forced to work 12 to 14 hours a day, even some all-night, with 19-to-20-hour shifts, often seven days a week, for wages as low as 6 ½ cents an hour. [62]

Let's consider what her White House biography page has to say:

> In 1973, Hillary became a staff attorney for the Children's Defense Fund, and in Arkansas, Hillary worked tirelessly on behalf of children and families. She founded the Arkansas Advocates for Children and Families and served on the board of the Arkansas Children's Hospital. [63]

So what are we to conclude about Hillary's authenticity? What kind of family values does Hillary really endorse? What kind of mother would allow such atrocities to occur on her watch? Is it not unreasonable to expect corporate board directors to be aware of the business operations and policies that dictate the profits they are themselves accountable for?

As karma would have it, the public is getting wise to her corporate love affair with Wall Street and biotech companies like Monsanto. Her main presidential campaign operative was a former Monsanto lobbyist. One *Washington Times* article refers to her as the "Bride of Frankenfood" quoting environmentalists in Iowa. "I was surprised because these women were really pushing for Hillary until they found out about the Monsanto connection and then they dropped her like a hot potato," says Iowa Democratic Party Chairman James Berge. [64]

Bernie Sanders Calls Out Monsanto

"I'll never forget this. I was invited by CBS, not a small company, to appear on television to talk about why I was opposed to bovine growth hormone. CBS then called me up and said, 'Well, Monsanto is threatening to sue us, so we can't go on with it.' They are very powerful."

– Bernie Sanders 2015 South Carolina Town Hall Meeting [65]

During the 2016 presidential race, Senator Bernie Sanders positioned himself as the only candidate willing to stand up to

Monsanto, publicly demanding accountability as the voice of reason within the confines of the GMO revolving door.

With the senator's backing, his home state of Vermont was first to pass a law requiring GMO labeling on food made from these ingredients. [66, 67] The senator wrote an amendment to the 2013 Farm Bill giving states the power to require GMO labeling. The amendment was defeated in the Senate 71 to 27. Sanders criticized the outcome saying, "An overwhelming majority of Americans favor GMO labeling but virtually all of the major biotech and food corporations in the country oppose it." He insists,

> The people of Vermont and the people of America have a right to know what's in the food that they eat. This should not be a controversial issue. People should have the right to know exactly what is in their food, and states should have the right to require that this information be made available to consumers on labels. This would be a win for everybody, except the biotech and food corporations who spend millions of dollars lobbying Congress. [68]

Sanders has always been a vocal opponent of such trade agreements as the Trans-Pacific Partnership, NAFTA, CAFTA and the Permanent Normalized Trade Agreement with China (PNTR). He urges lawmakers to make the right choice for America and consumers, because the secret policies of the TPP were not designed to benefit anyone but big business, because it was developed by industry, for industry.

Sanders maintains his record of dissonance on this disastrous and very top-secret legislation: "The TPP would make it easier for countries like Vietnam to export contaminated fish and seafood into the U.S. These trade agreements have ended up devastating working families and enriching large corporations.," wrote Senator Sanders. [69]

The GMO Turnstile

As their bankroll confirms, many former Monsanto executives have become accustomed to the government's open door policies with regard to our food supply and biological heritage.

Many of the top political figures entered the GMO regulatory arena with simply a law degree in tow, relying on industry-paid science as a guiding principle for their agenda.

Some major political players are:

Michael Taylor

Michael Taylor worked either for the Food and Drug Administration or the United States Department of Agriculture under every presidential administration since Gerald Ford, with the exception of George W. Bush.

Armed with a law degree from the University of Virginia, Taylor was hired as a staff attorney for the FDA in 1976. In 1981 he got a job practicing law with King & Spalding representing the Monsanto Corporation where he stayed until 1991. Then he received an invitation to work for the FDA as deputy commissioner for policy, a brand new position, and in 1994 he was named administrator of the Food Safety & Inspection Service at the USDA. Between 1996 and 2000, Taylor again worked for Monsanto as the vice president for public policy. He reappears at FDA in 2010, under the Obama Administration where he gets appointed deputy commissioner for the Office of Foods and Veterinary Medicine. [70, 71]

According to a telling article in the *Examiner,* Michael Taylor wrote a 1988 paper where he argued that the Delaney Clause could be interpreted to allow carcinogenic chemicals in food, as long as they were present in low amounts, displaying minimal risk. Former US Navy Staff Scientist Dr. Nancy Swanson says the Delaney Clause was an addition to the Federal Food, Drug, and Cosmetic Act of 1958. It was known as a "zero risk standard... one that prohibited any amount of food additive or pesticide found to cause cancer from being added to processed food," Swanson notes. The Delaney Clause, she says, was "repeatedly amended to allow for more and more exceptions." Then in 1996, the clause was completely abandoned as the Clinton Administration was allowing GMOs free market access to our food chain. [72]

Linda J. Fisher

From 1983-2003, Linda Fisher held high-ranking positions in the EPA under four different administrations beginning with Reagan and ending with George W. Bush. Fisher also worked as the vice president for Government Affairs for Monsanto. [74] According to DuPont's website, Fisher is the vice president for DuPont Safety, Health & Environment and the chief sustainability officer. She serves on the advisory committee for biotech foods at the USDA. Fisher has a degree from Ohio State University with a Master of Business Administration from George Washington University. [75]

Suzanne Sechen

As the primary reviewer for rBGH, Suzanne Sechen worked in the Office of New Animal Drugs from 1988-90, before going to the FDA, where she worked on several Monsanto funded studies for rBGH as a graduate student at Cornell University. [76]

Michael (Mickey) Kantor

In 1992, Michael Kantor acted as Clinton's campaign chair and was appointed US Trade Representative, serving from 1993-96, leading negotiations in the creation of the World Trade Organization (WTO). From 1996-1997, Kantor was the United States Secretary of Commerce. He was also a member of the board of directors for Monsanto and continues to work for them. [77]

Marcia Hale

The *Augusta Chronicle* reports that for four years Marcia Hale worked as a senior staff member in the Clinton administration until 1997, when she accepted the job of vice president for Monsanto Corporation overseeing "biotechnology and sustainable development around the world." [78]

Michael A. Friedman

Michael Friedman served as the acting commissioner of the FDA, for the Department of Health and Human Services under the Clinton Administration; then he was hired in 1999 as the senior vice-president for clinical affairs at G.D. Searle & Company, a pharmaceutical division of Monsanto. He also worked 12 years at the National Cancer Institute directing cancer research and therapy programs. He earned a doctorate in medicine from the University of Texas. [79]

Margaret Miller

As the chemical laboratory supervisor for Monsanto, Margaret Miller worked on rBGH safety studies. Following that she served as the deputy director of Human Food Safety and Consultative Services, New Animal Drug Evaluation Office, Center for Veterinary Medicine in the FDA. [80]

William Ruckelshaus

William Ruckelshaus operated as the EPA's first administrator under Nixon. He banned the general use of DDT on crops in 1972, then left the position to head the FBI as the director. Ruckelshaus returned to the EPA under Reagan in 1983 as the chief administrator. He resigned in 1985 and became a board member for Monsanto and several other corporations. [81]

David Beler

David Beler worked as the head of government affairs for Genentech, Inc. Then took a job functioning as the chief domestic policy advisor to Al Gore. Afterwards, he transitioned into the role of vice president of government and public affairs for Monsanto. [82]

Luther Val Giddings

Dr. Luther Val Giddings enters our scene as a biotech consultant for the World Bank. From 1989-1997, he performed for the USDA as a biotechnology regulator. He attended a working group on biosafety protocols in 1997 establishing his new role with the Biotechnology Industry Organization (BIO), a major biotech lobby group, while directing biotechnology policy studies at the Office of Technology Assessment for Congress. [82]

Clarence Thomas

From 1976-1979, Clarence Thomas represented Monsanto as their corporate lawyer. Since his appointment to the Supreme Court, Justice Thomas has participated in many legal cases involving his previous employer, while refusing to excuse himself from serious conflicts of interest. [83]

Donald Rumsfeld

Of course we've already mentioned Donald Rumsfeld with his long-standing political career. He was the US Permanent Representative to NATO from 1973-1974 and then White House Chief of Staff until 1975. You recall that he was Secretary of Defense under Ford and Bush Jr. and worked as the CEO for Searle Pharmaceuticals, now a Monsanto Company thanks, in part, to Rumsfeld. [84]

As we can clearly see the political agenda to date agrees that the public does not have the right to know what's in their food, nor do they have the right to choose foods they know are free of genetically modified organisms. How's that for transparency in the United States of America, *land of the free, home of the brave?* What are they hiding? (Keep reading).

Corporate Personhood

Through the corporate funding of the American Legislative Exchange Council, global corporations and a handful of state politicians are able to vote behind closed doors, rewriting state laws that govern your individual rights. These so-called "model bills" impact almost every segment of our lives, directing big benefits to huge corporations. This council claims corporations have "a voice and a vote" in relation to our state laws and our individual rights, however do we? [85]

The US Supreme Court essentially says corporations are people, at least in many important respects, as they dramatically expand their legal rights in the name of Corporate Personhood. [86] How is this affecting the rights of real human beings as political agendas sell us out to the highest bidder?

Contamination without Representation

Many believe that the GMO experiment is a blatant case of biological terrorism at its very core. We have Monsanto and various companies who own multiple patents on life and seek to control our genetic structure and the entire food supply. Where are the lines to be drawn?

With the mix and match structure of our genetic Rubik's Cube, it is my interpretation, that this will go down as the biggest ecological man-made disaster in all of history. Call it a premonition. I call it common sense.

Beneath the public radar there has been a silent infiltration of GMOs and glyphosates into our food supply with minimal testing and misrepresented results. This company reorganized nature on a genetic level and then, by all appearances, conspired with our own government to saturate our food supply without public input or opinion, much less, sound Environmental Impact Statements, labeling or meaningful regulations.

Our government aggressively promotes free market access for indiscriminate circulation of genetically modified organisms and has done so over the objections of half the world for the past two decades, essentially forcing contamination on the entire world. They actively attempt to cut off our ability to feed ourselves, in order to build a reliance on their remanufactured nutrition that is devoid of much of the nutrients that growing bodies need. How, by any stretch of the imagination, is this not a serious human rights violation?

The following is a summarized version of an article I wrote in response to the US House of Representatives, Committee on Agriculture hearing on GMO alfalfa deregulation in 2011. Upon watching the antics, it became abundantly clear that the agenda is, ultimately, full contamination of the entire food supply and that of other nations. My article was originally published online at *Salem-News.com* (87) and republished by prominent watchdog groups, like *GMWatch.org and GENET.*

. . . .

Note: Numbers in parenthesis are cue times from the original video.

. . . .

Genetically Modified Crops — Contamination Without Representation

November 17, 2011

April Scott Salem-News.com

(SALEM, Ore.)

The U.S House of Representatives, Committee on Agriculture held a formal hearing on genetically modified (GM) alfalfa on Jan. 20, 2011.

The hearing corresponded with an open 30-day comment period, designed to provide relevant testimony with regard to deregulation of genetically modified alfalfa.

The democratic process neglected to include a single organic or conventional farming representative. Throughout the two- hour hearing, various legislators publicly humiliated Secretary of Agriculture Tom Vilsack for even suggesting any compromise through talks with the organic and conventional communities. They all but ordered him to stand down his conversations with anyone but pro-GM enthusiasts (1:43:16).

Representatives left no seed unturned in honor of their allegiance to biotech crops and complete penetration into all foreign and domestic markets. In fact, Minnesota's Representative Collin Peterson referred to organic producers and consumers as "our opponents" [1](12:29).

Vilsack, even with his ties to Monsanto, was attempting negotiation with what they termed "so-called Option 3" containing a minimal stop-gap as an alternative to absolute contamination of organic and conventional alfalfa. In essence, planting barriers would have been implemented to maintain protective measures for the integrity of all seed varieties. Legislators blatantly mocked him and even pulled rank saying, that the Secretary of Agriculture does not have the authority to do anything but fully deregulate the crop without further ado. (35:38, 1:25:50, 1:29:15, 2:18:47)

It can be noted that Vilsack testified no less than three times that they we were in the midst of the 30-day comment period, and in his opinion, the talks among all sides were providing necessary elements worthy of analysis for all agricultural markets concerned. (29:00, 1:44:00, 1:51:54)

The theme of the hearing centered around the economic burden of GM farmers if full deregulation didn't go forth immediately (1:44:00). It was insisted by every representative that their loyalties were to the biotech community and that full deregulation was unquestionable without consideration for any form of barrier to protect other crops from cross-contamination.

In regard to preservation of non-GM crops, Texas Representative Michael Conaway begs the question, "how much of this is a definitional issue?" He questions organic standards and even insists that he "suspects that genetically engineered seeds will become the new organic" He blatantly suggests that legislative steps be considered to modify the language and thus re-define organic standards so that genetically modified crops can freely contaminate without restriction. Vilsack insists that it is merely a marketing issue and not an issue of health and safety. Conaway asks if we "are just 'hung up' on the phrase organic, meaning something we grew ourselves in the backyard with whatever?" (2:33:00).

Concern was expressed by a number of speakers that GM crops are promoted throughout the world as being no different than conventional crops, and if word got out that we established restrictive planting barriers, then it might be assumed that the GM crops were somehow different. That could put a damper on GM producers and their marketing potential. (30:45, 1:58:17, 2:18:47)

It was apparent, by the end of the one-sided discussion, that full deregulation and contamination remains unquestionable from the perspective of our democratic congressional leaders. In other words, it is most notably a flagrant case of contamination without representation. (87)

You could see the full-length video from the U.S House of Representatives, Committee on Agriculture forum on GM alfalfa, Jan 20, 2011 if it were still accessible. [88a]

Lucky for us, thanks to the video skills and quick reflexes of my friends at *GMO-FREE Portland* you can see an edited "in context" version of that hearing preserved at: [89]

https://www.youtube.com/watch?v=83gIyaEpWJY

In addition, I would like to give a big thanks to Jeff Kirkpatrick from *Ban GMOs Now* for locating the original hearing transcript. There is now a link to it under "GMO-Free Data Sources." [88]

World Food Prize Goes to Monsanto?

Monsanto is so pleased with themselves for commandeering the global food supply that they awarded themselves the World Food Prize, going to three of their own scientists, including one from Syngenta and another from Monsanto.

Maybe it's just a coincidence that Monsanto, Syngenta and another biotech giant DuPont Pioneer are the major sponsors of the prize in the first place? Is this not an obvious conflict of interest or some sort of code of ethics violation? [90]

Increased Crop Yields?

Biotech industry giants have long claimed that GE technology produces larger yields and therefore will lend itself better than conventional crops to feeding an overpopulated world. Jack Heinemann says otherwise. He is a professor of molecular biology at the University of Canterbury, New Zealand and the director of the Center for Integrated Research in Biosafety. Heinemann evaluated crop yields of three staple crops, measuring those outputs between 1985 and 2010. His published report "Sustainability and innovation in staple crop production in the US Midwest," shows that Western Europe has experienced yield gains at a faster rate than North America for all of the three crops he measured:

> I'm a genetic engineer, but there is a different [sic] between being a genetic engineer and selling a product that is genetically engineered—there's no evidence that [GE crops] have given us higher yields...the evidence points exclusively to breeding as the input that has increased yields over time. And there is evidence that it is constraining yields in the North American agroecosystem.

European nations have also reduced pesticides more than we have, he says. [91, 92]

How Much of Our Food is GMO?

Generally speaking we're seeing a loss of market options as biodiversity of traditional crop varieties are being wiped out by the biotech market in the name of progress. Farmers previously had the option to select from nearly 9,000 different corn varieties in 2005, although 57 percent of those were transgenic, farmers still had over 3,000 non-GE varieties to choose from. Just 5 years later, GE seed varieties took over the marketplace and remarkably non-GE seed options declined by two-thirds, making them considerably more difficult for growers to purchase. Other traditional non-GE crops like soybean and cotton were also experiencing dramatic reductions in market availability, with a mere 10 percent of soybean strains and 15 percent of cotton seed varieties left on the market, in 2010, for farmers to buy. [92] *USA Today* says that the International Service for the Acquisition of Agri-biotech Applications report shows, genetically engineered crops grown in the US make up about 95 percent of sugar beets, 94 percent of soybeans, 90 percent of cotton crops, 90 percent of papaya and 88 percent of the feed corn categorized as GMO. [93] Also, *Mother Jones* published a USDA graph in 2012 showing GE corn, soy and cotton as the top three GMO crops grown in the US that year. They illustrate the previous 12 years showing a 60 percent increase in GMO corn crop acreage according the graph. [94]

Huffington Post confirms GMO sugar beets have replaced the bulk of our traditional cane sugar in popular products like soda pop, snacks and other sweets that likely contain high fructose corn syrup (GMO) too. Canola and cottonseed oil are used a lot in processed foods, which are often GMO as well.

USDA list of the top seven GMO crops in 2012:

1. Corn: largest crop grown in the US for both animal and human consumption and for biofuels—88 percent of corn reported as genetically modified. *Time* reports 33 varieties of GMO corn approved for the marketplace.

2. Soy: second largest crop grown in US (after corn)—93 percent genetically modified, most often found in processed foods ex: hydrogenated oils, lecithin, tocopherol.

3. Cotton: 94 percent of cottonseed planted in the US was genetically engineered—used for products like margarine (hydrogenated oils), vegetable oil and shortening.

4. Papaya: 75 percent of Hawaiian papaya reported as genetically modified (2012).

5. Canola: estimated 90 percent canola crops grown in the US were transgenic.

6. Sugar beets: over half of sugar selling in America in 2012 came from sugar beets—90 percent of which were GMO.

7. Alfalfa: fourth largest crop grown after corn, soybeans, and wheat (USDA reports no genetically engineered wheat on the market). [95]

It's interesting to note, there have been no announcements for the approval of genetically modified wheat, yet unapproved glyphosate tolerant GM wheat showed up in a field growing in Oregon. Japan and South Korea suspended their wheat imports over concerns of the contamination in 2013. American wheat shipments were canceled that year. [96]

Dr. Martha Mertens from Institute for Biodiversity, a German federal agency, wrote the "Assessment of Environmental Impacts of Genetically Modified Plants." She explains, globally, there are many more transgenic plant species that have been released into the environment over the past several years. In Europe applications are submitted under what is called a "Deliberate Release Directive" for about 50 different plant species, which are transformed to express a variety of traits.

Dr. Mertens says in addition to the four main crop species being grown commercially and tested in field trials, other transgenic plants are also being tested including:

cereal crops such as wheat, barley, and rice, and broad-leaved crops (potato, sugar beet, tobacco, sunflower, and alfalfa). The range of species has been extended to vegetables (e.g. tomato, cauliflower, chicorée, aubergine, carot, pea, lettuce) and fruits such as melons, strawberries, and raspberries and even to wild plants (e.g. wild radish).

Even more, she reports applications for deliberate release of woody fruit species such as apple, cherry, plum, olive, orange, and forest trees such as poplar and eucalyptus. Transgenic flowers (e.g. carnation, marigold, petunia) are growing rapidly in countries around the EU. [97]

GMOs Flooding the Local Market:

- Corn
- Canola
- Alfalfa
- Cotton (cottonseed oil)
- Soy and soy lecithin
- Sugar from sugar beets
- Papaya
- Squash
- Honey (GMO pollen)
- Meat (GMO animal feed)
- Dairy Products (rBGH/animals)

GMOs Preparing for Market

- Salmon
- Rice
- Apples
- Oranges
- Potatoes
- Tobacco
- Pineapple

[98, 99, 100]

Potential GMO Hidden Ingredients

baking powder
canola oil (rapeseed oil)
caramel color
cellulose
citric acid
cobalamin (Vitamin B12)
condensed milk
confectioner's sugar
corn flour
corn masa
corn meal
corn oil
corn sugar
corn syrup
cornstarch
cottonseed oil
cyclodextrin
cysteine
dextrin
dextrose
diacetyl
diglyceride
erythritol
Equal
Food starch
fructose (any form)
glucose
glutamate
glutamic acid
glycerides

glycerin
glycerol
shoyu
sorbitol
soy flour
soy lecithin
soy milk
soy oil
soy protein
soy isolates
soy protein isolate
soy sauce
starch
stearic acid
glycerol monolete
glycine
hemicellulose
high fructose corn syrup (HFCS)
hydrogenated starch
hydrolyzed vegetable protein (HVP)
inositol
inverse syrup
inversol
invert sugar
isoflavones
lactic acid
lecithin
leucine
lysine
maltitol

malt
malt syrup
malt extract
maltodextrin
maltose
mannitol
methylcellulose
milk powder
milo starch
mono and diglycerides
monosodium glutamate (MSG)
NutraSweet
oleic acid
Phenylalanine
sugar (unless specified as cane sugar)
tamari
tempeh
teriyaki marinade
textured vegetable protein
threonine
tocopherols (vitamin E)
tofu
trehalose
triglyceride
vegetable fat

This list is provided as a courtesy of Institute for Responsible Technology. [101]

CHAPTER 2

....

Independent Science

"The safety of GMO foods is unproven and a growing body of research connects these foods with health concerns and environmental damage. For this reason, most developed nations have policies requiring mandatory labeling of GMO foods at the very least, and some have issued bans on GMO food production and imports."

—Dr. David Suzuki, geneticist

Scientists Unite

In 1999, 815 scientists from 82 countries signed an "Open Letter from World Scientists to All Governments Concerning Genetically Modified Organisms (GMOs)." The Institute of Science in Society published the full letter. The following is a summary of the main points:

The scientists report that they:

- "Are extremely concerned about hazards of GMOs to biodiversity, food safety, human and animal health and they are demanding a moratorium be put on the environmental releases in accordance with the precautionary principle."

- "Are opposed to GM crops that will intensify corporate monopolies, exacerbate inequality and prevent an essential shift to sustainable agriculture to provide food security and health throughout the world."

- "Call for a ban on patents of life-forms and living processes which threaten food security, sanction bio-piracy of indigenous knowledge and genetic resources and violate basic human rights and dignity."

- "Want more support on research and development of non-corporate, sustainable agriculture that can benefit family farmers all over the world." [1]

Subsequently in London, two dozen top scientists from seven countries bridging disciplines of agroecology, agronomy, biomathematics, botany, chemical medicine, ecology, histopathology, microbial ecology, molecular genetics, nutritional biochemistry, physiology, toxicology and virology, aligned themselves as the Independent Science Panel on GM during a 2003 public conference joining the UK Environment Minister Michael Meacher and 200 other participants. [1a]

The group released "The Independent Science Panel on GM Final Report." This was a four page summary presented for the conference, ahead of their final publication of "The Case for a GM-Free Sustainable World." This exposé called for a ban on GMO crops, to instead work to "advance sustainable agriculture." [1a, 1b] At the time, it was touted as the "the strongest, most complete dossier of evidence" ever compiled revealing problems and dangers associated with GMO crops, while highlighting the benefits of sustainable agriculture. [1a]

The researchers, "in light of new genetics," released the 2013 report "Ban GMOs Now" providing an in-depth view of the health and environmental hazards associated with modern GMO farming practices and outcomes:

> GM agriculture is a recipe for disaster...it is also standing in the way of the shift to sustainable agriculture already taking place in local communities all over the world that can truly enable people to feed themselves in times of climate change. [1c]

The Institute clearly takes a hardline approach on glyphosate use and exposure. More than 566 scientists from 71 different countries signed the group's 2015 manifesto calling on "all governments to ban glyphosate-based herbicides:" [1d]

> We, the undersigned international scientists and medical professionals, call on governments at all levels to ban the spraying of glyphosate herbicides. As professionals who have read the literature on glyphosate herbicides and their effects, we have concluded that they are causing irreparable harm. [And] In addition to human diseases, glyphosate herbicides are linked to more than 40 new and re-emerging major crop diseases. They are causing irreparable harm to the entire food web; including the plant kingdom, beneficial microbes that supply nutrients to our crops and soils, fish and other aquatic life, amphibians, butterflies, bees, birds, mammals, and the human microbiome. [1d] They further reveal, chronic exposure to glyphosate herbicides is associated not only with cancers but...infertility, impotence, abortions, birth defects, neurotoxicity, hormonal disruption, immune reactions, an unnamed fatal kidney disease, chronic diarrhea, autism and other ailments. [1d]

The Union of Concerned Scientists

Researchers and students from Massachusetts Institute of Technology (MIT) combined forces to create the Union of Concerned Scientists in 1969, with new efforts to empower and unite citizens with sound science and evidence to promote informed decision making in public health and safety, the environment and in matters of general well-being. [2]

After forming the Center for Science and Democracy, the Union continued its call for "scientific research to be directed away from military technologies toward solving pressing environmental and social problems." The Center itself maintains a heavy focus on challenging campaigns of misinformation and inappropriate influences on policymakers so to strengthen science-based health, safety, and environmental laws, while standing up for scientists who have been targets of personal attacks. [2] One Union report, "Genetic Engineering Risks and Impacts," reveals that from the very beginning researchers started voicing concerns about the potential for GMOs to cause allergic reactions in consumers. [2a]

In 1996, the Union reported, "....we do know of ways in which genetically engineered crops could cause health problems. For instance, genes from an allergenic plant could transfer this unwanted trait to the target plant." One example they offered was a university study where soybeans were crossed with a Brazil nut for animal feed. The process caused what researchers termed a "potentially deadly" allergic reaction in some of the test subjects who had allergies to Brazil Nuts: [2a]

> Unintended consequences like these underscore the need for effective regulation of GE products. In the absence of a rigorous approval process, there is nothing to ensure that GE crops that cause health problems will always be identified and kept off the market. [2a, 3]

The study "Genetic Engineering of Crops Can Spread Allergies, Study Shows" had the researchers at University of Nebraska reporting, "the first solid evidence that proteins that can cause potentially serious allergic reactions could be transferred to crops through genetic engineering." [3]

In 2013, the Union published a policy brief called "The Healthy Farm: A Vision for U.S. Agriculture" to promote ecologically sound farming methods, rather than the industrial farming complex, known for its risky approach to crop and soil management. [2b] You can access links to all of these reports under the "GMO-Free Child Data Sources," in Chapter 2.

It goes to show you that the scientific community, as a whole, does not stand behind the fractured policies and political structures concealed behind the façade of industry science and biotech dollars.

We have seen incredible upsurges in chronic illness around the country. *Reuters* says the number of Americans suffering from three or more chronic illnesses shot up from 13 percent in 1996 to 22 percent by year-end 2005, just for people 45 to 64. Even more shocking, it bumped up twice to 45 percent for those 65 to 79 and even rose from 38 percent to a whopping 54 percent for those folks 80 and older. When all were combined, the total number of people with three or more chronic illnesses in the US went from 7 percent in 1996 to 13 percent in 2005. [4] This is a significant increase that should raise the red flag for our nation's medical community.

Think about it, it was just nine years following the introduction of GMOs in 1996 when physicians began reporting huge spikes in such disorders as food allergies, asthma, autism, reproductive and digestive problems. [5] Regardless, it has been said that scientists nor doctors are able point a definitive finger at GMOs as the cause (due to lack of labeling and tracking), however it has been agreed upon by countless modern medical and scientific communities that the correlation is arguably high.

Outside of the health and safety implications and the GMO Rubik's Cube factors I explained earlier, there are in fact, many contributing elements to the downfall of the GMO human experiment. Let's see what the scientists have to say.

The Scientists

"Despite what the media and so-called "experts" proclaim, there are NO peer-reviewed scientific papers establishing the safety of GMO crops."

—Don Huber—former Purdue University professor and plant pathologist

Arpad Pusztai

I introduced readers to Dr. Arpad Pusztai in 2010 with my

Salem-News.com article "While We Were Sleeping...GM Food and the Brink of No Return." [6]

As an Eminent Scientist and fellow of the Royal Society of Edinburgh, Arpad Pusztai (Poos-tie) was the world's leading expert on plant proteins called lectins. Pusztai was well respected in his field for more than 35 years. working as a top-notch plant geneticist at Scotland's University of Aberdeen, Rowett Research Institute, the leading nutritional lab in the UK.

With three books and over 270 scientific papers he had the complete confidence of his colleagues and thus was awarded a 1.6 million pound contract from the Scottish Office to study GM foods. [6, 7] Convinced of their potential, Pusztai was widely recognized as the ideal person to lead this three-year research program that would become the standard in testing protocols for GMOs in the EU. But when he fed what he thought was harmless GM potatoes to his lab rats, things went quickly awry. [7]

Journalist Andy Rowell wrote the book, *Don't Worry, It's Safe to Eat."* He says there was, "...not a single publication in a peer-reviewed journal on the safety of GM food at the time..." and the project's methodology was thoroughly reviewed and cleared beforehand by the Biotechnology and Biological Sciences Research Council (BBSRC), the government's central funding body for the biological sciences in the UK [7].

Pusztai had a team of more than 20 scientists at three facilities tracking the project carefully. The researchers were shocked by the initial outcomes right from beginning:

> By late 1997 preliminary results from the rat-feeding experiments were showing totally unexpected and worrying changes in the size and weight of the rat's body organs. Liver and heart sizes were getting smaller, and so was the brain. There were also indications that the rats' immune systems were weakening. [7]

Official observations showed some concerning patterns in the health of the animals eating the GM foods:

stunted growth, impaired immune systems, bleeding stomachs, abnormal and potentially pre-cancerous cell growth in the intestines, impaired blood cell development, misshapen cell structures in the liver, pancreas and testicles, altered gene expression and cell metabolism, liver and kidney lesions, partially atrophied livers, inflamed kidneys, less developed organs, reduced digestive enzymes, higher blood sugar, inflamed lung tissue, increased death rates and higher offspring mortality. [6, 7, 8]

Reports say that the rats that ate GM potatoes had smaller livers, hearts, testicles and brains, damaged immune systems, with structural changes in their white blood cells, raising the risk of infection and disease compared to those rats fed the non-GM potatoes. [7, 9]

In a gripping book *Seeds of Destruction,* author F. William Engdahl illustrates how the scene got worse as the scientists began noticing damages showing up in the thymus and spleen, along with noticeably enlarged tissues, including the intestines and the pancreas. Plus they said that they found significant proliferation in the cells of the stomach and intestines, which could indicate future potential for cancer growth. The negative effects started showing up just 10 days in and remained persistent after 110 days, which is equivalent to 10 years for us humans. [8]

Dr. Pusztai agreed to talk about the results during a live TV interview in June 1998; a decision, he said, that would come back to haunt him. Director of the Rowett Institute Professor Philip James was present and in full agreement with the study content and the direction of the discussion during the broadcast. In fact, he congratulated Pusztai and commented on how well he had handled the interview questions. The Institute endorsed Arpad's work by sending out a press release: "A range of carefully controlled studies underlie the basis of Dr. Pusztai's concerns." [8]

The book illustrates the tense situation and what Pusztai announced to millions, during that Monday broadcast:

We are assured that this is absolutely safe. We can eat it all the time. We must eat it...there is no conceivable harm which can come to us. But, as a scientist...I find that it is very, very unfair to use our fellow citizens as guinea pigs. [8]

Pusztai said he was not allowed to provide specific details about his observations, however, "If I had the choice, I would certainly not eat it until I see at least comparable scientific evidence which we are producing for our genetically modified potatoes," he concluded. Within 48 hours everything changed, reportedly, following calls from Prime Minister Tony Blair's office to the Rowett Institute. Arpad was fired along with his wife who also had worked on the study, according to Engdahl's accounts. She was a highly respected researcher at Rowett for more than 13 years without incident. Her husband was warned not to speak with the press about his research under threats of losing his pension. All of his research was promptly seized and kept from public view. His team was dissolved and he was forbidden to talk to other members under threats of legal action. [7,8]

The Institute attempted to do major damage control, sending out several different press releases, each one contradicting the last. Finally they settled on a believable story saying Pusztai simply "confused" samples from GMO-fed rats with those of ordinary rats, who were, "fed a sample of potato that was known to be poisonous." Accounts say Pusztai was furious at their blatant disregard for the truth and their attempts to discredit his reputation with such falsehoods of basic error and incompetence that were simply unheard of within his level of expertise. [7. 8]

The media continued trying to further discredit him with outrageous claims, saying it was one of the "worst errors ever admitted by a major scientific institution."[8]. A follow-up audit was conducted on Pusztai's work that thoroughly disproved the accusations, exonerating him. Andy Rowell's narrative says that, "Rowett later shifted its story, finding a flimsy fallback in the claim that Pusztai had not carried out the long-term tests needed to prove the results." They said Pusztai was guilty of unprofessional conduct, because his work had not been peer-reviewed prior to the broadcast.

However, in spite of the controversy the research paper successfully passed the peer-review process by a sizable panel of scientists (larger than usual) and was subsequently published; and it was widely recognized as a valid and factual account within reputable scientific communities. The government started condemning the study's methodology, despite the fact they reviewed and approved all of his testing methodologies in the first place, before ever awarding him the funding for the project. [7. 8]

In February 1999, some 30 top scientists from 13 countries signed an open letter opposing the attacks in support of Pusztai's conclusions. The *London Guardian* ran the letter which triggered, "a whole new round of controversy over the safety of GMO crops and the Pusztai findings," Engdahl says.

Also some of the retired colleagues from the Institute, "privately confirmed to Pusztai that Rowett's director, Prof. Philip James, had received two direct phone calls from Prime Minister Tony Blair. Blair had made clear in no uncertain terms that Pusztai had to be silenced." Reports further indicate,

> Blair had initially received an alarmed phone call from the President of the United States, Bill Clinton. Blair was convinced by his close friend and political adviser, Clinton, that GMO agribusiness was the wave of the future, a huge-and-growing-multibillion dollar industry in which Blair could offer British pharmaceutical and bio-tech giants a leading role. [7. 8]

GMOs were the cornerstone of Blair's 1997 election campaign to "Re-brand Britain." Furthermore, he spells out that the goal of the Clinton White House was to make the 1990s "the decade of the successful commercialization of agricultural biotechnology products." This is said to have been confirmed through a senior staff member. [7,8]

The fact is biotech stocks in GM companies were soaring on

Wall Street in the late 90s. Under the circumstances, *it was asserted,* Clinton was not about to let some scientist in the UK sabotage his billion-dollar project, nor would his good friend Tony Blair allow for it either. [7.8]

To complete the final puzzle piece Pusztai's former associate Professor Robert Orskov, a leading nutrition scientist for Rowett for 33 years, told Pusztai that the initial phone call behind his dismissal came from Monsanto. Moreover, "Monsanto had spoken with Clinton who in turn had directly spoken to Blair about the 'Pusztai problem.'" Engdahl says if all this is true it means,

> The private corporation ... had been able to mobilize the President of the United States and the Prime Minister of Great Britain on behalf of its private interests. [And] a simple phone call by Monsanto could destroy the credibility of one of the world's leading independent scientists. [7, 8]

Pusztai's research was finally published in October 1999, in The *Lancet*, after a clear majority of scientific reviewers voted in favor of it completely validating its findings. Dr. Richard Horton received a "threatening" phone call from a senior official at the Royal Society saying, "his job might be at risk if he decided to publish the Pusztai study." [7. 8]

The Royal Society refuted the publication armed with an "unpublished and non-peer-reviewed study" of their own, by their own Pro-GMO scientists, trying to invalidate Pusztai's work nearly two years after they specifically condemned his study for the exact same reason. Dr. Pusztai pressured the Royal Society which finally admitted the research was still unpublished when they referenced it; they justified it because, "it had been discussed at international scientific conferences," so it was not an issue. Oddly enough, Pusztai's research was not given the same level of respect or consideration under nearly the same circumstances. His work too, had been presented at an international conference, prior to the Society's own review. [7, 8]

Rowell further criticizes the whole affair:

> The fundamental flaw in the...response is not that they try and damn Pusztai with unpublished data, nor is it that they have overlooked published studies [supporting Pusztai's concerns]...everyone agreed that more work was needed... that work remains to be undertaken... [a] scientific body, like The Royal Society, that allocates millions in research funds every year, could have funded a repeat of Pusztai's experiments.

To date, *no* body of research has attempted to reconstruct his study. [7, 8]

On the tenth year anniversary of the TV broadcast Arpad Pusztai came out, and publicly warned that we shouldn't underestimate the biotech industry with their political and financial hold on our politicians. He vowed to use all means at his disposal to expose the "shallowness" of industry claims, "and the lack of credible science behind them," while trusting in people's good common sense to see through the "falseness of the claims for the safety of untested GM foods." [7, 8. 9]

In 2009, the scientist and his good wife, Dr. Susan Bardocz, were presented with the Stuttgart Peace Prize for their advocacy for independent risk research and scientific integrity, along with acts of courage and undaunted insistence on the public's right to know the truth. [10, 11]

Gilles-Eric Séralini

Gilles-Eric Séralini is a French molecular biologist, whose two year research study followed the outcome of rats fed GMO corn and Roundup. Researchers say they recorded considerable liver and kidney damage, along with hormonal disturbances, after just four months in the rats fed GM corn, along with low levels of Roundup doses in their water everyday (well below levels allowed in drinking water in the EU). [12]

You might be surprised that the scientists report that their follow-up research showed that the rats developed tumors within the 6-month mark. Plus toxic effects were present in the feeding combinations when they ate corn and Roundup together, as well as when they ran special isolated tests with corn and Roundup fed to subjects alone. The researchers observed outcomes with higher rates of large tumors and mortality rates in most of the groups. [12]

GMOSéralini.org explains that the team's research endured meticulous examination and scrutiny with a four-month review by a variety of scientists, all before being published. In a move that was vastly condemned by hundreds of scientists worldwide the journal retracted the study, after making a key change in the editorial board which was heavily endorsed by Monsanto themselves. In addition, they say Marc Fellous the former Chairman of Biomolecular Engineering Commission of France was indicted in 2015, by the High Court of Paris facing charges of forgery. The case was also an important part of a libel trial that Séralini later won in relation to his study. The Biomolecular Engineering Commission is a group that approves GM crops for consumption and market sale. [12]

Séralini won a lawsuit against *Marianne Magazine* in 2015, after the High Court found them guilty of public defamation in the attempt to discredit his work. Their 2012 article falsely criticized the Séralini study claiming, "scientific fraud in which the methodology served to reinforce pre-determined results." [12] Still these deceptions continue to clang from the quire of online trolls as if the heavens have blessed their GMO souls.

Apparently, it was Henry I. Miller, an American lobbyist that made up wild accusations of fraud against Séralini in the first place. [13] His *Forbes* magazine article claims, "Scientists Smell a Rat in Fraudulent Genetic Engineering Study." [14] Miller is best known for his support of the big tobacco industry and for his direct intentions to discredit any evidence that would link tobacco and heart disease. [14]

However, *Environmental Sciences Europe* proudly republished the Séralini paper in 2015, following three rigorous peer review studies.

The updated version contains current information and up-to-date responses to previous criticisms.

In a letter to Séralini, the original journal admitted that they really found nothing "incorrect" about the results by the research team. The problem revolved around the "inconclusive" nature of some aspects of the paper. The team pointed out that there would be numerous studies retracted, or never even published, due to the inherent inconclusiveness of the subject matter, if that were indeed the issue in question. [15]

Here again, we see blatant examples of special favors being given to Monsanto and their biotech teams. But as the truth begins to bloom, the public is becoming increasingly aware of the risk factors that are presenting themselves in relation to the chronic dis-ease engulfing our nation.

Anthony Samsel and Stephanie Seneff

Dr. Anthony Samsel has extensively explored the toxicity levels of glyphosate. His background was established in public health, the Army Corps of Engineers and the Navy. He is a retired consultant from Arthur D. Little, and he did contract work for the EPA as well. His colleague Dr. Stephanie Seneff is a senior research scientist at MIT. Her focus is tied to biology and the relationship between nutrition and health. Since 2011, she has written over a dozen papers. [16]

Health Impact News reports, "Glyphosate Causes Cancer: EPA 'Trade Secret' Sealed Files Reveal Cancer Link Known Back in the 1970s." The article cites Dr. Samsel's research as a scientist and glyphosate expert. [16] Brian Shilhavy is the editor of *Health Impact News; he* spoke with Samsel in a recent interview about how his interest in glyphosate peaked while researching it as a farmer himself. Samsel says he was using coyote urine to scare off deer that were eating his crops, and he ran out. Instead, he decided to apply some of his own urine and discovered that it was very effective except it was killing the weeds. He didn't understand why. That led to another experiment with potted plants, where he ended up with same result the second time. That's when it hit him; he must have high levels of glyphosate in his body, and he needed to do something about it. [16]

Recently, Dr. Samsel described a set of EPA documents in his possession showing that Monsanto has known about the link between glyphosate and cancer since the 70s. The biotech community responded to the news by launching attacks on his credibility. [16] However, in early 2015 the International Agency for Research on Cancer (IARC) as part of the World Health Organization (WHO), released a scathing report slamming glyphosate as "probably carcinogenic," and asserting that it likely causes non-Hodgkin lymphoma and prostate cancer. The news rocked mainstream media, and Monsanto's bottom line continues to plummet. [17]

Dr. Samsel confidently agrees with that conclusion, taking it a bit further—glyphosate is not what we would term a *"probable"* carcinogen...it *is* a carcinogen based on those studies that have been hidden for years, classified as "trade secrets." [16]

The open access journal *Entropy* has positioned itself as an international leader and interdisciplinary "journal of entropy and information studies." Their publication of Samsel and Seneff's research exposes the truth that "...glyphosate enhances the damaging effects of other food-borne chemical residues and environmental toxins." That clearly means that other chemicals used in combination (intentionally or not) with the herbicide will increase toxicity levels further than what happens in isolation. We call that a synergistic effect. The same study shows glyphosate's "negative impact on the body is insidious and manifests slowly over time as inflammation damages cellular systems throughout the body." [18] Whoa! What did that say?! Let's think about that for a moment, because that my friend is a major focal point and perhaps one of the principle smoking guns in this controversy. That's because inflammation is the cornerstone of your body's protective talent. Some inflammation is perfectly normal and a vital part of the body's natural healing response. It is designed to increase healing at the site of injury or infection, but the problem is that chronic inflammation is at the (GMO?) root of all chronic disease including, Alzheimer's, arthritis, auto-immune disorders, cardiovascular disease, cancer, Type 2 diabetes, neurological diseases and the list is endless. [19] Is this not the current trend in consumers in the United States at this particular juncture, according to every available national healthcare statistic? Americans are plagued with a myriad of chronic diseases and biological malfunctions. This is no secret.

Following the *Entropy* paper, Samsel and Seneff have continued to collaborate publishing a series of four more papers together titled, "Glyphosate pathways to modern diseases (II-V): ...," with each one concerning a different aspect of glyphosate's toxicity. "Glyphosate II..." explains gluten intolerance and celiac disease through glyphosate contamination in wheat. [18a] "Glyphosate III..." focuses on glyphosate's chelation of manganese and the resulting health effects, including a very compelling link to known features of autism. [18b] "Glyphosate IV..." discusses multiple ways in which glyphosate could cause cancer. [18c] "Glyphosate V..." is probably the most exciting and disturbing of their series, as it provides a strong case for the possibility that glyphosate, acting as a non-coding amino acid analogue of glycine, can get into proteins by mistake during protein synthesis. In the paper, they show how this one feature alone could easily explain the rise in multiple modern conditions and diseases, such as autism, Alzheimer's, diabetes, obesity, rheumatoid arthritis, kidney failure and various cancers, through an insidious accumulation of damaged proteins throughout the body. [18d]

Dr. Samsel and Dr. Seneff have layered the evidence pool with what could be some major floatation devices among the sinking casualties of the GMO ship that hails us all.

David Suzuki

Dr. Suzuki is a geneticist and former professor at the University of British Columbia. According to the *David Suzuki Foundation* website, he is an award-winning scientist, environmentalist and broadcaster. He hosts radio and television programs explaining science to the average person. He received an E.W.R. Steacie Memorial Fellowship in 1992, as the outstanding research scientist in Canada under the age of 35. He held this honor for three years, along with 25 other honorary degrees in Canada, the US and in Australia. Dr. Suzuki has written 52 books, including a textbook titled *An Introduction to Genetic Analysis* (with A.J.F. Griffiths), which was recognized as being the most widely used genetics textbook in the United States. The scientist warns "we have no idea what the long-term consequences will be of these genetic manipulations on the public." [20]

In a 2001 CBS television interview, Suzuki told the host, "There is no way the health authorities can test all the possible combinations and permutations over a large enough population, over a long enough period" to be able to say with any assurance that they're harmless. And "by slipping it into our food without our knowledge, without any indication that there are genetically modified organisms in our food we are now unwittingly part of a massive experiment." [21] He says,

> The problem is this: geneticists follow the inheritance of genes in what we call a vertical fashion. What biotechnology allows us to do is to take genes from this organism and move it, what we call horizontally into a totally unrelated species; without regard to the biological constrains. It's very, very bad science. We assume that the principles governing the inheritance of genes vertically, applies when you move genes laterally or horizontally. There's absolutely no reason to make that conclusion. In a human being a mutation … can determine whether you're crippled or you die. Just because they're tiny particles, doesn't mean they're not potent… when you move a gene, one gene, one tiny gene… out of this organism into a different one, you change completely its context. And there is no way at the present time that we can predict how that's going to behave and what the outcome will be; in a civil society, we as consumers ought to be given the choice, whether we

do or do not want to become part of this massive experiment. [22, 23, 24]

Dr. Suzuki implicates enormous investments in the biotechnology paradigm and the fact that the investment must pay off for the investors. He says more than half the products are not being produced to taste better or for better nutrition. They are being developed to allow these plants to be "drenched with Monsanto pesticides." [22, 24]

Alexey V. Surov

In 2010, I reported on a joint experiment by Russia's National Association for Gene Security and the Institute of Ecological and Evolutional Problems, revealing hamsters fed genetically modified (GM) foods produce grandchildren that are unable to deliver fourth generation offspring. [26]

In my article, "GM Food....Feeding the Hungry or Population Control?" I explain that scientists monitoring the behavior, weight gain and birthrate of several groups of hamsters discovered, upon birth, the second generation had slower rates of growth and sexual maturity. The next generation was unable to produce. The scientists fed the hamsters for two years, over three generations, reporting that those fed the GM diet, and especially the group on the maximum GM soy diet, suffered some devastating outcomes. By the third generation most of the GM soy-fed hamsters had lost the ability to have babies; whereas the pups that were born, had slower growth rates and higher mortality than those that were not fed GMO soy. [26] Some of hamsters in the third generation, that ate GM feed, even had hair growing inside of their mouths. [27] (What's up with that?)

The *Huffington Post* says the study reveals 78 pups were born to the non-GM soy group, 52 pups were born in the control group and the GM soy-fed parents only had 40 babies and 25 percent of them died. The report shows a massive death rate in the GM-fed group that was five times higher than the 5 percent they noted among the control animals. Within the group eating high contents of GM soy, only one single female had babies. Although she had 16 pups, about 20 percent of them didn't survive. Surov says, "the low numbers in the F2 group (the third generation) showed that many animals were sterile." [28]

Consider this next time you pass three city blocks of infertility clinics—infertility has skyrocketed in the US with real indications of a populous reduction program, revealed only by seemly outrageous publications. In essence, if aspiring parents are even able to conceive a wanted child, perhaps we might see a day when their offspring will struggle to eat or verbally communicate, due to certain malformations, causing hair to grow in the mouth, like outcomes in the Surov study. Picture yourself the last time you found one stray hair in your mouth.

Nancy Swanson

Dr. Nancy Swanson worked as a staff scientist for the United States Navy and a physics professor at Western Washington University. She retired with five U.S. patents, 30 scientific publications and two books about women in science:

> Not only do the corporations own our governments, they now own science as well. Not only do they control the news via mainstream media, they now control the publication of scientific data. They are determined and relentless...to suppress evidence of harm from their products. They continually state that they want science- based discussions, but only if they get to choose the data. [29]

Dr. Swanson was curious if consumption of GMO crops was related to the rapid rise of chronic disease in Americans. She undertook a study comparing the percentage of GMO corn and soy crops planted, along with the amount of glyphosate applied to corn and soy, plotting out the increases over various time periods. Following suit, she overlapped the data charts to determine if there was any correlation between them and certain chronic diseases. [29] "The consumption of GMO crops or consumption of animals consuming GMO crops was correlated with incidence of or deaths due to organ diseases, cancers, and neurological diseases," she found. [29, 30] Her paper "Genetically engineered crops, glyphosate and the deterioration of health in the United States of America," was published in The *Journal of Organic Systems,* in 2014. In summary, the abstract shows,

> A huge increase in the incidence and prevalence of chronic diseases has been reported in the United States (US) over the last 20 years. Similar increases have been seen globally. The herbicide glyphosate was introduced in 1974 and its use is accelerating with the advent of herbicide-tolerant genetically engineered (GE) crops. Evidence is mounting that glyphosate interferes with many metabolic processes in plants and animals and glyphosate residues have been detected in both. Glyphosate disrupts the endocrine system and the balance of gut bacteria, it damages DNA and is a driver of mutations that lead to cancer. [30]

Swanson thoroughly scoured US Government databases for data files related to GE crops, glyphosate applications and disease epidemiological data: "Correlation analyses were then performed on a total of 22 diseases in these time-series data sets." [30] Dr. Swanson's study shows considerable associations between glyphosate applications, GE corn and soy planted in the US:

> [The] correlations show that the effects of glyphosate and GE crops on human health should be further investigated. [And] all of the correlations were greater than 90%, with autism and senile dementia at 99%. Intestinal diseases were correlated with the number of acres of Bt corn planted. Again, the correlations are all approximately 95%. [30]

The following is what her data shows:

GE Crops Grown in the US

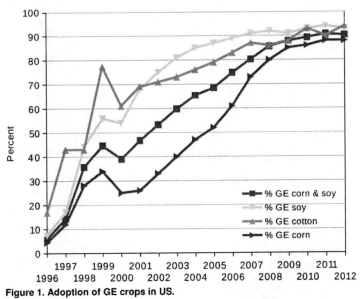

Figure 1. Adoption of GE crops in US.

Courtesy of Dr. Nancy Swanson & Dr. Les Berenson

Swanson, Leu, Abrahamson & Wallet Journal of Organic Systems, 9(2), 2014 ISSN 1177-4258 12

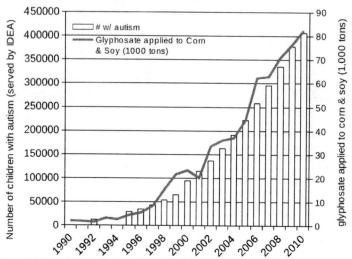

Figure 23. Correlation between children with autism and glyphosate applications.

Courtesy of Dr. Nancy Swanson & Dr. Les Berenson

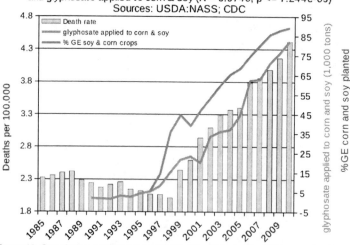

Figure 18. Correlation between age-adjusted End Stage Renal Disease deaths and glyphosate applications and percentage of US corn and soy crops that are GE.

Courtesy of Dr. Nancy Swanson & Dr. Les Berenson

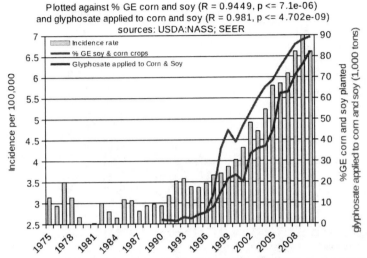

Age Adjusted Urinary/Bladder Cancer Incidence

Plotted against % GE corn and soy (R = 0.9449, p <= 7.1e-06)
and glyphosate applied to corn and soy (R = 0.981, p <= 4.702e-09)
sources: USDA:NASS; SEER

Figure 9. Correlation between age-adjusted bladder/urinary tract cancer and glyphosate applications and percentage of US corn and soy crops that are GE.

Courtesy of Dr. Nancy Swanson & Dr. Les Berenson

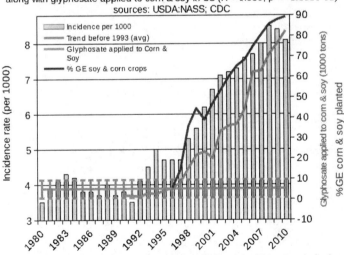

Annual Incidence of Diabetes (age adjusted)

plotted against %GE corn & soy crops planted (R = 0.9547, p <= 1.978e-06)
along with glyphosate applied to corn & soy in US (R = 0.935, p <= 8.303e-08)
sources: USDA:NASS; CDC

Figure 14. Correlation between age-adjusted diabetes incidence and glyphosate applications and percentage of US corn and soy crops that are GE.

Courtesy of Dr. Nancy Swanson & Dr. Les Berenson

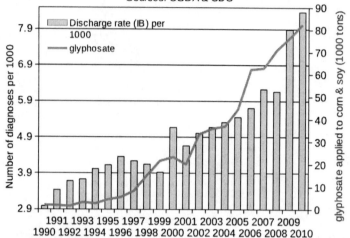

Hospital discharge diagnoses (any) of Inflammatory Bowel disease
(Crohn's and Ulcerative Colitis ICD 555 & 556)

plotted against glyphosate applied to corn & soy (R = 0.9378, p <= 7.068e-08)
Sources: USDA & CDC

Figure 20. Correlation between inflammatory bowel disease and glyphosate applications to US corn and soy crops.

Courtesy of Dr. Nancy Swanson & Dr. Les Berenson

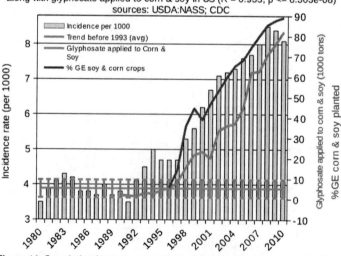

Annual Incidence of Diabetes (age adjusted)

plotted against %GE corn & soy crops planted (R = 0.9547, p <= 1.978e-06)
along with glyphosate applied to corn & soy in US (R = 0.935, p <= 8.303e-08)
sources: USDA:NASS; CDC

Figure 14. Correlation between age-adjusted diabetes incidence and glyphosate applications and percentage of US corn and soy crops that are GE.

Courtesy of Dr. Nancy Swanson & Dr. Les Berenson

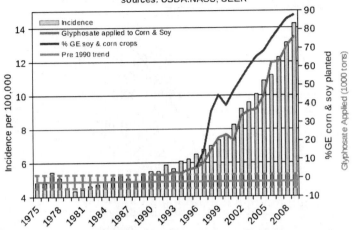

Figure 10. Correlation between age-adjusted thyroid cancer incidence and glyphosate applications and percentage of US corn and soy crops that are GE.

Courtesy of Dr. Nancy Swanson & Dr. Les Berenson

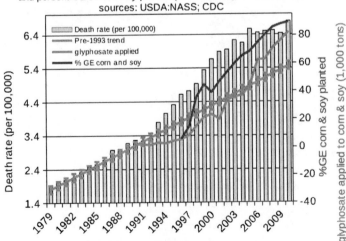

Figure 26. Correlation between age-adjusted Parkinson's disease deaths and glyphosate applications and percentage of US corn and soy crops that are GE.

Courtesy of Dr. Nancy Swanson & Dr. Les Berenson

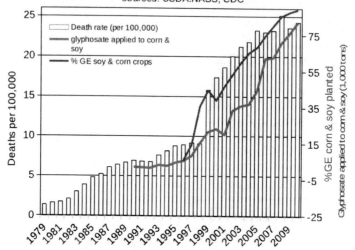

Age Adjusted Deaths from Alzheimer's (ICD G30.9 & 331.0)
Plotted against glyphosate use (R = 0.917, p <= 2.205e-07) &
%GE crops planted (R = 0.9373, p <= 9.604e-06)
sources: USDA:NASS; CDC

Figure 25. Correlation between age-adjusted Alzheimer's disease deaths and glyphosate applications and percentage of US corn and soy crops that are GE.

Courtesy of Dr. Nancy Swanson & Dr. Les Berenson

Dr. Swanson concludes,

> Some of the plots show a significant linear rise that began prior to 1990. Others show a peak in the 1980s, then a decline followed by another rise in the 1990s. Clearly, there are multiple factors involved. Though the data for glyphosate are only available beginning in 1990, glyphosate was first introduced in the marketplace in 1974. [30]

Don Huber

Don Huber is a plant pathologist and professor emeritus at Purdue University. He explains that GMO science is based on faulty concepts where "one gene controls one function":

> We know that isn't the case, we threw out that whole concept of genetics ... 50 years ago with the sequencing of the human genome, when we realized it's not one gene, one function; it's the spatial relationship between genetic material and the influence of the environment that determines what is produced. [31, 32]

Huber warns that genes do not operate alone; they work together and have many different features based on environmental conditions and the health and responses of the genome as a whole. [31, 32]

I think that when you re-manufacture our genetic code, in the words of Forest Gump, it's "like a box of chocolates. You never know what you're gonna get."

In January 2011, Huber advised the federal government about his discovery of a novel organism that has the potential of "causing infertility and spontaneous abortions in exposed farm animals." He expresses concerns about the health of humans and the animals we consume. He warns that the unnamed organism might be associated with over reliance on weed killers used on food crops.

Huber wrote a letter to the Secretary of Agriculture, Tom Vilsack. Huber asked the federal government to bypass deregulation of Roundup Ready crops, specifically the RR alfalfa. He cautioned Vilsack about the potential for this new microscopic pathogen to impact the health of plants, animals and probably even human beings. The letter thoroughly lays out his intentions, along with his colleagues around "moving the investigation forward with speed and discretion, and [to] seek assistance from the USDA and other entities to identify the pathogen's source, prevalence, implications, and remedies." [31,32]

Dr. Huber has over 40 years of experience as a top-level scientist in both professional and military segments, responsible for evaluations and preparedness for natural and manmade biological threats involving things like germ warfare and outbreaks of disease—"based on this experience, I believe the threat we are facing from this pathogen is unique and of a high—risk status. In layman's terms, it should be treated as an emergency." The tests confirm the lab results evaluating the presence of this unique organism in a wide variety of livestock that have shown tendencies towards spontaneous abortions and infertility patterns. The preliminary findings are the result of his ongoing research, replicated with the same results within a clinical setting: "appearance of this pathogen might be used to explain the accelerated incidence of infertility rates and spontaneous abortions over the last few years inside U.S agencies involving cattle, dairy, pigs, and horses." [31, 32]

Huber says there is recent data verifying infertility rates in dairy heifers running over 20 percent, with spontaneous abortions in cattle as high as 45 percent. One prime example, he notes, nearly half of the one thousand pregnant heifers, in the study, suffered spontaneous abortions after they were fed wheatlege. In comparison, over the same period, another one thousand heifers from the same herd were eating hay and were able to sustain all of their pregnancies. The researchers blame the wheat crops for high concentrations of this new pathogen, which they confirmed in lab results. [31, 32]

The researchers called for a multi-agency investigation involving the USDA, along with an immediate moratorium on planned deregulation of GMO Roundup Ready crops to determine any existing causal/predisposing relationships with glyphosate and/or RR plants, so they could potentially rule out any threat to human or animal health and any future crop production. [31, 32]

Given the seriousness of these assertions, Dr. Huber is by far one of the most prepared to make such allegations and determinations with 50 years of pathogenic studies. Dr. Huber clearly knows what is at stake and has continued to push back on the potential hazards involving use of these new crop technologies. [31, 32] The USDA ignored all of Dr. Huber's concerns and approved RR Alfalfa anyway. [31, 32]

Thierry Vrain

Dr. Thierry Vrain is a well-respected scientist formerly with the federal government of Canada. Designated as an official spokesperson to assure the public of the safety of GMO foods Vrain believed very much in their potential. After careful research and reconsideration of the evidence Dr. Vrain changed his stance, sending a cautionary letter to the Health Minister of Canada and describing his concerns about the use of glyphosate-based Roundup on food crops. [33]

I had a rare opportunity to speak with Dr. Vrain, in the summer of 2015, about his renewed perspectives on GMOs and what he sees as a serious cause for concern regarding the broad use of glyphosate-based herbicides, in particular. He cautions regulators about the use of this toxic herbicide. the resulting chemical pollution and its antibiotic effects that impact the microbiome of consumers.

In his letter to the Canadian Minister of Health, Vrain points out,

> Animal feeding studies proving the safety of GMOs do not include testing for the safety of glyphosate. None of them mentions the residue levels of glyphosate in the feed. Meanwhile...independent studies in various countries published in the last 5 years have ascertained the impact of glyphosate on various cellular enzymes and organs of animals and of human cells.

Roundup is "sprayed on many non-engineered crops with the intent to kill them right before harvest," Vrain says in the letter. The problem is the antibiotic patent describes its effectiveness for killing bacteria at 1 ppm, he notes. [33, 34]

Vrain introduced me to the Séralini study which we will examine further. It concludes that glyphosate is a well-known endocrine disrupter at just ½ part per million. [35] The endocrine system is important, because it's the collection of glands that produce your body's hormones. It regulates your metabolism, growth and development, tissue function, sexual function, reproduction, sleep and mood, among many other things. It comprises the pituitary gland, thyroid gland, parathyroid glands, adrenal glands, pancreas, ovaries (in females) and testicles (in males). [36]

Vrain illustrates a review of medical literature showing a link between celiac and other diseases related to imbalances in the microbiome that are "fully explained by the antibiotic properties of glyphosate." He also warns about direct toxicity in animal cells because "glyphosate binds to metals indiscriminately, and not just in plant cells." Glyphosate, he criticizes, "bio-accumulates in the plants and...animals that eat the plants. Furthermore, he says the chemical, "accumulates in the lungs, the heart, kidneys, intestine, liver, spleen, muscles, and bones ... and chronically ill people have higher residues in their urine than healthy people." [37]

In his public presentations Vrain frequently references studies showing proteins made by engineered plants are different than what they should be. He vocally asserts that the GE technology used to insert a gene can result in damage to those proteins. He continues to point to scientific literature full of studies proving, "engineered corn and soy contain toxic or allergenic proteins." Vrain directly maintains, "GE technology is based on a naïve misunderstanding...that relies on the notion that each gene is coded for one single protein." The Human Genome Project, Vrain affirms, proved this hypothesis wrong back in 2002. [38] What does that mean? It clearly indicates that biotech scientists are holding firm to outdated concepts to justify what they know are faulty conclusions about how genes function and perform within the context of the entire genome.

Dr. Vrain continues to oppose the idiocy surrounding this obsolete science which perpetuates the foolishness behind the idea that genes operate apart from one another. In all actuality, they very well know and have known for some time that they have no control over the synergistic effects of the genetic structure, once they've remodeled it.

Stanley Ewen

Dr. Stanley Ewen is one of Scotland's leading experts in tissue diseases. As a histopathologist for 29 years he is concerned that the cauliflower mosaic virus, used in GMOs, could increase the risk of colon and stomach cancers. Ewen worries for the health of citizens living near GM crop trials, suggesting contamination could hasten the growth of malignant tumors. He told the *Sunday Herald*, "I'm very concerned that people who rely on local produce might be endangering themselves," He says the cauliflower mosaic virus shows up as a "promoter" in GM foods. He compares it to a tiny engine that drives the implanted genes to express themselves. Not only that, he points to the risk of potential infection from the virus that could be acting as a "growth factor" in the stomach or colon, encouraging polyp growth. "The faster and bigger they grow, the more likely they are to be malignant," he adds. [39]

Ewen confirms, "It is possible cows' milk will contain GM derivatives that can be directly ingested by humans as milk or cheese." In addition, he believes there may be the potential for GM DNA to affect colonic and stomach lining, causing growth factor effects that could accelerate cancer formation in those organs; although, he notes, that it is yet to be proven. [39]

Irina Ermakova

Irina Ermakova Chief Neuroscientist at The Institute of Higher Nervous Activity and Neurophysiology Russian Academy of

Science, Moscow. She made major headlines in 2005, announcing her findings on lab rats and their offspring after they were given a diet containing glyphosate-tolerant GM soy. Concerns were widely raised when some of the pups, born to the GM soy group, suffered low survival and/or stunted growth. Within three weeks of birth, she says, over 55 percent of the rats from the GM soy group died, in comparison to 9 percent from the non-gm group and around 7 percent from her control group: [40] "When male rats were fed GM soy, their testicles actually changed color—from the normal pink to dark blue." [41]

Ermakova is no stranger to scientific methodology and study protocol. She has participated in countless international conferences while completing numerous joint investigations with scientists in Czechoslovakia, UK, USA, and Sweden. In addition, she's published 123 scientific papers. [42]

Ermakova revealed her findings at the Scientists for a GM FREE Europe conference in Brussels:

> many things went wrong for rats fed genetically modified soybeans. They became more anxious and aggressive; there was a high mortality of rat pups born to the females in the first generation, disturbances of reproductive functions, and pathological changes in the internal organs of males and females.

When Ermakova fed rats GM soy flour they suffered five times higher infant mortality rates than those fed on conventional soy feed. [43. 44, 45]

The paper, "Experimental Evidence of GMO Hazards" details the GM dietary influences on the physiological state and behavior of Wistar rats and their offspring when fed GM RR soy. The team analyzed the physiological state (weight, size and so forth), reproductive functions, the rate of mortality, and behavior of rats and their offspring. [45]

Dr. Ermakova was invited to reveal her primary findings at a Biotech conference, where she asked their scientific community to replicate her study. They never did. Instead, they went on the attack. Her boss advised her not to do anymore GMO research—her samples were stolen from her lab and someone started a fire on her desk. One of her colleagues even said, "maybe the GM soy will solve the overpopulation problem." To top it off, at the end of her study, Ermakova says she found out that the supplier of the animal feed started using GMO soy in the formula and so "all the rats were now eating it." After two months, she checked in with the lab members who told her that the infant mortality rate had jumped to over 55 percent. [46]

The American Academy of Environmental Medicine (AAEM) called for additional independent studies on the safety of GM crops. Ermakova's findings played a major role in that decision. Her research has prompted regulatory agencies in several countries to review their own approval of GM foods. Although it would only cost a few thousand dollars to replicate Ermakova's research, the biotech community never has. [46]

V.A. Shiva Ayyadurai

MIT Scientist and Systems Biologist, Dr. Ayyadurai's new study calls out Monsanto's claims of "equivalence" and the entire GMO approval process used to determine its safety for human and animal consumption. He says the federal standard is flawed and he proves it. This study is the first of its kind, a systems biology analysis representing the final outcome of three previous scientific papers, published in *Agricultural Sciences* and *The American Journal of Plant Sciences*. The study concludes that the process of genetic modification in soy disrupts the natural processes of the plant and begins production of formaldehyde which is a known carcinogen. [47. 48]

Dr. V.A. Shiva Ayyadurai and his team used a digital system to integrate 6,497 in vitro and in vivo laboratory experiments from 184 scientific institutions across 23 various countries. In that, they discovered significant formaldehyde production, along with a dramatic depletion of glutathione which is an essential antioxidant that the body needs to complete the process of detoxification. [47. 47a, 48]

Inhibiting detoxification has disastrous results on human health with damages to the metabolic processes of the body. With that we would see massive epidemics of cancer and chronic disease, which is what we are seeing in every state of the union. This should be considered a public health emergency. Dr. Ayyadurai affirms,

> The results demand immediate testing along with rigorous scientific standards to assure such testing is objective and replicable. It's unbelievable such standards for testing do not already exist. The safety of our food supply demands that science deliver such modern scientific standards for approval of GMOs. [47. 48]

Former EPA Senior Scientist Dr. Ray Seidler says,

> Dr. Ayyadurai reveals a new molecular paradigm associated with genetic engineering that will require research to discover why, and how much formaldehyde and glutathione... and what other cellular chemicals relevant to human and animal health, are altered We need the kinds of standards Dr. Ayyadurai demands to conduct such research...formaldehyde is a known class 1 carcinogen. Its elevated presence in soybeans caused by a common genetic engineering event is alarming and deserves immediate attention and action from the FDA and the Obama administration. Soy is widely grown and consumed in the U.S., including by infants fed baby food products, with 94% of soy grown here being genetically engineered. [47]

Dr. Ayyadurai put out a press release offering up his ten million dollar building in Cambridge, Massachusetts, if Monsanto could prove his conclusions wrong: "If this is what it takes to bring the truth to the American people, then I am more than willing to do it." He criticizes the whole fast-track market approach, which it would have been invalidated if this study would have been used for the safety assessment criteria for GMOs in the first place. [47]

Once again, this demonstrates the deficiencies in the current approval process. It clearly appears, as though, they are putting the public and our children at greater and greater risk for cancer and chronic disease, within the confines of this mass feeding experiment.

Michael Antoniou

In 2015, Dr. Michael Antoniou a scientist at King's College London, shared his results from a peer-reviewed study proving that Roundup is toxic at chronically low doses. The paper concludes that even within the levels permitted in drinking water in the EU, it can damage the liver and kidneys of rats who consume it. [49]

The report says, "alterations in gene function were found indicating such diseases, as fibrosis (scarring), necrosis (areas of dead tissue), phospholipidosis (disturbed fat metabolism), and damage to mitochondria (the centres of respiration in cells)." [49] The paper was published in the *Environmental Health Journal* showing levels of glyphosate-based herbicides alter the gene function of over 4000 different genes in the kidneys and livers of rats. The scientists also re-analyzed the gene expression profiles in liver and kidney tissues from the Roundup-treated rats in Seralini's long-term feeding study. The researchers figured out the gene expression changes, seen in the new analysis, confirm the liver and kidney pathologies, exactly as suggested by the original anatomical and biochemical (blood and urine) findings in the Séralini study. The report concludes that the dose of Roundup, administered in this study, was about half the amount of pure glyphosate permitted in the drinking water in the EU, which is 20,000 times less than those allowed in Australia and another 14,000 times lower than those in the USA. The authors add that long-term Roundup exposure....at an ultra-low and environmentally relevant dose, "can result in liver and kidney damage with potential significant health implications for animal and human populations." Dr. Antoniou says,

> The findings of our study are very worrying, as they confirm that a very low level of consumption of

Roundup weedkiller, over the long term can result in liver and kidney damage. Our results also suggest that regulators should re-consider the safety evaluation of glyphosate-based herbicides. [49, 50, 51]

Antoniou teamed up with scientists John Fagen and Claire Robinson creating Earth Open Source to help restore grassroots agriculture and science driven food and farm policy. In 2012, the team released "GMO Myths and Truths" with over 600 citations, most of which were from peer-reviewed journals. The report concludes,

1. Genetic engineering is not precise or predictable, nor has it been shown to be safe. The GE techniques can lead to the unexpected production of toxins or allergens in the food that are unlikely to be spotted during regulatory checks.

2. GM crops, including some already in the food and animal feed, show clear signs of toxicity in animal feeding trials, most notably pointing to disturbances in liver and kidney function and immune responses.

3. "GM delivers more pesticide use but little else." Plus, "when many people read about high-yielding, pest- and disease-resistant, drought-tolerant, and nutritionally improved super-crops, they think of GM. In fact, these are all products of conventional breeding, which continues to outstrip GM in producing such crops. The report contains a long list of these crop breeding successes." [49, 50]

4. GM will "not feed the world" and viable alternatives do exist. [49,50]

FarmingUK says the report,

should open up the debate at a high level on the benefits

of GM crops and be essential reading not just for policy makers. The questions raised in this report are too numerous and serious to be simply disregarded. [And] what makes it even more difficult to ignore is the credentials of the authors concerned, these are not your light-weight anti-everything tree huggers but acclaimed scientists. [51]

The scientists published a 2nd edition in 2014, which is available for download at: earthopensource.org.

Andrés Carrasco

Andrés Carrasco is an embryologist with Argentina's Ministry of Science. He reveals the results of his research on the effects of Roundup on amphibians, suggesting that the herbicide can cause "defects in the brain, intestines, and hearts of (amphibian) fetuses." Moreover he reports that the amount of Roundup used in GM soy fields was around 1,500 times more than what he used on amphibians in his lab that created the defects he observed. Carrasco says the study was inspired by the experience of desperate peasant and indigenous communities suffering from exposure to toxic herbicides used on the GM soy fields throughout Argentina.

A 2009 article in *Grain* states,

> Three days after the interview, the Association of Environmental Lawyers filed a petition…calling for a ban on the use and sale of glyphosate until its impact on health and on the environment had to be investigated Five days later the Ministry of Defence banned the planting of soya in its fields. This sparked a strong reaction from the multinational biotechnology companies and their supporters. [52]

Reports say they, "mounted an unprecedented attack on Carrasco, ridiculing his research and even issuing personal threats." *Global Research* says Carrasco recalls four men arriving at his laboratory that were being extremely aggressive. He says they were attempting to interrogate him and obtain details of his study. "It was a violent, disproportionate, dirty reaction...I hadn't even discovered anything new, only confirmed conclusions that others had reached." Following, Argentina's Association of Environmental Lawyers filed a petition calling for a ban on Roundup, and the Ministry of Defence banned GM soy from its fields. [52. 53]

Judy Carman

Dr. Judy Carman Epidemiologist and Associate Professor of Health and the Environment for Flinders University, Australia, published a pig study in 2013 titled, "A long-term toxicology study on pigs fed a combined genetically modified (GM) soy and GM corn maize diet." [54, 55] Simon Lauder reported in an ABC interview that Carman's researchers raised two sets of 84 pigs on different diets at a commercial piggery. One group ate GM corn and soy; the other ate a non-GM diet. [54] The researchers, "chose pigs because they have a similar digestive system to humans, and because some of the investigators had been observing reproductive and digestive problems in pigs fed GM crops." [55] The doctor observed two significant outcomes in the GM-fed pigs; the first was related to the weight of the uterus, in the females, which was 25 percent heavier, compared to those that were fed conventional non-GM feed. The second finding showed a level of severe stomach inflammation in the GM-fed pigs that was much higher than in the non-GM fed pigs. Overall, the levels were 2.6 times higher in the GM-fed pigs. In addition, they report,

> Some of the investigators had previously seen a reduced ability to conceive and higher rates of miscarriage ... where sows were fed a GM diet, and a reduction in the number of piglets born if boars were used for conception rather than artificial insemination. [Also] higher rates of intestinal problems in pigs fed a GM diet, including inflammation of the stomach and small intestine, stomach ulcers, a thinning of intestinal walls and an increase in haemorrhagic bowel disease, where a pig

can rapidly "bleed-out" from their bowel and die; these findings are both biologically significant and statistically significant. [And] key findings were not reflected in the standard biochemistry tests that are done in GM feeding studies, probably because standard biochemistry tests provide a poor measure of inflammation and matters associated with uterus size. [55. 56]

Dr. Carman says she has been repeatedly attacked and intimidated and recounts that pro-GM scientists have threatened disciplinary action and even circulated a derogatory letter, sending it to officials in the government and the university. [57] *Sustainable Pulse* spoke with one of the study's coordinators, a crop and livestock advisor named Howard Vlieger:

For as long as GM crops have been in the feed supply, we have seen increasing digestive and reproductive problems in animals... farmers have found increased production costs and escalating antibiotic use when feeding GM crops. In some operations, the livestock death loss is high, and there are unexplained problems including spontaneous abortions, deformities of new- born animals, and an overall listlessness and lack of contentment in the animals. In some cases, animals eating GM crops are very aggressive...given the scale of stomach irritation and inflammation now documented. I have seen no financial benefit to farmers who feed GM crops to their animals. [56]

Biotech Ruse Refuses Real Science

Jeffrey Smith submitted a written testimonial to the French courts, in November 2010, in support of Professor Séralini. It details formal attempts to hush scientific data from independent scientists while trying to block research efforts on biotech products. Two researchers Marc Lappé and Britt Bailey discovered considerable decreases in cancer fighting isoflavones in GE soybeans. The seed vendor Hartz refused to provide further samples for testing. [57]

Smith says Allison Snow a plant pathologist for Ohio State University found notable side effects in GM sunflowers. She reveals that the seed companies prevented her from further study by refusing to supply her lab with GM seeds or genes. [57]

The editors of *Scientific American* hammer on the fact that virtually no independent studies are being conducted that potentially could find problems:

> it's impossible to verify that genetically modified crops perform as advertised—that is because agritech companies have given themselves veto power over the work of independent researchers.... user agreements have explicitly forbidden the use of the seeds for any independent research. Under the threat of litigation, scientists cannot test a seed to explore the different conditions under which it thrives or fails.....they cannot examine whether the genetically modified crops lead to unintended environmental side effects.

They confirm that GE seed research is still being published, although it is purposely set up in a way,

> only studies that the seed companies have approved ever see the light of a peer-reviewed journal...experiments that had the implicit go-ahead from the seed company were later blocked from publication because the results were not flattering. [58]

Scientific research is not just being restricted in the US. In Japan, a scientist requested GM soybeans that were under government review, for animal feeding studies. DuPont refused to grant samples for the study. Furthermore, after Professor Bela Darvas discovered GE corn harms endangered species, Monsanto blocked supplies of the corn so the doctor couldn't review them, and they distributed a false and misleading report about his research findings. [57]

Smothered Science and Ecological Terrorism

Dr. Charles Benbrook Executive Director of the Board of Agriculture of the U.S. National Academy of Sciences says that he has personally spoke with dozens of scientists who,

> had to contend with this backlash and these counter attacks that the industry unleashes on scientists that they view as a threat. The majority of them get out of the field...will not put themselves, or their families, or their career at that kind of risk again. [57]

A researcher in Turkey collected seeds to assess the scope of GMO contamination in the country. *Turkish Daily News* says that just before her testing was complete they re-assigned her to a different department and denied her access to her lab. [57] Luckily, this shift just may have saved her research career from a severe outcome—just ask other scientists that have been brazen enough to report GMO crop contamination to people that should care.

Ignacio H. Chapela

Dr. Ignacio Chapela a microbial ecologist at University of California, Berkeley found indigenous corn varieties of maize had been contaminated by GMO pollen. Johannes Wirz defines the situation in the "Case of Mexican Maize" for the *Nature Institute*, featuring Chapela's scientific investigation centering around 60 native varieties cultivated in the remote mountains of Mexico known as the "heartland of maize diversity." The paper says that it is likely the GM corn was coming in from the US and being planted illegally in the country, adding that imports of GM corn had been under moratorium since 1998, and so it had no lawful business or trade across the southern border. [59]

Let's consider this: For thousands of years corn maize varieties have been the cornerstone of Mexican heritage. Hispanic farmers have maintained the world's oldest seed strains, containing multitudes of genetically diverse types that have been contaminated through cross-pollination with Monsanto's GM varieties. Generations upon generations of seed cultivation and storage have been utterly destroyed by this contamination. Despite protective measures, GM corn continues to be shoved across the Mexican border, landing on tabletops for unsuspecting consumers to eat and plant. This trespass has taken place without the knowledge or consent of the Mexican people, sound familiar? Keep in mind that Hispanic cultures develop rich relationships with their food, often eating and sowing the seeds from meals, as part of the normal cycle of daily living.

When Dr. Chapela submitted his research observations to the journal *Nature* he informed the Mexican government as a courtesy. This was a move that he would later regret. Wirz speculates:

> One might have expected that those companies that sell GM-corn to growers would have been disconcerted by the publication of this article. Although, it wasn't the case because Arthur Einsele, public relations chief for the biotech company 'Syngenta', stated that the mixing of foreign genes with the land varieties was not a concern. He even suggested that the mixing could contribute usefully to the diversification of domestic plants (quoted in Dreesmann 2001). [59]

Chapela's work still leaves little doubt about the state of GM contamination in the country, but at the time, it was direct threat to official plans to introduce GM corn to Mexican markets. Reports say he was surprised when he was called in for a meeting with the director of the Commission of Biosafety and GMOs. The director was furious about the journal submission, demanding that it be withdrawn immediately before publication, Chapela says. The official tried to intimidate and threaten the doctor, even cautioning him that they knew where his kids went to school.

Chapela even says he got a letter threatening to hold him responsible for any damages affecting the agriculture and economy as a result of his publication. It didn't stop there either; two women, he recounts, Mary Murphy and Andura Smetacek started unveiling a smear campaign against him, posting disparaging messages about him on a biotech industry list-serve which was distributed to more than 3,000 scientists. [60] The posts falsely claimed that Chapela's research was biased and that his paper had not been peer-reviewed. They said he is "first and foremost an activist," and his paper was published in collusion with the environmentalists.

Hundreds of other messages were being spread about, repeating and exaggerating the same non-sense allegations. The biotech list-serve went out of their way inundating the journal with a vicious smear campaign demanding Chapela's research be retracted. UC Berkeley received letters attempting to convince them not to grant Chapela his tenure. And although he had the overwhelming support of the university and his department, the international biotech lobby proved too powerful; Chapela's tenure was denied, but returned to him eventually after he filed a lawsuit.[60]

Investigators later examined the email characteristics of the letters from Murphy and Smetacek. The *Guardian* reports that the names were both fabricated by a public relations firm working for, guess who? That's right, Monsanto; you guessed it. Some of Smetacek's emails also showed the internet address of *gatekeeper2.monsanto. com*, proving to them that the server was owned by Monsanto. [60]

The universal protocol of the biotech pawn, almost always, involves a standard of attack on genuine science to suppress the facts, regardless of any extent they have to go to in order to maintain a shell of legitimacy.

Dr. Chapela has been deeply disturbed by the calculated pressures, and the "de facto ban," he says exists on world scientists today who are "asking certain questions and finding certain results." He emphasizes that "It's very hard for us to publish in this field. People are scared." He reveals that young scientists, "are not going into this field precisely because they are discouraged by what they see." [60]

The science journal *Nature* condemns the attacks occurring on researchers studying GMO feeding outcomes; regular assaults orchestrated by a "large block of scientists who denigrate research by other legitimate scientists in a knee-jerk, partisan, emotional way...not helpful in advancing knowledge and is outside the ideals of scientific inquiry," criticizes writer Emily Waltz. [57, 60]

Researchers repeatedly complain that Monsanto refuses to grant permissions to independent scientists for GMO based feeding studies. No legitimate analysis can be performed or published on any transgenic product without Monsanto's express permission and provision of those products. Monsanto rarely grants this authorization to those seeking its permission. [58] They know, if you can't track it, you can't control it. Perhaps they fear the mounting evidence disrobing the deceit of the entire biotech industry.

Sue Kedgley

New Zealand Parliament Member Sue Kedgley testified before The Royal Commission of Inquiry into Genetic Modification (RCIGM) in 2001:

> I have been contacted by telephone and e-mail by a number of scientists who have serious concerns about aspects of the research ... and the increasingly close ties that are developing between science and commerce ... convinced that if they express these fears publicly, or even if they asked the awkward and difficult questions, they will be eased out of their institution. Perhaps we could set up human clinical trials using volunteers of genetically engineered scientists and their families, ... they are so convinced of the safety of the products that they are creating and I'm sure they would very readily volunteer to become part of a human clinical trial. [53, 57. 60, 62]

During a 2006 podcast interview Kedgley told producers of the Canadian radio show "Deconstructing Dinner" that there are,

> so many loopholes and flaws in the current regulatory regime for testing the safety of genetically engineered

food….a regulatory- free façade which enables food producers to claim that their products have been properly tested and ….that genetically engineered foods are safe.[62]

Biologist Phil Regal from the University of Minnesota, also appeared on the program after testifying before the Royal Commission, where he said, "People who boost genetic engineering are going to have to do a mea culpa ….ask for forgiveness like the Pope did on the inquisition—we made a mistake. Let's start over." [62]

Upon the constructs of our kitchen table it is imperative that we consider the vast amount of sound scientific data and analysis being held hostage by corporate manipulation and mainstream media influences. The extensive demonstrations of commercial and scientific fraud are ramming us down a rabbit hole of soiled evidence and back room exchanges that completely disregard pertinent matters of public safety and corporate intent.

Mad Science and the Recombinant Bovine Growth Hormone (rBGH)

Six Canadian Government scientists testified before a Senate committee in 1998, that they were pressured by superiors to approve the rBGH drug, after documents were stolen from a locked file cabinet. They said Monsanto was trying to bribe them, with millions of dollars, to pass the drug without any further testing. [64]

The documentary film, *Seeds of Deception,* reveals the tests were being skewed to the point that they were purposely intent on showing rBGH injections would not interfere with fertility in animals. The film says the FDA leaked documents showing researchers were using cows, for the study, that were pregnant before the injection was ever administered in the first place. [65]

FDA Veterinarian Ricard Burroughs was the lead reviewer in the approval process of recombinant bovine growth hormone (rBGH). Since he was the only member of the FDA team with dairy herd experience he was charged with writing the primary protocols to evaluate the safety of rBGH for cows. [64. 65]

Burroughs himself says the drug, "was approved prematurely without adequate information," and even the FDA officials "suppressed and manipulated data to cover up their own ignorance and incompetence." He maintains that he exposed the science behind the studies, because it was really well outside the expertise of the agency's employees; so rather than admit they were in over their heads, "the Center decided to cover up inappropriate studies and decisions." [65]

Burroughs criticizes the fact, like any other drug, FDA doesn't conduct these tests themselves. It's really the drug maker that is responsible for the studies and for relating the results; but Burroughs charges that they "would come in and try to negotiate the protocols to water them down." Ultimately, after they presented their findings, he was totally shocked that "they just went out and skewed the data." One such example, he offers, was Monsanto's claim that only a handful of cows developed udder infections; whereas the documents reveal, actual numbers topped 9,500. Moreover, the infected cows were often removed from the company's studies completely. Burroughs demanded further testing but was fired in 1989: "I was told that I was slowing down the approval process."

Later, his former boss from the FDA testified that Burroughs was set up. He was allowed to rejoin the agency eventually, although after reinstatement he was not permitted to see any of the rBGH data again, and they made his life so miserable that he quit the position. [65]

The *Huffington Post* reports that the Canadian Government criticized the FDA's approval of the drug, in what is known as the "Gaps Analysis Report," while illustrating omissions, contradictions, weaknesses and significant gaps in the FDA approval process. The analysis concludes the "1990 evaluation was largely a theoretical review taking the manufacturer's conclusions at face value. In addition, "no details of the studies nor a critical analysis of the quality of the data was provided." They say that since rBGH is a hormone, "its chemistry should have prompted more exhaustive and longer toxicological studies in laboratory animals." The report too, reveals that because these studies weren't conducted, "such possibilities and potential as sterility, infertility, birth defects, cancer and immunological derangements were not addressed." Also the FDA "improperly reported" data from the feeding study and arrived at false and unsupported conclusions regarding safety. [66]

Furthermore, the FDA was forced to admit they overlooked a significant antibody study with 20-30 percent of the rats developing clear antibody responses to the drug. The Canadian report asserts that some of the male rats had thyroid cysts and changes to their prostate glands, which was not investigated. [66]

Promotion in motion

A telling report from KGW in Portland, Oregon said that Tillamook County Creamery Association in Oregon, the second largest block cheese producer in the nation, condemned Monsanto because it pressured members, around 147 farmers, to reverse their decision not to use rBGH in their cows to boost milk production. The Association described Monsanto's tactics as "an aggressive intrusion." [63, 67]

The European Network of Scientists for Social and Environmental Responsibility (ENSSER)

The ENSSER released a public statement declaring, "no scientific consensus on GMO safety." The ENSSER first published the blaring criticism in late 2013, in response to what they say were "claims from the GM industry....that there is a 'scientific consensus' that GM foods and crops are safe for human and animal health and the environment." The statement refers to the claims as "misleading," adding that "the claimed consensus on GMO safety does not exist." One of authors Dr. Angelika Hilbeck, the chair of ENSSER says, as well as receiving the endorsement of the peer reviewers at the journal, the statement has also been peer-reviewed and transparently endorsed by more than 300 scientists and experts from relevant fields of inquiry.

At the top of the list appears a quite unexpected signature by Dr. Belinda Martineau, a former member of the Michelmore Lab at the UC Davis Genome Center, who helped get the first GMO to market.

Dr. Martineau declares,

I wholeheartedly support this thorough, thoughtful and professional statement describing the lack of scientific consensus on the safety of genetically engineered (GM/GE) crops and other GM/GE organisms (also referred to as GMOs). Society's debate over how best to utilize the powerful technology of genetic engineering is clearly not over. For its supporters to assume it is, is little more than wishful thinking.

Dr. Judy Carman Director of the Institute of Health Environmental Research in Australia, signed the statement testifying,

Of the hundreds of different GM crops ... approved for human and animal consumption ... few have been thoroughly safety tested—it is not possible to have a consensus that they are all safe to eat—at least, not a consensus based on hard scientific evidence.

Professor Elena Alvarez-Buyllla is the coordinator of the Laboratory of Molecular Genetics of Plant Development and Evolution, Institute of Ecology, in Mexico. She endorsed the statement, voicing strong concerns over widespread GM contamination cornering the Mexican maize industry: "... sweeping claims that GM crops are substantially equivalent to ... non-GM crops are not justifiable. GMO releases, can threaten the genetic diversity on which food security depends ... globally." And furthermore,

Such decisions with broad implications for society should not be made by a narrow group of self-selected experts ... whom have commercial interests in GM technology, but must also involve the millions of people who will be most affected; in Mexico we have an ongoing uncontrolled experiment ... in which GM genes are allowed to cross-breed with native maize varieties. The inevitable result will be genetic alterations with unpredictable effects.

One co-author of the statement E. Ann Clark is a retired associate professor at the University of Guelph in Canada who criticizes the fast track approval process:

Groupthink is perhaps the best way to characterize claims of scientific consensus on the safety of GM crops. This phenomenon ... refers to the irrational outcomes that result when pressures to conform within a like-minded group degrade mental efficiency, reality testing, and moral judgment. Consensus claimers manifest striking consistency with ... groupthink, including illusions of invulnerability, collective rationalization, and suppression of dissent. The reality is that there is no consensus on GMO safety. Strident and incessant claims of such a consensus must not override the urgent necessity for well reasoned and conducted research into the safety of GM crops.

Jack Heinemann a well-respected professor of genetics and molecular biology at the Centre for Integrated Research in Biosafety, University of Canterbury, New Zealand, also co-authored the statement stating:

Public confidence in GMOs will not increase as long as some scientists try to keep the public and other scientists from asking legitimate questions about their safety, efficacy and value. Even if all questions ... were answered tomorrow, that would not mean that future products should be exempt from questioning and thorough testing. Instead of shouting, 'Don't look here, we have a consensus already', we should address the cause of public mistrust; by embracing open discussions of GMOs ... from a variety of points of view, acknowledging and including the true diversity of scientific opinions. [68]

Abusing Nature

Biotech designs are crossing more than kingdoms in pursuit of genetic recognition; one such horrific example illustrates this case in the extreme, genetically modified glow in the dark pets. Yes, rabbits, pigs, sheep and your family cat are now among the glowing. [69]

These are the story lines of fiction writers gone awry and science has taken its bow, mocking nature and the very core of our existence. Their promises to feed the world were, in fact, a façade of epic proportions designed to restructure nature (something that is inherently free and part of your birthright as a human) and sell it back to you.

Genetic Transfer and Promoter Genes

Can these transgenic genes become part of our own human physiology, making us, in essence, GMO human beings? For years, regulators and the biotech industry have claimed that GMOs would not create a horizontal gene transfer in humans or animals. Research is telling us a whole different story.

GMO DNA:
- Is in the digestive tract of sheep fed GMO feed;
- Is taken up by the animal's organs and,
- Is in the milk and meat.

The Institute for Responsible Technology reports that the only human feeding study ever published shows portions of the soy Roundup Ready (RR) gene being transferred into the gut bacteria, where researchers believe it might have continued to function. [70, 71]

Before her death in 2016, Dr. Mae Wan Ho was a prominent geneticist and vocal critic of genetic engineering who warned us:

> transgenic DNA typically contain genetic material from bacteria, viruses and other genetic parasites that cause diseases as well as antibiotic resistance genes that make infectious diseases untreatable. Horizontal transfer of transgenic DNA has the potential ... to create new viruses and bacteria that cause diseases and spread drug and antibiotic resistance genes among pathogens. [71]

A study published by the National Institute of Health (NIH), *PubMed*, hones in on the central issue:

> As genetically modified (GM) foods are starting to intrude in our diet concerns have been expressed regarding GM food safety. Animal toxicity studies with certain GM foods have shown that they may toxically affect several organs and systems. The review of these studies should not be conducted separately for each GM food, but according to the effects exerted on certain organs. The results of most studies with GM foods indicate that they may cause ... hepatic, pancreatic, renal, or reproductive effects and may alter the hematological, biochemical, and immunologic parameters. However, many years of research with animals and clinical trials are required for this assessment. [72]

Note: PubMed is a free public resource, established and maintained by the National Center for Biotechnology Information (NCBI), at the US National Library of Medicine (NLM), which is located at the National Institutes of Health (NIH).

Countless researchers continue to repeat the warnings,

cautioning us about the potential of horizontal gene transfers with the use of transgenic DNA in our food supply. Science clearly indicates the potential for it to open the doorway to new viruses and disease. In addition, many scientists express deep concerns that the promoter genes in GMOs may be waking up dormant genes in our kids (and us) that have long been latent or asleep, genes like cancer and autism. [73, 74] Everybody has disease and genetic tendencies lurking around their body that they don't want swimming in their gene pool, and the last thing we want to encourage is their reproduction. Researchers admit they have no control over those genes that are promoted and those that are being suppressed. [73, 74]

Our children are most likely suffering as a result of this process, yet the science is being hidden from us to protect Monsanto's shareholders and the reputations of those involved. Meanwhile, governments around the world are choosing sides with or without the benefit of knowledge-based science and independent facts, provided by researchers that are not bound to stockholder pockets and corporate intimidation. The *real* war on science is taking a global toll on public health, the environment and the decent scientists fighting to protect the integrity of their scientific standards.

Honest researchers are being bullied into suppressing valuable evidence that would essentially minimize the public health risk, silently perpetuated upon global families that don't understand the consequences of consuming these transgenic foods and the toxins that embrace them, because, the science is being suppressed to protect the *principles of poison.*

CHAPTER 3

·····································

Principles of Poison

Pesticide use in the United States began around 1945. Now more than one billion pounds of weed killers, insecticides and fungicides are used each year in the US. Over 1,000 chemicals are registered in about 20,000 products, used mostly for agriculture, but frequently sprayed in public places, offices and hospitals. [1] Glyphosate-based Roundup, the most popular herbicide (pesticide) was used originally as a de-scaling agent before Monsanto bought the patent in 1969. [2] In 2000, Monsanto's glyphosate patent expired leaving it wide open for a host of other glyphosate-based products to be sold by around 40 other producers under a variety of trade names.

Dr. Robert Kremer, a 32-year veteran microbiologist for the USDA, explains how glyphosate destroys plants, particularly by inhibiting enzymes that are involved in the making of the plant's amino acids. Glyphosate breaks down something called the shikimate pathway (she kih mut) in the plant and that blocks proteins that the plant needs to survive. [3]

Researchers know that glyphosate is a powerful chelator, meaning it binds to the nutrients in plants, draining the calcium, manganese, iron and zinc out of the plant making them bio-un-available, causing cell damage and plant death. [3]

Like all living species, our body depends on the use of these metals to survive, and although humans don't have a shikimate pathway like plants, our gut bacteria do. [3] In Chapter 4, we'll explore the consequences of this matter in the brain and behavior of our children.

From the beginning of the GMO "Green Revolution" in 1996, to the end of 2008, our US farmers sprayed an additional 383 million pounds of this herbicide on crops, compared to what they had in previous years prior to the release of GMO seed crops. [4] In almost direct proportion to its overuse, farmers are widely out-smarted by advancing super weeds developing intelligent cycles of resistance to these chemicals. Farmers have noticed that the more resistant weeds become to their herbicide, the more chemicals they have to apply to get the same results. This behavior has led to the development of yet more toxic herbicides to combat advancing weed invasions. [5]

Why not Roundup the Antibiotics?

The overuse of antibiotics has become a hot topic because they've discovered that they create some much bigger problems in humans, animals and the environment than they ever expected.

Glyphosate is known as a very efficient means of killing bac-teria. Both good and not so good microorganisms are destroyed by its powerful effects, so it was patented as an antibiotic in 2010. [6] Studies show that the pesticide becomes part of the cellular struc-ture of the plant and therefore simply can't be washed off the food. We eat the plant, and the chemical destroys our living gut bac-teria which is where scientists say about 80 percent of our immune system resides. [3, 7] This bacterial kill-off deeply affects the produc-tion of essential hormones like tryptophan and serotonin...which is why researchers say that we are seeing massive increases in chronic diseases like diabetes in our children and the general population. [8]

The Environmental Working Group (EWG) reports, "Monsanto's GMO Herbicide Doubles Cancer Risk." The article explores studies by the International Agency for Research on Cancer (IARC) looking at the potential for cancer-causing properties in glyphosate. The world's top experts in cancer research took a comprehensive look at the latest research, concluding that the chemical glyphosate is "definitely carcinogenic to animals in laboratory studies and that human exposure is linked to a higher risk of developing blood cancers such as non-Hodgkin's lymphoma."

The same researchers also re-validated their 2014 conclusions of a meta-analysis...several studies showing occupational exposure to "glyphosate has been found to double the risk of one blood cancer, non-Hodgkin's lymphoma, and increase the risk of a related cancer, multiple myeloma." [9] In addition, they emphasize the cancer studies showing farm workers are at increased risk of multiple myeloma, by as much as 70 to 80 percent when they are exposed to glyphosate. [9] In response to these alarming outcomes, California decided to add glyphosate to the state's list of known carcinogens and require Roundup products have a warning label. [10] Monsanto is suing the state to prevent this landmark decision.

German researchers found high concentrations of glyphosate in urine tests of humans and dairy cows for a study published in January 2014, in the *Journal of Environmental & Analytical Toxicology*. The study concludes, "The presence of glyphosate residues in both humans and animals could haul the entire population towards numerous health hazards." [11] Plus, "Glyphosate was detected in different organs of slaughtered cows including intestine, liver, muscles, spleen and kidney." And even though Monsanto claims the herbicide washes out of the body via the urine, after it is consumed, researchers found that "Chronically ill humans have significantly higher glyphosate residues in urine than healthy humans." [12]

In 1999, Monsanto defined the "extreme level" of their chemical herbicide as 5.6 milligrams per kilogram of plant weight. [11]

Meanwhile, Norwegian scientists found a massive 9 milligrams of Roundup per kilogram, on average, in the tests they ran on GMO soy. The scientists concluded that whenever we eat GM soy we are taking in a considerable dose of Roundup along with it: [11, 12]

> Roundup Ready [GE]-soy may have high residue levels of glyphosate ... and also that different agricultural practices may result in a markedly different nutritional composition of soybeans .... lack of data on pesticide residues in major crop plants is a serious gap of knowledge with potential consequences for human and animal health. [11, 13]

A 2008 study in *Chemical Research in Toxicology*,

> confirms that the adjuvants in Roundup formulations are not inert. ... the proprietary mixtures available on the market could cause cell damage and even death around residual levels to be expected, especially in food and feed derived from R (Roundup) formulation-treated crops. [14]

Another telling report from *PubMed* says that several studies have identified glyphosate's potential to create adverse health effects in humans as an endocrine disrupting chemical. Endocrine disrupting chemicals are known to cause developmental disorders, birth defects and cancer tumors, this report confirms. [15, 16] The study appears in *Food and Chemical Toxicology* an international journal, confirming that "Glyphosate induces human breast cancer cells growth via estrogen receptors." [15, 16]

In 2015, World Health Organization (WHO) a specialized agency of United Nations (UN) concerned with international public health, took a bold stance for the truth, declaring glyphosate the active ingredient in Roundup, probably causes cancer. [17,18] Professor Christopher Portier co-authored the report. The World Health Organization's International Agency for Research on Cancer's (IARC) report concludes glyphosate is a *probable carcinogen*. Portier presented the outcome at the Soil Association meeting in

London. Reflecting on the conclusions of the report he confirms, *"glyphosate is definitely genotoxic. There is no doubt in my mind."*

The Soil Association has over 27,000 members calling for a UK wide ban on glyphosate use on wheat during the pre-harvest stage. [19] A 2015 press release from the Association quotes Dr. Robin Mesnage, from the Department of Medical and Molecular Genetics at Kings College, on results of the comprehensive new analysis:

> Glyphosate is everywhere…in our food and water. The lack of data on toxicity of Glyphosate is not proof of safety and these herbicides cannot be considered safe without proper testing. We know Round Up… contains many other chemicals which, when mixed together are 1,000 times more toxic than Glyphosate on its own. [19, 20]

"The Dose Makes the Poison"

Authors of the book *Our Stolen Future* heavily criticize one underlying assumption directing the system of chemical-safety testing, which is, "the dose makes the poison." Toxicology risk assessments are designed to look for adverse health effects from compounds over a range of high-to-low doses until they establish certain standards of exposure, assuming that the chemicals that are more toxic at high doses are much less dangerous at lower levels. For decades, the assumption was that these guiding principles were protecting the public from undue exposure from compounds known to be toxic.

Leading author of the book Theo Colburn was an environmental hero and scientist working to educate people about the hazards of endocrine disrupting chemicals, until her death in 2014. She said it has been traditionally argued, what is known simply as *background* levels of contamination, aren't cause for much concern. However, despite any doubts, new evidence has surfaced combining studies of toxicology, developmental biology, endocrinology and biochemistry that sufficiently determines that this assumption has been dreadfully wrong. The safety standards protecting public health were built upon a foundation of false beliefs, according to Colborn. In addition, she said researchers spotted two central themes that appear to invalidate the primitive practice known as "the dose makes the poison:"

- Sensitivity to contamination is very different at all stages of life—a low dose may present no risk to an adult but the same dose can cause severe outcomes to a developing fetus.

- Dose-response curves...used to measure the contamination show that low levels of a contaminant actually cause greater effects than the higher levels, when exposer happens during the same stages of development. [21]

These emerging patterns indicate a need for continued research and advanced studies in order to adequately protect human and animal health from food and environmental toxins, and the serious health outcomes that our society is facing.

Argentina Agriculture—Map of Cancer

One key study was commissioned by the mayor of a little town called Monte Maíz, Cordoba, Argentina, to study cancer in local populations. The *Guardian* reports that the Physicians Network of Sprayed Towns started mapping cancer incidence in 2010. [22] The study coordinator Dr. Medardo Ávila-Vázquez, a pediatrician at the National University of Córdoba, worked alongside several academic groups to publish the report in February 2015. UNC medical students and physicians conducted a thorough epidemiological census:

> After 18 years of systematic sprayings....respiratory problems are much more common and are linked to the application of agricultural poisons, as is chronic dermatitis. Similarly, during fumigation, epileptic patients

convulse much more...depression, immune and endocrine disorders are more frequent...high rates of miscarriages... and consultations for infertility in men and women have significantly increased. Herds of goats... in some areas record up to 100 % of abortions [miscarriages] or premature deaths due to malformations linked to pesticide exposure. Increased thyroid disorders and diabetes are also detected in local people....more and more children are born with defects in these areas, especially if the first months of pregnancy coincide with the time of spraying. Down's syndrome, spina bifida, myelomeningocele (neural tube defect), congenital heart disease, etc. are diagnosed more frequently...during some years, at triple the normal rates, and directly linked to increased pesticide applications around the towns. [23, 24, 25]

The scientists were disturbed by what they found; the crop-sprayed towns actually showed a significant change in causes of death. According to the data reports from civil records offices, "over 30 % of deaths are from cancer, while nationwide, the percentage is less than 20%...."[23] The team says the year significantly concurs with the expansion in the use of glyphosate and other agrochemicals, used in large amounts in Argentina. These areas report spikes topping, "[an] 858 % increase in the toxic agrochemical use," the report says. [23] Furthermore, in May 2014, Córdoba's Ministry of Health published the data from its cancer registry which affirms, "the most intensive agricultural areas, deaths due to cancer exceed by 100% those in the city, and by 70% the provincial average." [23]

A second study was announced in 2015, at the 3rd National Congress of Doctors for Fumigated Communities, Buenos Aires. The researchers detonated an explosive discovery within the world of women's hygiene—85 percent of tampons, cotton and sanitary products tested contained glyphosate (including many popular brand names). The study's head researcher Dr. Damian Marino adds, "all of the raw and sterile cotton gauze analyzed in the study showed evidence of glyphosate." [27, 28] Surprisingly, he says the original purpose of the study was not to test cotton gauze or tampons: "There is a basic premise in research that when we complete testing on our target we have to contrast it with something 'clean,' so we selected sterile gauze for medical use, found in pharmacies." His team had no idea what they would find. [29]

Dr. Ávila-Vazquez reacted to the unexpected outcome:

> The result of this research is very serious, when you use cotton or gauze to heal wounds or for personal hygiene uses, thinking they are sterilized products, and the results show that they are contaminated with a probably carcinogenic substance. [29]

Endocrine Disrupting Chemicals (EDC)

The World Health Organization (WHO) published a report in 2012 titled "Endocrine Disrupters and Child Health." Essentially, the paper defines the endocrine system as being in charge of regulating your metabolism and bodily functions. It illustrates how "endocrine glands secrete hormones that act on their target organs through cognate (related) receptors. The targets are in many cases also endocrine organs that secrete hormones..."

The endocrine related organs are your skin, liver, kidneys, and the largest part is the digestive system with the stomach and small intestine. Working in conjunction with the nervous system the endocrine system is highly engaged in regulatory activities to assure that your body functions properly. It's made up of a complex group of glands and hormones. You could think of it like the body's chemical communication system, sending messages back and forth from cell to cell. [30, 31] These messages have been brought to you by your body's hormones. They act as Mother Nature's chemicals; hormones like estrogen, testosterone, insulin and many more, move through your bloodstream, flowing from cell to cell to facilitate a whole myriad of human functions that you don't even notice are going on. The endocrine system embraces a variety of services for you covering reproduction, stress management, behavior, insulin levels, metabolism and development of the brain, body and sexuality etc. [30, 31]

The World Health Organization (WHO) has categorized some pesticides among serious endocrine disrupting chemicals defined as "substances that alter one or more functions of the endocrine system." {30] Hundreds of research studies have looked at endocrine disruption in the body and how it affects the central nervous system, the immune and metabolic systems, along with many of our glands and organs. This is serious business for the body and for our medical communities struggling to manage expanding healthcare costs. [31]

Despite being narrowly defined as a reproductive-developmental issue, endocrine disruption can have dramatic effects on the body as a whole. Research suggests that many health outcomes resulting from endocrine malfunctions may not manifest themselves for years, maybe decades and can also be passed on through reproduction. The industry studies conducted for regulatory purposes of glyphosate used fairly high doses and reported the inability to detect these effects. However, as noted earlier, studies show the underlying problem is that EDCs do not act like typical poisons where higher doses have the potential to create higher toxicity levels. [32]

According to the Detox Project, compiled results from numerous peer-reviewed studies, show glyphosate:

- Alters hormone levels in female catfish and decreases egg viability;
- Disrupts the production of the steroid hormone progesterone in mouse cells,
- Creates disturbances in reproductive development in rats," "after exposure during puberty,"
- Prevents action of, "androgens [in human cells], the masculinizing hormones, at levels up to 800 times lower than glyphosate residue levels allowed in some GM crops used for

animal feed in the USA. DNA damage was found in human cells treated with glyphosate herbicides at these levels. "

- Disrupts the action and formation of estrogens ...the "first toxic effects... at the low dose of 5 ppm and the first endocrine disruption at 0.5 ppm—800 times less than the 400 ppm level authorized for some animal feeds."

- Increases "proliferation of estrogen-dependent breast cancer cells...at a level permitted in drinking water in the EU."

- Shows, "severe organ damage and...increased incidence of mammary tumours in female animals ... using diluted levels "14,000 times lower than allowed in drinking water in the US."

- Is an "endocrine disruptor through its toxicity to human cells in vitro at levels permitted in drinking water in Australia. The endocrine disruption occurred through a mechanism of toxicity to the cells, making them unable to produce...progesterone."[32]

In 2013, the EPA raised the amounts of glyphosate allowable in oilseed crops, including concentrations in flax, sesame and soybean from 20 ppm to 40 ppm. It also increased levels for sweet potatoes, up from 0.2 ppm to 3 ppm and carrots from 0.2 ppm to 5 ppm, multiplying quantities in these foods by a whopping 15-25 times. The change affected numerous types of produce and animal feed. Glyphosate contamination in cereal can now be as high as 30 ppm, with levels topping 100 ppm in animal feed and soybean plants register as much as 20 ppm, according to the new law. [33, 34]

EPA Glyphosate Evaluation

In 2015, Dr. Nancy Swanson reported on EPA evaluations of 271 injury reports from glyphosate exposure between 2002 and 2008. The paper says, "Exposures were primarily reported from people who had sprayed glyphosate in their yards and gardens" [35] . The EPA reported the following:

- "98 (36%) cases of neurological symptoms,—seizures, unconsciousness, neuropathy, dizziness, tremor, malaise, anxiety, slurred speech, loss of coordination, numbness & tingling, lethargy, confusion and difficulty concentrating;
- 80 (30%) cases of dermal symptoms—blisters, lesions, hives, rash, redness, swelling, peeling, burning, itching and soreness,
- 13 (5%) cases of gastro-intestinal symptoms—vomiting, nausea, abdominal cramps, blood in urine & stool, and diarrhea,
- 28 (10%) cases of upper-respiratory symptoms—fluid and blood in lungs, pneumonia, bronchitis, sore throat, congestion, sinusitis, coughing, choking, shortness of breath, difficulty breathing and heavy breathing,
- 39 (14%) cases of ocular symptoms—corneal abrasion, redness, burning, swelling, itching, blurred vision;
- 10 (4%) cases of some combination of the above; and 2 cases of no adverse symptoms..." [35]

Why not Bt Toxin?

You may recall from Chapter 1 that Bt corn is developed using a gene from soil bacteria called Bt (Bacillus thuringiensis); this produces the Bt toxin within the plant itself. The toxin bursts the stomach of certain insects killing them.

It's estimated that 65 percent of the corn grown in the United States is Bt corn. [36] Feeding studies clearly show why consumers are rejecting this synthetic food substitute with a self-contained toxin factory inside every little kernel.

Séralini reports his lab rats were fed one of Monsanto's Bt corn varieties, called MON 863. The rats experienced an activation of their immune systems, showing higher numbers of basophils, lymphocytes and white blood cells. I think we can safely conclude that this is a clear indicator of an allergic response due to the toxic nature of the Bt corn itself. [37]

The *International Journal of Biological Sciences,* in 2009, published the Séralini results, "A Comparison of the Effects of Three GM Corn Varieties on Mammalian Health:"

> Our analysis clearly reveals for the 3 GMOs, new side effects linked with GM maize consumption, which were sex- and often dose-dependent...associated with the kidney and liver, the dietary detoxifying organs, although different between the 3 GMOs...other effects were also noticed in the heart, adrenal glands, spleen and haemato-poietic system [with] signs of hepatorenal toxicity, possibly due to the new pesticides specific to each GM corn. [Plus] unintended direct or indirect metabolic consequences of the genetic modification cannot be excluded. [38]

Let's take a moment to examine briefly what the hematopoietic system is and why it's important to consider toxicity levels. The hematopoietic system is made up of the tissues and organs that are involved in the production of blood. They include your bone marrow, spleen, tonsils and lymph nodes. [39] These toxins invade our organs, wreaking havoc, which is a particular cause for concern within the bodies of developing fetuses and children.

Dan Charles a reporter for National Public Radio (NPR) revealed, "Insects Find Crack in Biotech Corn's Armor." The story aired problems that continue to surface with Monsanto's Bt corn and the insects they are designed to kill: "The scientists who called for caution now are saying 'I told you so,' because there are signs that a new strain of resistant rootworms is emerging... Iowa, north-western Illinois, and parts of Minnesota and Nebraska, rows of Bt corn have toppled over, their roots eaten by rootworms."

Entomologist Aaron Gassmann with Iowa State University, high-lights the problem farmers are facing and Monsanto is denying, in "Field-Evolved Resistance to Bt Maize by Western Corn Rootworm," a paper detailing studies on insects he collected from various fields. He reported that the bugs had a greater-than-expected ability to tolerate the Bt toxins from the plants. [40] Reading this reminded me of Jeffrey Smith's candid warnings during our interview:

> We're getting a much higher dose of Bt toxins than ever before in our lifetime. It also turns out that the Bt spray, the biotech industry and regulatory agencies have declared completely benign, according to peer-reviewed published studies, indeed is not; it's linked to immune responses in humans and animals, as well as tissue damage in the intestines. Bt corn has also been linked to immune responses and other things in carefully controlled studies; and the Bt toxins are known to poke holes in human cells in laboratory studies and, therefore, we are concerned that products with Bt-toxins will not only cause immune system problems but also gastrointestinal and potentially permeable gut... Bt toxins were found in the 98 percent of pregnant women tested in Canada and getting to their unborn fetuses, possibly going through the holes they created in the intestines. Once in the blood, according to a study on mice, it might be toxic to red blood cells. If it gets into the blood of unborn fetuses, which it does, it might get into their brain because there's no blood brain barrier. We might have holes and toxins in the brain of the offspring of that generation.

Also, Smith criticizes the lack of safety testing:

> The only human feeding study ever conducted on commercialized GMOs showed the Roundup Ready gene inserted into GMO soybeans transferred into the DNA in bacteria living inside our intestines and might have contained a defunction, we don't know if the Bt toxin gene similarly transfers, if it does, it might be part of our intestinal flora, which might explain why 93 percent of

the pregnant women in the Canadian study tested positive for having it in their blood, because they may have been producing it in their own intestines. It's a horrible thought and yet it might be true, it may be colonizing the gut bacteria. [41]

How about instead of practicing the archaic models of the *principles of poison*, we adopt a more favorable approach to humanity and the health of our global environment? Should we not institute a rational approach, perhaps built on a foundation of common sense and reliable action, rooted in the health and safety of our children and our children's children? What would that approach look like?

The Precautionary Principle

As a reasonable nation should we establish the guidelines of the *precautionary principal* in a logical approach to experimental food intended for public consumption? Let's examine this sensible methodology:

The Precautionary Principle as defined by the UNESCO COMEST may direct a more intelligent route for mankind:

When human activities may lead to morally unacceptable harm...actions shall be taken to avoid or diminish that harm. Morally unacceptable harm refers to harm to humans or the environment that is:

- Threatening to human life or health, or
- Serious and effectively irreversible, or
- Inequitable to present or future generations, or
- Imposed without adequate consideration of the human rights of those affected. [42]

The judgment of plausibility should be grounded in scientific analysis. Analysis should be ongoing so that chosen actions are subject to review. Uncertainty may apply to, but need not be limited to, causality or the bounds of the possible harm... [42]

So far, this gage has not been utilized as it should be. In light of these clear-cut indications, using our children as a barometer for our lack of safety standards is not practicing good stewardship of our role as a nation or as parents. And by far, it's not doing our children any favors. Wouldn't you imagine those in charge of our health care systems would be up in arms over the increasing costs associated with treating a country plagued by chronic disease, or is this perhaps a benefit to our new government controlled sick care system? Does the formula *more sick = more money*, make good economic sense for Wall Street?

I believe the point is well made. Americans have clearly suffered a massive uptick in chronic diseases since GMOs and their companions made their way to our dinner table. Whatever happened to America the *superpower*? How will this contribute to a healthy population, capable of sustaining development of a fine nation? Perhaps this is a case of *survival of the fittest* and self-protectionism for the corporate agenda?

The competitive edge once boasted by America is sinking down a slippery slope of GMO sludge that is bound to end in disaster. You can't very well build a sturdy pedestal of *American superiority* (insert eye roll here) on the backs of a sick population. What are the benefits of running a sick care system? (Money, money, money!)

Why is Monsanto Suing our Farmers?

Countless hard-working farmers all over the world have gone bankrupt fighting wrongful lawsuits condemned by Monsanto, after GMO seeds made their way onto their private properties contaminating their own conventional crops. One such case, involves a Monsanto lawsuit filed against Canadian Farmer Percy Schmeiser in 2000. The judge, in short, concluded that it ultimately didn't matter how genetically altered seeds got onto to his private lands and contaminated his crops. The decision established a dangerous legal precedent, determining that even if the seeds blew off a truck, were carried by the wind or perhaps simply brought in by birds or wildlife...the farmer still had infringed upon Monsanto's patent rights, and therefore, was legally liable for damages. Percy, like so many other farmers named in Monsanto lawsuits, says he has never planted a GMO seed on his farm; yet he was forced to destroy all of his crops and seed storage.

Consider that many farmers are growing seed varieties cultivated by their forefathers. When they get contaminated by GMO varieties, by no fault of the farmer, they are virtually worthless. Then Monsanto comes along and sues them. This is bad for farmers, bad for consumers and good for Monsanto. Generations of our farmers have nurtured their crops and even risked their lives to import, cultivate, maintain and safeguard the quality and purity of our agricultural heritage. Like those of other nations, our seeds are a central part of American history and our vibrant culture. This massive contamination is really a travesty against the very fabric of our nations and the lives of every citizen. This is a matter of ecological terrorism and the principal culprits are allowed to continue the crime unpunished.

The Big Bad Truth

The *Associated Press* exposed contracts showing that Monsanto is purposely squeezing out competitors, controlling smaller seed companies and protecting its control over the multibillion-dollar market for genetically altered crops [44].

The report quotes Neil Harl an agricultural economist at Iowa State University who has studied the seed industry for decades:

We now believe that Monsanto has control over as much

as 90 percent of (seed genetics). This level of control is almost unbelievable...and makes it possible for them to increase their prices long term. And we've seen this happening the last five years, and the end is not in sight. [44]

Chemical Deceptions

A staff writer for The *Washington Post* shocked the nation, in 2002, when he uncovered years of deceptive practices by Monsanto. Michael Grunwald exposes the truth behind the chemical giant with "Monsanto Hid Decades Of Pollution—PCBs Drenched Ala. Town But No One Was Ever Told." The article explains that Monsanto produced the now infamous PCB chemicals until 1977, although they had been fully aware of the potential to cause health issues, since a 1937 Harvard study found "prolonged exposure could cause liver damage and a rash called chloracne." They even put out company memos, the story says, acknowledging, "systemic toxic effects."

Applied as industrial coolant, PCBs were used in electrical equipment, adhesives, newspaper print, carbon paper, paint, deep fryers and bread wrappers. PCBs were finally banned in 1979, after the EPA classified them as "probable" human carcinogens. [45]

Grunwald says that for around 40 years they produced these industrial chemicals at a local factory where Monsanto routinely and secretly released toxic waste into a community creek in Anniston, Alabama. They also dumped millions of pounds of PCBs into open-pit landfills. He points out that the town's poor people ate the dirt calling it "Alabama clay," which they would cook up to add flavor to it, he says. Unaware of the contamination the locals continued to swim, fish and even baptize their children in the polluted waters. It's revealed that thousands of pages of Monsanto documents, many bearing warnings like *CONFIDENTIAL: Read and Destroy,* show that "for decades, the corporate giant concealed what it did and what it knew," charges Grunwald.

Documents show, in 1966, Monsanto hired Denzel Ferguson a Mississippi State University biologist to perform research studies around its chemical plant in Anniston. The report details how he brought in several tanks of bluegill fish and put them into Snow Creek. This is what he described to Monsanto about the conditions he found: "All 25 fish lost equilibrium and turned on their sides in 10 seconds and all were dead in 3½ minutes." [45] "I've never seen anything like it in my life," remarked Mack Finley a previous Ferguson graduate student—now aquatic biologist at Austin Peay State University.

George Murphy was another grad student with the project: *"their skin would literally slough off, like a blood blister on the bottom of your foot...it was like dunking the fish in battery acid."* [45]

Ferguson personally said he recorded serious issues with the "extremely toxic" wastewater flowing directly into Snow Creek right from the Monsanto plant and then reaching into the bigger Choccolocco Creek, where he also found similar aquatic "die-offs." The measured outflow, he reported "would probably kill fish when diluted 1,000 times or so." The book says that Ferguson warned Monsanto advising them, "since this is a surface stream that passes through residential areas, it may represent a potential source of danger to children." He continued to insist that Monsanto stop dumping their untreated waste and clean up the area. Monsanto didn't listen, in fact, they continued to hide the matter from the public. Monsanto appointed a special committee, in 1969, to silence the bubbling controversies over their PCBs, at the time, worth $22 million a year in revenue. Their two main objectives, Grunwald reveals, from the first meeting was to "permit continued sales and profits" and "Protect image of . . . the Corporation." [45]

Two years before, Grunwald says, researchers in Sweden established that PCBs were a growing threat to the global environment, after they identified traces of the chemicals throughout the food chain and in the birds, fish, pine needles and shockingly in their own children's hair. Meanwhile, PCBs were starting to show up all over the US in our nation's fish, shrimp, oysters and our bald eagles too. Dairy farmers in Maryland and Georgia were surprised to find them in their milk. Florida blamed the chemicals for a large shrimp kill. Even the company's own tests on rats, chickens and dogs showed unfavorable outcomes: "The PCBs are exhibiting a greater degree of toxicity than we had anticipated," the committee chairman confessed. The fish analysis was even worse. "Doses which were believed to be OK produced 100% kill." The chairman, reportedly, pushed company consultants to provide more "Monsanto-friendly" results, however they responded, "we are very sorry that we can't paint a brighter picture at the present time."

Amidst the uproar, the books says meeting documents demonstrate that one option, as a committee member noted, was to "sell the hell out of them as long as we can." A second option on the table was to immediately stop making them. Instead, members recommended what they saw as the "responsible approach," which was an incremental phase out of their PCB products, once they could sufficiently develop viable alternatives. The intention was to sustain, "one of Monsanto's most profitable franchises" for as long as possible while managing to "reduce our exposure in terms of liability." Committee charts show that they plotted out graphs to weigh out the risk factors related to "profits vs. liability over time." Does this sound like a company that has our best interest at heart? [45]

Finally, Grunwald imparts, one company funded study found out PCBs cause tumors in rats. Monsanto ordered that study's conclusion be altered from "slightly tumorigenic" to say "does not appear to be carcinogenic." He says, a confidential memo was sent out saying, "We can't afford to lose one dollar of business." [45]

Suing Monsanto

Currently there are dozens of lawsuits pending in our nation's courts (and around the world) naming Monsanto as the principle defendant, as they are struck down by humanity from all corners of the globe, as the wounded rise upon mountains of accusations fraught with counterfeit trade claims, deceptive practices and subsequent harm.

In the wake of lawsuits, filed in both New York and California, *Reuters* says, "Personal injury law firms ... are lining up plaintiffs for what they say could be 'mass tort' actions against agrichemical giant Monsanto that claim the company's Roundup herbicide has caused cancer in farm workers and others exposed to the chemical." The lawsuit against Monsanto states that they "led a prolonged campaign of misinformation to convince government agencies, farmers, and the general population that Roundup was safe." The article quotes attorney Michael McDivitt whose Colorado-based law firm represents 50 plaintiffs. McDivitt is confident because "we can prove that Monsanto knew about the dangers of glyphosate." In addition, he says, "there are a lot of studies showing glyphosate causes these cancers."[46]

In the midst of these lawsuits, The Center for Biological Diversity sued the Environmental Protection Agency, in February of 2016, for failing to provide requested records regarding its approval of extremely toxic, Enlist Duo. Also known as 2,4-D, the so-called Agent Orange pesticide which is deemed to be highly toxic to a broad variety of plants, mammals and birds, with considerable harmful effects observed in the health of humans too. In 2014, the Center filed a public records request under the Freedom of Information Act, for which the EPA has yet to fully comply.

The lawsuit seeks to obtain full disclosure around why the chemical was approved in the first place. Lori Ann Burd Environmental Health Director for the Center says, "the public has a right to essential information to illuminate why the agency made the decision to approve this dangerous pesticide cocktail in light of its potential environmental and human-health impacts...[And] after two years of stalling, sending only heavily redacted records, and ignoring our appeal for information, EPA has left us with no choice but to go to court to obtain the records on this deadly chemical." [47]

Principles of Poison—at Odds With Human Rights

Force-feeding the population without knowledge or consent simply violates the core of American values. By far, it's the epitome of unpatriotic and treasonous activity undercutting the health, security and credibility of our entire nation.

They are undermining our freedom of choice and our role as parents, whose voices should be ringing from the rooftops condemning the bio-technical re-creation of our planet, the food and the cavalier attitude in which it was thrust upon an unknowing public, for over two decades. Although Americans are beginning to awaken from the GMO sugar slumber to realize it isn't the same food as Grandma used to eat, we continue to be led by the tongues, like lambs to the slaughter with our young in tow.

With their history of repeated acts of deception can Monsanto really be trusted, along with our misguided politicians to make diligent decisions affecting the health of humans worldwide? Does this not have catastrophe written all over it?

Update: A new study has been released called "Glyphosate – Unsafe on Any Plate." Independent lab tests have found "alarming levels" of glyphosate in many popular brand-name cereals and snack foods. The highest levels were detected in Original Cheerios (1,125.3 ppb) which was recently labeled GMO-Free. The second highest readings came from Stacy's Simply Naked Pita Chips by Frito-Lay (812.53 ppb). Belief it or not, the lowest levels were registered in Trix Cereal (9.9 ppb) and Goldfish Colors (8.02 ppb). You can access the full report under "GMO-Free Data Sources," Chapter 3. [48]

CHAPTER 4

....

The GMO Gut-Brain Connection & the Big Fail

"Our bacteria manufacture most of our B vitamins—B6, B9, and B12, which is cobalamin—essential to our neurology (brain). Bacteria also manufacture vitamin K and some of your vitamin C. We have a symbiotic relationship with these bacteria. We help them and they help us. They take the food and they don't just break it down and obliterate it to unrecognizable things. They dismantle the food, and they utilize everything that's in the food."

Dr. Anthony Samsel

The "Second Brain"

Your gut does so much more than digest your food. The gastrointestinal system contains around 100 million nerve cells, scientists have termed the Enteric Nervous System (ENS). It has also been called your "second brain." The ENS is a complex system that even responds to your emotions and experiences, sending messages back and forth to your central brain via your neurotransmitters. Researchers say the conditions in the gut really reflect in the decisions of the brain and body, so much that your overall well-being depends on the health of your gastrointestinal system. The gut contains thousands of beneficial bacteria that work in your favor, regulating your hormone production, immune responses, toxic elimination and your mental health—absorbing the vitamins and minerals your body needs. [1, 2]Your gut health is vital to how your brain is running, how you feel and how you respond to your daily life. Ditto and double for young developing minds. Don't forget that as we move forward in our work.

The Human Microbiome Project (HMP)

The Human Genome Project (HGP) and Human Microbiome Project (HMP) both made some miraculous discoveries that have changed everything they thought they knew about how the body functions, and how it interacts with other life forms in our environment and within our own body. The human microbiome is a whole new world of science that we have only begun to explore. These concepts are rapidly changing the pharmaceutical paradigm, putting into context what so many professionals have long suspected, and that is the consumption of a myriad of chemical compounds over extended periods of time have resulted in the destruction of our health and now we know why.

Researchers have discovered that we are made up of a bacterial microcosm, running our little hormone factories like metabolic machines with miniature soldiers fighting for our survival all the livelong day. [3] With this new science they are gaining a wider perspective on this important interaction and its co-dependent relationship between us humans and our bacterial colonies that are at the very core of our existence.

We will explore the microbiome further and the outcomes that relate directly to the health and functioning of each and every one of us and our children.

Researchers have recently discovered that we are made up of about 100 trillion cells of living bacteria that are perhaps even more evolved than we are. (Insert deep breath here). Only about 10 percent of our cells are actually human. They classified about 10,000 species of microbes, some of them science has never seen before. These microbes, they say, have more than 8 million genes—over 350 times the number of human genes that you and I have. [3, 4, 5, 32]

Studies identify different types of human flora throughout the entire body including various colonies existing in the brain, lungs, mouth, digestive tract, skin, genitals and of course in the gut, where they found entirely different species living together in colonies—interacting with all of the others, as one complete system, these microbial creatures are essentially in charge of our every move. [3]

Have you ever heard of the gut-brain connection? Whatever happens in the gut, also happens in the brain. The importance of this vital connection has taken us out of the scope of conventional medicine. The gut is, in fact, a central powerhouse of bacterial action, connected to the moment-to-moment chemical reactions in your brain that are affecting every thought and behavior right now.

You will find out shortly what you can do to repair this delicate internal relationship. Like you, your child responds to the calls and battles of the gut-brain response system and the sooner you address any imbalances the better.

Glyphosate and the Shikimate Pathway

Glyphosate is marketed as being harmless to humans and wildlife. Since we're not plants and we don't possess the Shikimate Pathway like algae, fungi, bacteria and plants, it is reasoned that the chemical is safe to use on food crops. One significant problem, scientists are pointing out, is our gut bacteria do possess these vital pathways. [6]

In plants, glyphosate works by disrupting the shikimate pathway, used to produce a special group of amino acids that the plant needs to exist. Those are phenylalanine, tyrosine, and tryptophan. These amino acids are termed aromatic (though they say it has nothing to do with how they smell). They are necessary for the plant's day-to-day survival. [7] Humans require these aromatic amino acids be present in the diet every day, along with eight more amino acids. Arginine, histidine, isoleucine, leucine, lysine, methionine, threonine and valine are very vital. Without them we see a breakdown in the body's protein structures affecting vital organs. [8] As noted, the shikimate pathway does exist in your gut bacteria, which is defined as a central aspect of the body's ability to function and maintain itself.

Your gut bacteria has a symbiotic relationship with your body, digesting food, synthesizing your vitamins, regulating immunity and monitoring detoxification, plus so much more. Anything that comes along and disrupts the performance of the shikimate pathway in our gut bacteria has the strong potential to cause serious harm. [9]

Glyphosate the Antibiotic

Glyphosate was patented as an antibiotic because of its ability to destroy bacteria. Some bacteria, as we discussed earlier, have developed natural barriers to antibiotics. Throughout a series of evolutionary developments they've been able to outsmart scientists. Bacteria have been out-evolving us in novel ways for some time now. One prime example, is the ability to release what can only be described as a pheromone type substance, attracting other bacteria both like and unlike themselves. In essence, they send communication messages back and forth with the ability to completely download one another's information, and they can pass it on to their own offspring during reproduction about every 20-minutes. They don't even need the internet. This leaves them countless opportunities to outwit us. [10]

These paradigm-shattering discoveries are forever changing the landscape around how science characterizes the intelligence of the microscopic ecosystems of our planet and our bodies. Of course this offers us new insight as to why humanity continues to suffer ever-increasing threats of epidemics and diseases in light of modern advancements. Antibiotic resistance propels these challenges to new levels for our medical communities as they overlook the obvious repercussions of GMO/glyphosate consumption as a common denominator.

I think we can all question the fact that our regulators still insist that it's okay to consume all of these mixtures of GMOs, pesticides, antibiotics, food additives, along the mercury and aluminum in the vaccines that are serious neurotoxins. These toxins lurk in processed foods, and they circulate from your child's gut through the blood and directly into the brain. Once these neurotoxins enter the brain tissue they accumulate there and stay trapped. Plenty of studies confirm that these highly toxic combinations are a central theme behind the skyrocketing autism rates and the myriad of chronic diseases appearing in our populations.

The recent changes in our food supply and farming practices affect both our health and that of the microscopic world around us. We are one system completely interdependent on one another for our survival. Science has been so busy trying to outsmart Mother Nature by destroying weeds, insects and diseases and taking on the bacterial colonies, we now have a genuine man-made threat to human existence that has gone far beyond the borders of our nations to destroy us one gut at a time.

In Chapter 2, I introduced you to Canadian Scientist Dr. Thierry Vrain who works tirelessly to educate the public about what he, Dr. Don Huber and other scientists have discovered about the hidden dangers of GMOs and glyphosate and what they are doing to our health. Both Dr. Vrain and Dr. Huber have presented a mountain of evidence, causational relationships, and sound science that cannot be justifiably disputed by Monsanto, the FDA or the medical community.

During our 2015 conversation, the good doctor expressed critical concerns around the use of glyphosate on food crops just prior harvest and its antibiotic effects on the human microbiome. He even indicated to me that the hazards from glyphosate use in our food supply might be more worrisome in regards to our health than the GMOs themselves. Vrain revealed that Monsanto was hoping to market the chemical as a pharmaceutical and so they re-patented it as an antibiotic, because it not only kills insects and weeds but also our gut bacteria at just one part per million (ppm). The patent includes an extensive list of bacteria that is easily and effectively destroyed by this pervasive antibiotic. [11]

Antibiotics Destroy the Microbiome

You remember the Human Microbiome Project (HMP), where they classified the microbiome as a new organ with billions of living bacteria in your gut and body? Well, Dr. Thierry Vrain explains why that is so relevant:

> There are more nerves connecting your brain to your gut than anywhere else in your body. This is where your neurotransmitters originate and 100 percent of your serotonin comes from. This is the central hub of your immune system. Without proper levels of serotonin, one of the major neurotransmitters in the brain, our children are at high risk for depression and mental illness.

Now it all makes sense; the prevalence of ADHD, autism and asthma in our children is a clear indication of the sad state of their gut bacteria and the detriments of our environmental/ farming practices, under the constraints of the *principles of poison*. When your gut isn't healthy, it directly affects your immune system. An over-reactive immune system will show up as allergies in the body. It begins to over-respond to what it perceives to be intruders and so the immune system gets all excited, attacking everything incoming, including the food that it needs to survive and the body's tissue itself. Autoimmune diseases result in this way.

Your child's gut bacteria are being bombarded by glyphosate from their food, air and water. The cost of these damages on their health is inconceivably astronomical. Everything is all inter-connected within the systems of the body, and every action creates a complete and total reaction throughout the entire body. That is why we must take a holistic view of the damage and the cure.

I have serious concerns that I've seen the repercussions of this damage in my own children, grandchildren and those around me. Parents, nowadays, are submerged in the battle to find and rescue their real children underneath the myriad of suffering and disconnected symptoms.

In his presentations, Dr. Vrain sites feeding study outcomes showing damaged microbiomes:

> *The epidemic of gluten intolerance and celiac disease, really has little to do with the gluten and a lot to do with the glyphosate that has been sprayed on cereal crops* [now 30 ppm] *over the past 15 years, and that has damaged our microbiomes. One molecule of glyphosate damages the microbiome of bacteria and impairs the CYP enzymes, and you become toxified.*

The doctor says that we have 57 of these CYP enzymes that are the first lines of detoxification in the body. Glyphosate impairs these enzymes and damages the microbiome causing inflammatory diseases, cancer, autism, and many of the diseases that have become prevalent in recent decades. [13]

Studies like that of Dr. Samsel and Seneff show how glyphosate inhibits these enzymes. Vrain reports that they *"suggest that glyphosate's suppression of CYP enzymes," coupled "with its antibiotic effect on the human microbiome is involved in the etiology of the many chronic degenerative and inflammatory diseases that have grown to epidemic levels since the advent of the Roundup Ready technology."* [13]

Dr. Vrain explains how farmers spray the plants and the chemicals absorb it right into their plant cells. Roundup binds to the plant's minerals, depleting the food of these essential minerals and micronutrients that are vital to our body's day-to-day functioning, making them bio-unavailable, meaning that your body can't use them.

Meanwhile in 2013, as you might recall, the EPA raised the legal limits of allowable glyphosate in our food and water. [13]

Allergies, Asthma, ADHD and Autism

Food allergies go hand in hand with autism and ADHD. These epidemics have been on the rise over the past two decades, and research is finally catching up with what many parents and physicians have been observing in their children for years.

Dr. Kenneth Bock works with what he calls the "4-A disorders." Allergies, asthma, ADHD and autism are all interrelated issues, according to Bock. He is well respected for his solution-based treatments that expose the root causes of these challenging disorders. In his book *Healing the New Childhood Epidemics* Bock shares over 25 years of clinical achievements, confronting toxicity levels in the brains and bodies of his young patients. He points to the culprits as heavy metal pollutants in food, in the environment, and in vaccines, along with environmental and food toxins (pesticides). These are often combined with a genetic predisposition, nutritional deficiencies and metabolic imbalances, says the doctor. They all clash into what he calls the "perfect storm." This is wreaking havoc on the digestive and immune systems within these vulnerable children.

Bock says that categorizing autism as a psychiatric disorder is a diagnostic error. It's a medical problem he characterizes as a neurotoxic disorder. He also notes that babies born with autism are an extremely rare phenomenon. These children are being bombarded by toxins from the time they're born. That exposure, he believes, blocks the neuro-pathways of the brain and that is how we explain the dysfunction in the processing and reasoning seen in both ADHD and autism.

Bock dissects the connection between allergies, asthma, ADHD and autism clearly indicating that:

- All four disorders are characterized mainly by an overload of toxicity in the brain and body, which in turn causes the metabolism to malfunction.
- Nutritional deficiencies block the body's natural processes and impede detoxification of its systems.

- Intolerances and allergies to food and environmental factors cause harm to the brain.
- Allergies often contribute to full-blown autism, ADHD and asthma.
- There is a powerful link between the cause & recovery.

Bock reveals that addressing the root causes of the brain and body's toxicity, will over time, bring about recovery for each of the "4-A disorders," depending upon the effectiveness of the approach. With so many of the same causes and overlapping symptoms resulting in different outcomes, Bock shows parents how to become a true "medical detective" in search of what works best for their child.

Bock distinguishes how different each child can be and his methods need to be tailored to fit individual needs as the following indications are present, which most often are:

- Food allergies with neurological consequences
- Inflammation of the brain and gut
- Severe nutritional deficiencies
- Viral infiltration of the brain and gut
- Autoimmune attacks on body and brain
- Immune system over-activity & under-activity
- Under-nourished muscle tissue

Bock says that these children often suffer a wide array of inter-related health problems, due to these disorders, along with food and environmental sensitivities, gut inflammation, behavioral and learning challenges. Dr. Bock approaches this as a collection of significant symptoms, that if paid attention to, will present the entire picture for the parents and medical professionals. This picture reflects many children on the spectrum, which Bock says includes ADHD. [14]

The *Quarterly Review of Biology* published "The Function of Allergy: Immunological Defense Against Toxins," by Margie Profet. She reveals that when a body becomes overwhelmed by toxins and unable to cleanse itself, it starts to defend itself with allergic reactions. She further describes the body's response as an evolved defense mechanism, designed to expel toxins as fast as possible via vomiting, itching and/or sneezing to prevent circulation of the intruder. [15]

Profet implicates these toxic exposures saying, they can trigger a whole host of allergies causing other health related problems. She says this is not something we see in typical children. Normal kids are not supposed to be plagued by food allergies, and if we dig a little deeper we discover a myriad of dysfunction among their fine and gross motor skills, along with rage, depression, attention deficit, sensory issues, hyperactivity and learning disabilities, she discloses. [15]

The food allergy epidemic increased sharply throughout the 90s' in U.S children, as well as in the UK, Australia and Canada. This sudden surge was confirmed by hospital records and validated by the growing number of schoolteachers reporting significant upsurges in the percentage of severely allergic children in their classrooms. [16]

In 2007, CDC reported:

- Approximately 3 million children under 18 years old (3.9 percent), have had food or digestive allergies within the last 12 months;
- Children with food allergies are 2-4 times more likely to have other related issues like asthma, compared with children without food allergies;
- From 2004-2006, there were an estimated 9,500 children (under 18) admitted in the hospital due to food related allergies. [16]

A 2012 CDC report showed autism in 1 in 88 children surveyed in the US. This marked a 78 percent increase over the previous five years and 1,000 percent over the previous four decades. [17] A second CDC account, from the same year, shows compiled reports for just those children born in 2004, identifying 1 in 68 with an official diagnosis. The information was compiled by the Autism and Developmental Disabilities Monitoring (ADDM) Network. In Chapter 6, we will delve further into these results.

Before the early 20th century, there were no references in the medical books or journals for the term allergy. It became used to describe reactions to serum concoctions that were being administered, via syringe, during *medical experiments* with the first vaccines. Children undergoing these first trials (many without parental consent) often fell violently ill. In 1906, pediatrician Clemens von Pirquet described symptoms in patients, he dubbed "altered reactivity" or allergy. [18]

Furthermore, the term "anaphylaxis," meaning "against protection," was used first by Charles Richet in 1913, describing the health conditions he created in his lab animals, undergoing his research experiments with early immunizations [18].

According to a 2011 report, 64 percent of children diagnosed with ADHD are actually experiencing a hypersensitivity to their food. This report was published in the *Lancet*, by Dr. Lidy Pelsser of the ADHD Research Centre in the Netherlands. She writes that "the disorder is triggered in many cases by external factors — and those can be treated through changes to one's environment." [19]

The children were put on a special elimination diet in an effort to detect which foods were causing the issues. "After the diet, they were just normal children with normal behavior," Pessler says proudly. Tendencies towards distraction, temper tantrums and even forgetfulness subsided in the students. Teachers and the doctors began to report notable changes, "in fact, they were flabbergasted," Pessler reports. Some teachers didn't believe it; one called it a miracle and others thought it was strange "that a diet would change the behavior of a child as thoroughly as they saw it." [19]

Dr. Jackie Wood is with the Department of Physiology at Ohio State University. She reports that it "seems the higher brain tries to protect the gut, by sending messages to our cells for the release of histamine, a substance that produces inflammation ... this is protective mode by the brain in an effort to prepare the gut for surveillance." [20]

With allergies the body is in a constant state of hyper-awareness looking out for offenders that may or may not be harmful or even real. The body begins to treat everything as if it's an attacker of sorts; putting it into a perpetual cycle of response and repair. Because we have co-evolved with our beneficial microbes, without them, we are vulnerable to inflammatory disorders. This hyper-action in the body begins a cycle of inflammation to restore balance as needed. [21, 26]

In her *Psychology Today* article "Food, Inflammation and Autism: Is there a link?" Dr. Victoria Dunkley warns, "food sensitivities may trigger delayed symptoms anywhere from two days to several weeks after ingestion. Because offenders may cross the blood brain barrier, they can cause changes in mood, behavior and cognition." [21]

Now your beginning to understand the depth of what we are talking about here. Dunkley further proposes that, "elimination diets are often helpful at discovering whether your child has a food sensitivity...by removing the food in question (e.g. gluten or dairy) for at least two weeks then reintroducing the food item and noticing any adverse reactions..." She also says that we can look for a notable reduction in ASD symptoms once the offending food is taken out. [21]

In Chapter 8, we'll talk more about the elimination diet with within the context of GMO detoxification methods.

ADHD Drugs and the Gut-Brain Connection

In a September 2015 interview, Zen Honeycutt, founder of Moms Across America and vocal mama bear, spoke with author John Gray, Ph.D. As a prominent doctor and relationship expert, Gray is probably most well-known for his best-selling book *Men are from Mars, Women are from Venus*. [22]

Dr. Gray has done extensive work with parents and their children to help them overcome the challenges and symptoms of ADHD and autism. Topping the list as the most common "psychiatric" problem among American children, ADD/ADHD affects 2-4 million kids in the US. Gray says one in three boys (sometimes even one in five) per classroom has ADD/ADHD. Girls are affected by it much less frequently. He has major concerns surrounding the high number of our children taking drugs like Aderol and Ritalin. He describes research showing these drugs can cause brain damage and neurological malfunctioning, in some children. [22]

Gray talks about a specially targeted study by Harvard researchers that found Ritalin decreases vital blood flow to a part of the brain that controls movement and attention, called the putamen. This discovery characterizes the enormous hazards involved in the pharmaceutical approach to ADHD and how it is affecting our kids. It proves that these drugs, in many cases, can make bad symptoms significantly worse. Often these are the issues they are designed to alleviate in the first place. Five out of the eleven boys in the study, Gray says, had reduced blood flow to this imperative part of the brain, following the Ritalin dose. [22, 23]

Dr. Gray, like Dr. Kenneth Bock, also encourages proper detoxification, supplementation, various lifestyle adjustments, along with behavioral and nutritional support, which should be used to help correct these issues and address the underlying causes standing at the root of the problem. [14, 22, 24, 25] Gray objects to the epidemic being masked behind big media that perpetuates public confusion through propaganda and advertising campaigns intended to boost corporate profits for the drug companies. He expresses deep concern that parents are not getting the right messages regarding these conditions, especially surrounding the fact that there are many effective ways to resolve them outside of the Western pharmaceutical paradigm. [22]

All this is leading to the perpetual suffering of our children, but Dr. Gray assures us that good quality supplementation, along with the right nutritional protocols are equally effective to Aderol and Ritalin, without the unwanted side effects of the methamphetamine like substances. [22, 25]

Chemical Chaos and Dopamine Performance

In effect these ADHD drugs are speed, signaling the brain to artificially release the chemical dopamine, says Dr. Gray. There are many concerns that this leads to depletion of this very important neurotransmitter, making the problem worse in the long run. [22. 25] Gray hopes that we will, ideally, look to find more effective ways to help our youngsters access their dopamine, outside of drugs and the inappropriate behaviors attached to these disorders. For example, risk-taking behaviors are a pattern in these children being, unwittingly, used to pump the brain and body with dopamine. The body needs it and sends demands to the brain. Say your hyperactive little one is jumping on the couch and you firmly tell him to stop. Think of the rush he gets by doing it anyway. They don't know it, but what's what they're after.

Dopamine is a very specialized neurotransmitter, an information super highway, carrying messages throughout the body. It is what keeps us focused, on task and motivated to do what we need to do in this world and our ADD kids really struggle with this stuff. [22, 27] Dopamine is the brain's pleasure and reward center, as well as the impulse control unit that allows us the ability to work for long term goals without giving up. People with higher levels of this brain chemical tend to be more competitive, aggressive, and exhibit more self-control than those with more reduced amounts. As the supply dwindles, it can wreak havoc on the brain performance and capacity of your child to maintain any sort of acceptable behavior, in light of these shortages. Deficiencies have been linked to such things as addictions, criminal behaviors and even Parkinson's, obsessive-compulsive disorder, schizophrenia, autism and of course ADHD. [28, 29]

Little brains are not aware of why they are acting out or even why they crave that negative attention. They are simply responding as a matter of impulse, within in that chemical response system, triggered by the natural shortages. They are meeting their needs the only way they know how; cause a disturbance, get a dopamine boost. The cycle has to be completed one way or another. If one form doesn't work, then another way will be found. Boredom is a critical factor behind many troubled days. So we, as parents, need to help them foster better ways to not only stimulate dopamine production, but improve all of the body's functions. But how, you ask? Are you ready? It's a process, not an event. There's that phrase again.

Find (then add) What's Missing

Although similar, each child is slightly different. The body's biological makeup, the genetics and the environment, along with so much more are at constant play here, and that's why cookie cutter approaches generally won't work.

Something Gray notes, cannot be overstated, and that is the significance of addressing what has been absent in your child nutritionally. [22, 24, 25] Let's be clear about this, it doesn't make you a bad parent or neglectful; however, it is likely that your youngster is deficient in something—it's the nature of the food these days. Most of us are suffering from the critical insufficiencies of the modern food supply. Nothing is perfect, not even organic—though it is the very best option we have, unless we are able to grow and sustain our entire food chain ourselves, which is unlikely. I encourage you to do the best you can with what you have to work with.

Deficiency could be considered the central theme of childhood in contemporary living. Modern children get cheated with poor nutrition, too little sunshine and exercise, distracted overworked parents who are overwhelmed, too stressed out and often too grouchy, to live up to their true parenting potential. Kids get "rewarded" with an abundance of sugar, synthetic food-like substances, video games and a media bombarding them with lies and misrepresentations of reality. Society's priorities are not a family first approach.

Modern parents are understandably swamped by the demands of daily life and raising kids in the 21st century. Food producers are taking full advantage of that disconnect, while programing our children with commercials designed to attract, confuse and engage little minds.

The best advice is to avoid products that have commercials, better yet, avoid commercials all together. Boxed goods and processed foods are often full of GMOs. They are nothing more than synthetic substances that the body does not recognize as nutrition. Although they make life more convenient, they are seriously lacking in the necessary nutrients and complete minerals that developing brains and bodies need to perform normally.

All operative factors rely on the gut-brain connection to support themselves. Neglecting this vital relationship is not wise, if you want to address the negative influences affecting the health and functioning of your young child. At the same time, making up for what has been missing for the them (and you) nutritionally will not only prevent the problems from getting worse, but will work in their favor to assist in healing the gut-brain connection and ultimately the child. [20, 22, 25] As the issues are addressed and deficiencies corrected the other puzzle pieces of the disorder can begin to correct themselves, as a clearer more genuine picture of your child emerges from behind the smoke screen of daily symptoms.

There is an enormous amount of nutrient dense whole food options to choose from. Feeding the kiddos sources of compact, nutritionally bioavailable, living foods (fruits and vegetables) with all their high functioning enzymes and essential minerals, will start to make up for what has been missing and will likely help to resolve a good deal of the health issues in you and your child.

Of course, it is important to have any suspected deficiencies properly diagnosed by a medical professional, and then addressed with whole foods and quality GMO-Free supplements in order to correct the situation.

Glyphosate, Destroying Us One Gut at a Time

As we discussed in the last chapter, glyphosate-based Roundup is sprayed on GMO crops and non-GMO cereal grains (wheat and oats), sugarcane and beans. With its antibiotic action, it kills our beneficial gut bacteria, which is instrumental in the production of many important brain chemicals like serotonin and dopamine along with their precursors. The hard truth is that glyphosates in the food, air and water are wiping us out one gut at a time and probably causing our cancer epidemic too.

Babies naturally inherit their beneficial bacteria from their mothers, who pass it on as part of the microbiome, during the birth process (through the birth canal) and during breast-feeding naturally. In this way, it has been carried forth from generation to generation, spanning thousands of years of human evolution and bacterial changes advancing into this complex system, which is called our microbiome.

Most of us know there are special combinations of probiotic strains the body needs for digestion and to maintain these bacterial ecosystems. When our beneficial gut bacteria are out of balance, the environment becomes ideal for growing mold, candida and other harmful organisms in the gut. That is why you crave certain foods. It feeds your bad microorganisms and allows them to thrive and get stronger, while aggravating the problem more and more. The bad bacteria in your child's gut feeds on sugar and that is why your child craves it. [22, 26]

Dr. Gray reveals that the problem lies in harmful patches of fungus living inside the gut. "They devour the sugar as it devours them from the inside out and under normal circumstances…we could fight off those bad bacteria. The system, however, is way out of balance. The bad outweighs the good and is setting kids off in a spiral of dysfunction that has them suffering in magnitudes like never before." [22] Gray does a good job illustrating this misbalance in the gut and its connection to brain behavior, pointing to issues of vitamin D deficiencies that are common in kids these days. Your body, he reveals, uses vitamin D in about 3000 different ways. Our children, he says, aren't getting enough sunshine and so they lack the vitamin D they need, on a daily basis, to maintain these vital exchanges. You might be surprised to find that this essential nutrient is in charge of calcium absorption in the brain. [24] When we don't have enough vitamin D it hinders the release of calcium from the neurons, which is causing brain cell death, Gray explains.

This can cause brain cell death; you read that right. In order for your body and your bones to use the calcium properly, you have to have adequate levels of vitamin D. The doctor insists that glyphosate prevents this whole vitamin D process from taking place. He recommends that children get a minimum of 15 minutes in the sun, every day, *without sunblock.* He suggests supplementing vitamin D during particular seasons and for those who don't get enough exposure. [22]

Gray, like many practitioners, recommends replenishing the gut with quality probiotics, especially because moms typically don't have the healthy microbiome to pass on to their offspring anymore. He blames decades of antibiotic misuse, glyphosates, and other reckless practices that have completely undermined our ability to pass on adequate immune functioning to our offspring; this he says, inherently leaves our kids vulnerable to the diseases and illnesses that are the misfortune of this generation and those to come. [22]

Dr. Gray points to studies on children that have completely overcome ADHD, following the removal of foods containing glyphosates, in combination to adding vitamin D supplements to the daily diet. Of course, he correctly notes, every little body is different so other things may need to be added (or removed). [22, 25]

Gray mentions something that really resonates with me, "if your child has good, lean muscle mass, yet is struggling with ADHD, along with learning and behavioral challenges, studies show that just adding a good form of Omega 3s is going to be more effective than any of the drugs." For fast results, Gray recommends Liposomal vitamins that allow the body to better absorb and utilize them. Grape seed extract and high doses of Liposomal vitamin C, he notes, have also shown to be very effective in children with ADHD. Gray says we can give children as much as 1,000-2,000 milligrams a day of Liposomal vitamin C, without the risk of diarrhea or stomach problems. [22]

In Dr. Grays extensive work with autistic children, he discloses that patients seem to benefit dramatically from taking pre-digested proteins in superfood shakes, which are super minerals that stimulate amino acids. He also says that beverages containing lemon and Aloe Vera have been a major part of the healing process too. [24]

Scientific American reports, "research suggests that as many as nine out of 10 individuals with the condition also suffer from gastrointestinal problems such as inflammatory bowel disease and "leaky gut." [31]

Michael Spector, an award winning journalist for The *New Yorker,* puts it into a perspective that we can all understand with his poignant article "Germs are Us." He illustrates how the problem has gotten out of hand in a matter of a few generations. He sums it up well with the misuse of not only antibiotics, but also the excess use of antibacterial products that we (as a country) use to sanitize our lives. Germaphobes beware; when you kill the bad guys, you take the good guys down with them. They are your little helpers; there for your protection and you need them fighting for you and your kids to keep your family healthy. They are essentially in control of that little immune system (and yours) and the fewer beneficial microbes we have available, the more vulnerable we are. [30]

Encouraging use of antibacterial products, on a regular basis, is probably not the wisest approach. [30] I avoid using antibacterial products on my kids and grandkids because I know the long-term consequences aren't worth the short term fix. A little soap and water still does the trick and leaves us healthier in the long-term.

"The impact is hard to dispute," admits Spector, using an example of an American born in 1930, he says, they could expect to die by the age of sixty. Today though, our life expectancy is around seventy-nine years. Generally speaking, we've seen a significant reduction of infectious diseases here in the US. Things such as better standards of nutrition, access to clean water, and of course antibiotics brought about major leaps in life expectancy, says Spector. [30] At the same time, we need to recognize the complete effect on our environmental health, both externally and internally, when we decide to utilize such radical disturbances as antibiotic treatments. This decision should not ever be taken lightly, if we want to continue to restore the body's abilities and functions that help keep us in a balanced state of wellness.

Spector notes, "By the age of eighteen, the average American child has received from ten to twenty courses of antibiotics. Forty-three million courses were dispensed in 2010 alone, and throughout the developed world children receive, on average, at least one such treatment every other year." [30]

'Those drugs have saved countless lives, and it is very important that we not lose sight of that fact," says Dr. Martin J. Blaser, the chairman of the Department of Medicine and a professor of microbiology at the New York University School of Medicine. Logically speaking, he reveals, "Whenever they are used, though, there is collateral damage. And we are only now fully learning how severe that damage has been." [30]

Spector introduces Dr. Andrew Goldberg Director of Rhinology and Sinus Surgery at the University of California, San Francisco Medical Center. The good doctor recounts a surprising story about one of his early patients and a stubborn ear infection. The guy, he says, was seen many times for a chronic infection in just one ear, although they tend to occur in both sides, he adds. The doctor says he followed standard practices, prescribing several rounds of different types of antibiotics and antifungal drops. Even with the repeated treatments the man's ear did not clear up. [30] Unexpectedly one day the man came back into his office, saying that his ear had healed up completely. The doctor confirmed there was no sign of the pesky infection and wanted to know how he did it, assuming one of the antibiotics finally worked for him.

Dr. Goldberg recalls thinking the guy was nuts when he told him that he had taken wax from the good ear and put it into his bad ear. Within a few days, it was fine, the guy revealed. Dr. Goldberg said he never gave it a second thought, until he began to study the cause of common ear infections.[30] Here he thought the guy was foolish to suggest something so simple, like putting wax from one ear to the next, could possibly resolve a chronic infection in the ear or anywhere else.

Goldberg learned a valuable lesson that day, and that is our earwax carries many different kinds of bacterial species that could have easily destroyed the infection in his bad ear:

> It was actually something like a eureka moment... I realized that this patient was the perfect experiment: a good ear and a bad ear separated by a head. That guy wasn't crazy; he was right. Clearly he had something protecting one ear that he then transferred to the other ear. Drugs didn't cure him. He cured himself. [30]

Dr. Goldberg also expresses concern about the overuse of antibiotics. Chronic sinusitis is one of his research specialties, which is listed as the fifth most popular reason people take antibiotics to begin with. Goldberg and his associates were surprised to uncover the fact that someone with sinusitis, typically has about nine hundred strains of bacteria inhabiting their sinus passages. Amazingly, they estimate that healthy people have more like twelve hundred. He says, "...other elements of the bacterial community are keeping the infection in check. Those microbes are the equivalent of the good earwax. And for eighty years we have done everything in our power to get rid of all of them." [30]

Arizona State University researchers measured 50 different microbial by-products in the feces of autistic children and compared them with those in healthy children. They found significant differences in the levels maintained by the two groups. Scientists say that they don't understand the significance of these differences in the development of ASD, or whether or not they are the result of the condition or rather a direct cause. [31]

More and more researchers say autism spectrum disorders (ASD) could be caused by abnormal gut bacteria from a damaged microbiome. This dramatically affects the everyday health and functioning of these children. There is also a ton of evidence to support that restoring the proper balance of gut microbes could ultimately relieve many behavioral symptoms, plus the digestive distress seen in many of these ASD children. [18, 31]

Italian researchers have completed microbial intestinal comparisons in healthy kids vs. those with autism. They report that they discovered several different and even altered numbers of intestinal bacterial species, including drops in a specific type that supports good intestinal health. [31]

In Defense of Food, best-selling author Michael Pollan, reveals in a *NY Times* article *"Some of My Best Friends Are Germs."* He explains, he was invited to the BioFrontiers Institute at the University of Colorado, in Boulder, to participate in a new citizen-science initiative, called the American Gut Project. He took part in a lab microbiome sequencing experiment where researchers collected and analyzed his bacterial genome from samples taken from his tongue, skin and intestines. In an effort to map the genetic structure of the species within, hundreds of bacterial types were collected from numerous individuals and family members in order to get a better idea of the inner workings of these uncharted foreign communities, taking up residence in the human body and their implications on human and animal health. [32]

Pollan says, within our "second genome" structure, scientists identified hundreds of bacterial species that call us home, carrying forth genetic information in coded messages that influence the health, possibly even more than the genes you inherited from your parents. The difference, he indicates, may lie in the potential to reshape and even re-cultivate this "second genome," in spite of beliefs that inherited genes are more-or-less fixed for life. [32]

Currently, researchers are looking into the possibility of transferring bacterial colonies from one gut to another in an effort to determine the likelihood that they can successfully reconstruct a healthy microbiome in the new source to replace damaged communities. If accomplished, these transplants have the potential to completely overhaul the entire medical paradigm in how we treat all ranges of illnesses and chronic diseases. [30, 32]

Samples taken from baby diapers helped scientists track the bacterial colonization in the gut—a process that begins shortly after birth and continues to gradually shift and change, they say, with the inclusion of breast milk and then again with the introduction of solid foods and weaning. This microbial transformation continues until around the age of 3, when the baby's gut begins to resemble that of an adult, much like the parents. Pollan further explains that breast milk contains elements that are both "pre-biotic" (food for microbes) and "pro-biotic" (beneficial bacteria). Infant formulas do not take these vital aspects into account; researchers say bottle-fed babies lack optimal colonization in the gut. [32]

In addition, babies born C-section (about 1/3 of American children) don't acquire the vaginal and intestinal microbes from the birth canal. The researchers discovered that these young bacterial communities more closely resemble those of the mother's (and father's) skin. This is far less than ideal, and they say it could be a good indication of why we are seeing significantly higher rates of allergies, asthma and autoimmune disorders in these children. Without proper access to a good assortment of microbes at birth, their immune systems may fail to develop properly. "The way we live now, we are losing these organisms, and each generation arrives with fewer than the one before," Dr. Blaser says. [30, 31, 32]

Research is starting to present the advantages of transferring missing bacterial colonies manually, after birth, with a method known as "vaginal seeding" and the results, so far, look largely promising. [33] Another area of research that looks favorable, although it may not sound charming, is known as "fecal transplants." This involves introducing a healthy person's gut microbiota into a sick person's gut so that the good bacteria can take over and propagate. [30, 32]

Scientists use the word "microbiota" to refer to all of the microbes in a single community, whereas the term "microbiome" refers to the collective genes.[30} Experts have had a good amount of success with this transfer method against an antibiotic-resistant pathogen that kills 14,000 Americans a year. [32]

In another study, researchers took obese mice and transplanted into them the intestinal microbes from lean mice and surprisingly, they lost weight. In the Netherlands, a similar study on humans analyzed the outcomes of transferring donor species from lean individuals to the guts of male patients suffering from metabolic syndrome. Researchers reported staggering improvements in the recipients' sensitivity levels to insulin, which is important for metabolic health. It showed that the new gut microbes were somehow influencing their metabolism. [32]

Spector also talks about studies led by Peer Bork, of the European Molecular Biology Laboratory, in Heidelberg, Germany. They found that people can be classified by types of bacterial species that are ruling the gut. Humans, they discovered, tend to fit into one of three groups they call enterotypes, based on their microbial makeup. They note that the impact of this information can be compared to the discovery of the four blood types in human evolution. The potential for these findings to lead to new and better treatments for chronic illness is enormous and very exciting. [30]

Justin Sonnenburg, a microbiologist at Stanford, proposes that we begin to think of our body as "an elaborate vessel optimized for the growth and spread of our microbial inhabitants." In other words, we are essentially slaves to their micro-bacterial wants and whims, linked forever in a communal relationship of co-protectionism. We can't live without them and they can't live without us. [32]

Pollan says that this shift in thinking couldn't have come a moment too soon, in consideration of the war efforts besieged upon our bacterial colonies in the form of antibiotics, deficient diets and environmental toxins in the past century. Scientists are referencing this as the impoverished "Westernized Microbiome" as they consider organizing a rescue project termed "restoration ecology" to mitigate the situation to save our deficient guts. [32]

When we don't have enough of the "right" kind of species, imbalances tend to appear and take over in these colonies. They call that loss of diversity, which could result from an over-abundance of the "wrong" kind of microbes, outnumbering the good ones. This loss of diversity may have strong influences on a wide range of chronic diseases, infections and even obesity. [30, 31, 32] Researchers believe these vital communities may play a critical role in training and regulating our immune systems in order to accurately recognize the difference between friends and enemies, without overreaching to the panic button like everything is a threat. Allergies and autoimmune diseases prominent in Western culture may be the result of severe damage to this primordial relationship in which we co-evolved. [30, 31, 32]

"Consumption of hyperhygienic, mass-produced, highly processed and calorie-dense foods is testing how rapidly the microbiota of individuals in industrialized countries can adapt," Sonnenburg adds. [32]

The scientists note that the lower biodiversity problems of the West are likely due to overuse of antibiotics, pesticides and processed foods (cleansed of all bacteria, good and bad) and lack of exposure to bacterial sources in dirt and in daily living. Americans may live a more hygienic lifestyle, but as one researcher pointed out, "Rural people spend a lot more time outside and have much more contact with plants and with soil," so their gut bacteria are much more diverse than here in the West. They also discovered, generally, that the more rural populations do tend to be exposed to infectious disease and have lower life expectancies than the Western cultures, but with our lack bacterial diversity, that could justify why they also have lower rates of chronic diseases.[32]

National Institutes of Health summarized Dr. Seneff's research outcomes covering "Diminished brain resilience syndrome":

> Exposure to certain environmental chemicals, particularly glyphosate... may disrupt the body's innate switching mechanism, which normally turns off the immune response to brain injury once danger has been removed. Deficiencies in serotonin, due to disruption of the shikimate pathway, may lead to impaired melatonin supply, which reduces the resiliency of the brain. [34]

Furthermore, Seneff concludes,

> Depletion of certain rare minerals, overuse of sunscreen

and/or overprotection from sun exposure, as well as over-indulgence in heavily processed, nutrient deficient foods, further compromise the brain's resilience. Modifications to lifestyle practices, if widely implemented, could significantly reduce...neurological damage.[34]

What Next?

So far we've seen how GMOs and glyphosate chemicals have become prevalent in our communities and throughout the food supply. Although they are nearly impossible to avoid 100 percent of the time, any effort that you make now will surely get the ball rolling so you can begin to make your own comparisons, based on your own experiences, before and after the changes have taken hold. People tend to notice positive shifts in their digestion, sleeping patterns, moods and energy levels relatively quickly. I've heard about significant improvements occurring in as little as two-to-three days and as much as seven-to-ten days, after the switch. We're not talking half-way here. We're speaking of the whole organic enchilada. Now, I know I said it's a process not an event... and I mean that, but we're at a point in our relationship (you the reader, me the guide) where I can be blunt with you, and you will understand that my approach is for the good of your health and longevity, along with that of your offspring. Since you are still with me, I won't hold back in confessing to you the hours, days, years and tears that I have put into avoiding this whole GMO food affair, that I consider to be the detriment of our existence, life on this planet and that of our ecosystems.

It takes time to fully take hold of your course and see for yourself what these changes can mean for you and your family. Everyone is different and the experiences do overlap some, but all appear to have their own unique set of circumstances, timelines and outcomes. That is why it is important to begin the work of tracking all of our symptoms, both individually and collectively as a population.

In addition, we need to follow the line of our repair efforts, so we can begin to see the forest in spite of GMO trees. Perhaps your cleanup efforts start paying off and you begin to see your son or daughter feeling better; so you jot down a few journal notes every day or week to follow your progress. You will be glad you did and you will have a much clearer, long-term picture of what works and what doesn't. Let's say it together, you don't know where you are, if you can't see where you've been.

You might consider sharing your experiences to help others with their GMO-Free transition. You could also contribute testimony to further the scientific cause, for no other reason than to insist that "they" call in to question the validity and safety of the GMO feeding experiment. With this information, we (as a nation), should take a long hard gaze at the real necessity and our utter obligation to demand a new approach to the food, health and safety of our people and our children. As I noted earlier, the common sense methodologies of the precautionary principle may be our best lines of defense.

If nothing else, I am confident that I have demonstrated in this text how the chains of evidence prove that we are bound to a planetary experiment without our knowledge or consent; and that we owe it to our citizens and our children to step back and take a more thoughtful approach to the food we eat and feed our children. For the sake of our children's health and society as a whole, we must take care to reverse the damages and the agricultural structures that brought us here. If we want to mitigate the current circumstances dragging down our economy and restore the health of our children, we will buck this GMO food system and replace it with one that works. This is a grave matter of public importance and responsibility, a great deal of which is affixed to the barcodes of the biotech agenda.

Parents, scientists and doctors all over the world are deeply disturbed by the situation and the negative outcomes they have witnessed time-and-again in themselves, those they serve and in those they love. Chapter 5 is packed with powerful testimony, illustrating incredible stories of transformation by several families, through the eyes of moms. These are real-life narratives of suffering and subsequent recovery, due to a total overhaul of the diet and what I like to call their family's "food-style."

When we develop a state of mindfulness around what we eat and what we feed our children, we begin listening and responding to the true needs and calls of the body. In this way, we begin to cultivate the crucial relationship between ourselves and our food; that absolutely needs to happen to maintain this new existence, while communicating the same for our youngsters. Feeding your body what it demands for basic survival is the most essential part of being human. There really is not anything more important or more worthy of your time or attention, on a day-to-day basis, when it comes to your health and that of your kid's.

Let's meet several GMO-Free families that are committed to these dietary changes after overcoming a variety of health challenges directly related to the food they ate. We'll see how they're empowering their tykes and teens to navigate the contaminated food supply, while nurturing the delicate relationship between the brain, body and the being.

From here on out, I encourage you to keep your eyes open for GMO-Free tips, tricks and tools that will incorporate easily into your world to help you transition your family in ways that work best for you and your budget.

You will notice that none of these families are rich by any standard. They are your average parents trying to make organic ends meet.

CHAPTER 5

············

GMO-Free Testimony

············*Jennifer*············

We have two kids. Our son is five and our daughter is three. I have a wonderful, supportive husband. We grew up in Alaska together and then moved to Washington State.

Our Story

My son was born in 2009; shortly after, he became severely colicky. It didn't matter what we did; it didn't get any better. He would just cry all the time. You couldn't lay him down to sleep; you had to hold him constantly. He had lots of mucous in his stools, acid reflux, and always seemed to be in distress. They tried putting him on special types of formulas, but it didn't help. The doctors said that some babies are just colicky, and he would have to grow out of it.

I gave birth to my daughter, 2 ½ years later. She was 8 lbs., 10 ounces, happy and healthy, but within a couple of days, she started having these episodes where she would struggle to breathe. It was really scary, and no one knew what was going on. We took her to Children's Hospital in Seattle. They stuck cameras up her nose to look down her throat and found that her vocal cords and her esophagus were very red and inflamed. They thought it could be food allergies. They put me on a really restrictive diet of no peas, no beans, no legumes, no meat, no dairy, no eggs, and no soy. But it didn't seem to help at all. The doctors continued to do tests including swallow studies, upper GIs, and an MRI when she was about 4 weeks old, even thinking she had a deadly condition with fluid on her brain. Those were the scariest days of my life. We were lucky the MRI looked wonderful, so we crossed that off our list, but the sleepless nights continued.

When she was about 4 ½ months old, I had lost so much weight from the restricted diet that doctors suggested I put her on special formula. I stopped breastfeeding, and things got much worse, not better. The episodes became more frequent, lasting longer, sometimes as long as 12-16 hours with her struggling to breathe. The weeks and months dragged on, as we saw teams of different specialists. One tried to tell me that the worst-case scenario was that if she passed out from lack of oxygen then hopefully her vocal cords would relax, and she could start breathing again. That was no reassurance because we lived a half hour from our local hospital and over 2 hours from Seattle Children's. I hardly slept for months. I was just terrified she would stop breathing and die in her sleep.

Her pediatrician had decided we should try a medication for acid reflux. It was not her first choice, because once you put an infant on it, it is very hard to get them off. But because nothing was working, we were down to last resorts. Unfortunately, it didn't help; so we were back to square one, and now she was stuck on this medication, because she was too sick to take her off. We had an amazing team of doctors. Her pediatrician even referred her case to a doctor who had flown in to present at a medical conference. We would always get our hopes up when a doctor thought they had an idea of what was going on, but in no one ever did figure it out.

An Answer

When she was 10 ½ months old, I ran across some moms on the internet who had sick kids. They were telling their stories about cutting out GMOs.

She had started to refuse her formula and didn't want to eat. I think she knew it was making her sick. I brought all the information I found to our pediatrician and told her I wanted to try and go GMO-Free. The doctor said, why not, nothing else is working. That day, I went out and bought organic whole milk, organic fruits and veggies and organic baby rice and oat cereals. It was actually the first time she had ever had dairy. I also started making my own homemade baby food. Within two weeks, she started getting better, and her breathing episodes disappeared, and my daughter began to breathe normally, without struggling and gasping for air. I anxiously watched over her, relieved that the episodes had stopped, but still terrified that they would return at any moment. Luckily they never did.

When we first started switching over our diet, I wanted to make sure everything was GMO-Free, not necessarily organic, because we hadn't gotten there yet.

One day we had tuna for lunch, and afterward she had diarrhea for 3 days. I couldn't figure out what it was. Then I looked and figured out there's soy in the tuna fish. After trial and error, we realized that she was sensitive to soy, even if it's organic.

I have a family of four and I try to keep our grocery budget under $500 a month; it is doable. Right now, we're on a restricted income, but it's what we have to work with so I can stay home with my kids while they're small. I try and buy a quarter of a grass-fed organic beef from a local farm, as we are able, and I keep it in the freezer. My husband also hunts, so when he can get a deer, it really helps.

The truth is, I don't think twice about paying more for organic food. We had wonderful health insurance and the amount that we spent on doctors, tests and hospital bills in that first year of her life was so much, that we could have eaten organic until she was 18 without any limits on our food budget. Yes, a gallon of organic milk is around $6 a gallon, and the non-organic milk is only $1.99, but that includes all the toxins and chemicals that are in the animals are feed, and that goes straight into the milk.

I would encourage all pregnant and breastfeeding moms, to check out all the new studies that are coming out on human breast milk and the amount of pesticides that are showing up in it. Unfortunately, all that goes right into your child. It's not worth it.

GMO-Free Life

Once you get started on your GMO-Free journey and your family starts feeling better, you will spend a lot less on some things like anti-acid medications because your digestion will improve and you won't need them anymore. Moms will do anything to make their kids feel better! It's just a matter of wrapping your mind around the thought that you are spending more money for quality food right now, but you will make up for it with fewer doctor visits and medication.

I've always been a really big bargain shopper. I still am, just with organic food now. At first, it was really hard to adjust to the price difference, but now I don't think twice about it. You have to take into consideration how many school and work lunches you are packing every day because the cost of organic lunch meat and other packaged lunch items can be pricey.

You also have to take into account how much you're cooking from scratch. Whole foods are your best bet, both nutritionally and cost wise. Some families opt for cooking every meal from scratch and obviously that is the healthiest way to feed your family. Of course, that's not always possible for many busy and working families. That's why it's important to read labels and ingredients.

I feed my kids the typical breakfast of eggs and hash browns or breakfast burritos. Perhaps we'll have honey butter toast, fruit, and oatmeal. We also eat a lot of homemade yogurt - which you can freeze, by the way, and make into yummy frozen yogurt pops also! Sometimes we eat organic cereal, but not as much as we used to. It's pretty much the same breakfast everybody else has. For lunch, we do a lot of different things, like soups, sandwiches, cheese and crackers, fruits and veggies. Lunch can be hard when you're on the go, and can become a big struggle where I feel like we get stuck in a rut sometimes. When that happens, I go onto Pinterest to get new ideas.

One great tip is to keep a veggie tray in your fridge. When you get home from shopping, cut them up and put them in the veggie tray. It can be a life saver with little kids. We all know when they get hungry, they want food now. They don't want to wait for you to make it; when you're running late, you get home, and it's already dinner time, then you still have to make something from scratch. It might be an hour and a half before it's done. You can just pull out that veggie tray and put it down on the table. It fills them up and keeps them occupied while you are cooking and they end up eating all their veggies before the rest of the meal. It's really one of those staple things. Of course, you can do fruit and other stuff too. But I do find that veggies work best, because if your kids are like mine given the option, they will eat all the fruits first.

I keep things on hand like frozen homemade muffins that you can pull out when you need them, and they defrost fast. You can do the same thing with cake. I will make a birthday cake, and if there are leftovers, I will cut it into portion sizes and freeze it. Then if we're going to a birthday party, I grab a slice out of the freezer, and by the time we get there it's thawed. That's where I have the most struggle, BBQs, birthday parties, social events in general. You don't want your child to feel left out. It's a really big deal that they feel included.

As you travel down this road, you likely rethink your food containers, as well. You don't want to spend all of this money for your kid's food and then pack it into toxic containers that are going to leach chemicals into it.

My son was almost 3 years old when we made these changes. It was a little harder for him. There was a transition period in the beginning, where we were taking it slowly, but when I realized that everyone was getting better, I went full force. He was having fewer issues and was feeling generally less upset. I was having fewer digestive problems with my IBS. The more improvements I saw, the harder I worked to change our habits. Eventually, we ended up going completely organic and then we saw, even more, improvements.

Before the change, I noticed, my son would push food away when he was little. I would encourage him to eat it thinking it was healthy for him, but I think he intuitively knew it wasn't good for him and so he refused to eat it. The kids are really amazing; if they see something that they really want, they will ask me if it's organic. If I say no, they just put it back. They know that they feel better when they eat good, healthy, clean food. They like to ask a lot of questions, like where different foods come from and how they are grown. My 3-year-old is also really good about avoiding soy.

If someone gives her something she'll bring it bring it to me and ask if it's okay to eat it.

Honestly, there are things that my kids won't eat when I get them from the store; a perfect example is grape tomatoes, when we grow them I have to constantly tell them to stay out of them until they're ripe. They love eating out of the garden, especially the stuff that they grow themselves, harvest and pull right off and stick in their mouths! It's really so exciting for them, and they will eat more when they're able to pick it themselves.

Bear in mind that you have to set a good example - I never really liked raw carrots myself, but they are a really good and healthy snack, so I would cut them up for my son; he would never really eat them. Then my dad came to visit, and they walked in the garden together talking about how good carrots were. They pulled some up and ate them. He's been eating them ever since, and he loves carrots. Eating by example is a big thing and making sure both parents are on the same page is essential. Even if you don't like something, don't say you don't like it, out loud.

I have also really learned the importance of reading labels. I never read labels before this! I knew to stay away from diet stuff. I got really bad headaches from Aspartame, but other than that I wasn't reading labels before this all started, so I was kind of a disbeliever. People will try to argue with me about it, but you can't argue with your child getting better or you getting better. Getting diarrhea after almost every meal is not normal. Having bloating and stomach pains, acid reflux, dealing with allergies and hives, these things are not normal.

If I eat GMOs I get the IBS symptoms again and a lot of bloating, diarrhea and stomach pain sometimes within 15 minutes of eating it. It's almost like having food poisoning.

When my daughter was little, she did get soy a few times when well-meaning folks handed her a cracker or some other thing you wouldn't think even had soy in it. Many people didn't know what a GMO was, and most processed products have GMO soy in them. When she gets it, she gets stomach pains and diarrhea.

The number of people on acid blockers is astronomical. People are starting to just think that it's normal, and it's not!! And once people start to switch and then move forward, they'll start feeling better and be like,

"Wait a minute, there is something to this." That's the big thing; people can try to say "Oh' it's not true," but you know that you're feeling better, and your kids are feeling better too. That's what really matters. I know how overwhelming it can seem in the beginning, but once everyone starts feeling better, you'll embrace it, more and more. I find that it really makes it easier to talk to other organic moms and see what they're doing. Always try new things, so you don't get stuck in a rut.

On the Go

Very rarely we'll eat away from home and even then, most of the time I bring our food. It's very hard to find an organic or GMO-Free restaurant. Often even if they tell you that they have organic or GMO-Free options, they are very limited. Maybe just the salad bar is organic. In the last few years, we have seen a few more organic restaurants in Western Washington where we live. One of the restaurants is all organic and soy-free. We can take the kids there, and everybody gets to have anything they want from the menu! It's really an amazing experience because we've never been able to do that before.

There are two different ice cream shops in Ballard that cater to the organic customers. They make completely organic treats, sorbets, and ice cream. It's also all soy and allergen free. My daughter had her first peanut butter cup there, last year. (Typically, they have soy lecithin in them). It's really an amazing feeling to walk into a dessert place, and let her pick out whatever she wants without fear. It's exciting when you discover you have new options. It's becoming more frequent as this lifestyle becomes more mainstream. I've also noticed, as it becomes more main-stream, you have to be careful too. A lot of the big corporations aren't in it for the right reasons and have started getting more and more into making organic products. I've started to pay more attention to reading the labels, every time I shop, regardless of whether I've been buying that product for a couple years and think it's safe. Corporations will merge and change hands; then they change the ingredients, looking for cheaper ways to cut corners - leaving you thinking it's still the same stuff, when indeed it is not. Food manufacturers can be very tricky, slipping in ingredients that are less wholesome and nutritious. They will say and do anything to increase their bottom line. Lying and false advertising is just the beginning of the food pyramid scheme. Just because it says Non-GMO or even organic doesn't mean that you can be a mindless-type consumer, even when paying more for them. I say this from personal experience, not out of judgment, because you will be misled, you are being misled.

I pay particular attention when big companies start buying out little companies; they start taking shortcuts with the quality of ingredients they use. If you pay attention, you will find that some of the ingredients actually change.

The Power of Many

If you can find someone that's just raising a couple cows, someone that is doing grass-fed and using Non-GMO grains, you can buy meat from them and usually get it quite a bit cheaper, than you can in the grocery stores. This community often works in a trade and barter environment in order to close the circle of need for everyone.

Get in Touch

You should to ask a lot of questions, call companies, read labels, talk to your grocer, farmers and neighbors. Share ideas, recipes, advice and support one another. That's what it takes.

It is important to get in touch with your food system. Find out who is making it and what their business model looks like. Take a gander at their website. Do they have a contact number? Take 5 minutes and have a conversation with them. It does make a difference. Note, if they are they open about their practices or are they guarded?

You are a busy parent without time to hop down every rabbit hole that you see. I understand, that is why we (the *cleanfood* movement) have been out here doing the work for you, as much as possible. In Chapter 7 you will find several organic and natural food search tools to help you find local producers you can trust.

This has been a grass-roots efforts with an ever-changing landscape that keeps us on our proverbial toes, and that's why it's so important to talk about this, establishing teams and connecting over this. We can all help each other further this essential journey to raise happy, healthy GMO-Free children in world, that is not entirely suitable. After all, it does take a village. I know that now more than ever.

Julianna

I'm 45 years old and I have two boys; they are 13 and 16. We live in Michigan. I graduated college - went straight into manufacturing and worked many, many years in automotive and transportation manufacturing. I always had high-stress jobs. I had a lot of meetings, and I ate whatever people brought in. You just don't think twice about it.

Our Story

Both of my boys were born C-section. They both had what I thought were normal health issues. One had frequent ear infections, and the other one had allergies. I think that's kind of the normal story for most people.

I had migraine headaches by the age of 12, and by my late to mid-30s, I started getting sicker and sicker. It just progressively got worse. It's not like I had a major diagnosis, I just didn't feel good, ever. I had days where I barely functioned.

In 2001, I had my son but I don't think at that point, I really realized how bad I felt and I thought 'hey, well everybody feels bad.' Looking back, everyone I knew complained about frequent colds or headaches or my joints hurt or I'm too tired to run with my kids. Everyone complains about one or more of those sorts of things. It started to become normal in society like illness is normal. When you feel like this and you can barely get out of the chair, you look at a marathon runner and think, "I don't know how that person does that." I would take my boys to the playground and find myself a shady place to sit down. I wanted to go hiking with them and other stuff, but I just couldn't. I was working 70 hours a week and I would just eat my way through the day, kind of mindlessly. I was so stressed out and I never put the puzzle pieces together.

We've been told, at least this is true for most people, this is what you eat. You eat whole grains; you drink milk. You feed your kids cereal in the morning, because that's what the commercials tell you to do and it's fortified with all those nutrients. They made it healthy; they put protein in your Cheerios or whatever. They go to school and see cheeseburgers and chicken nuggets, and you want your kids to do what everybody else is doing because it's easier and your kids want to fit in.

I was going along like this, I had my yearly checkups at the doctors and I had several surgeries, including five abdominal surgeries in the course of seven years and I felt old. I would get up in the morning, barely able to get out of bed. It took me 45 minutes to get my muscles going for the day. I had to make notes so I could remember everything I had to do that day - I had no memory. I went to the eye doctor and he put me in bifocals, and I'm thinking, "My goodness I'm 34; am I going to be blind by the time I'm 70?" There were always those little thoughts. The pieces never really fit together to show the whole picture of what was really going on.

There was also my son that would go to bed fine and then wake up like he was sitting next to a cat. We had no carpet in our house; he was on allergy meds which weren't working any longer. I couldn't figure it out, what kept triggering these allergies. They weren't seasonally induced. I remember posting on *Facebook*, "Can someone recommend a good allergist? My son's nose is driving me crazy."

A good friend of mine had been telling me for about two years, "You need to look at going gluten free."

I thought, "What you mean I can't live without bread, are you kidding me? What am I going to feed everybody?" She recommended we go see her allergist that does an acupuncture and allergy muscle testing thing. She said, "She might be able to help you figure out what is going on." I made appointments for both of us to see her, and she told me that my son had issues with gluten and corn… and she told me I had issues with gluten, onions, tomatoes and vinegar. I looked at her and thought, "I live off chiliburgers and pickles. What's left to eat when you take all that away?" I was committed for my son's sake, not my sake, to get him to stop sneezing. That poor kid was desperate, and so I came home and told my husband, "Alex and I are going gluten free. I don't know what that means but were doing it." The first thing I did was cut bread out. I had done the Atkin's Diet, and that taught us that you don't need bread for a ham sandwich. You take your ham, and you roll it up with cheese and lettuce and eat it. I said to my son, "Your sandwich is now a ham roll-up." We started exploring other options out there; most of the bread is really gross. He didn't care for them, so I didn't really buy much. Then I started *Googling*. This was probably six years ago now. From then, until now, there has become significantly more information available.

It was in that research that I initially discovered genetically modified foods. I was saying to myself, "Why is this a problem anyway? Everybody eats gluten. It's everywhere you go." So, when I first heard of GMOs I wondered, "What the heck is that." I started doing the research and poking around on the Environmental Working Group (EWG) website and started reading some other resources on there. Then I watched *Food, Inc.* I watched that whole movie with my jaw on the floor, thinking, "What are they feeding us?! What are they trying to do to us?" I don't understand why they think it's okay, feeding us chemicals they know cause infertility and cancer. I just don't get that.

I told my family that I was going to do everything I could to get rid of the GMOs. The fact is that they have never proven them to be safe; they tell you they're safe but they never have proven it. There have been no long-term studies, and they change them every single year. Before you put it in our food supply, it should be tested. Right? But it's never been tested. And so, I added all those pieces together and for me....ya know, I've had this argument with some people that I know that say, "Well it's never been proven to be unsafe," and to me that is the opposite of the right argument, because I want to know that it's safe. And if there's any risk at all, I need to do what I can to avoid that risk until they prove it safe. If they prove it safe and I'm satisfied, then fine. They've never proven it safe and they're not even trying to. In fact, they're trying to hide it from us which also ticks me off, because I feel like we really need to take responsibility for ourselves; that means we need all of the information in which to make an informed decision, and you can't, if you don't know what it is. You can't make an informed decision, so for me, it was a protection issue.

I don't know that it's safe; I don't want my kids eating it, and when we cut it out of our diet we started to see significant improvements.

My oldest child is a good example, born 11 pounds, 6 ounces; but then he dropped off the growth chart by the time he was one year old. He was below the growth chart and he stayed there. As you do with your kids, you measure their height and keep track to measure how they're growing. I have a chart on the wall to measure his growth; and when I took gluten out of his diet, he sprouted four inches in five months. I started asking why … and a good friend of mine has three kids that are celiacs. She said her daughter did the same thing, because there's such a problem with absorption of nutrients.

When the gut is so inflamed, they call it leaky gut, and you can't absorb nutrients that way; your body doesn't digest food properly… you don't have the fuel to grow properly. That affects each kid slightly differently. Some kids, it's a physical growth issue; some kids, it's a mental growth issue, a neurological issue and/or an immune system issue. Sometimes it's pieces of all of them. When you look at the rise of illness in kids, it's grown exponentially in the last two generations. We are looking at third and fourth generations of kids fed genetically modified, nutrient-deficient diets. They don't get enough sunshine. They don't drink enough water. They eat too much sugar; and guess what we get, the illnesses that we're dealing with now. We have 8-year-olds dealing with Type I diabetes. Cancer is the number one killer of children under age 15. We have an epidemic of allergies, ADHD, and asthma. The things the kids are struggling with, we now consider normal. We call it normal for our kids to be sick.

You know, I was like everybody else … *Okay, so the doctor says this is good, and the commercials say "Yeah, drink milk! It does a body good." My kids are supposed to drink milk to get calcium.* I didn't question any of that - (that's true with most everybody), until I realized that there was such a strong connection between what we were eating and what we were struggling with as a family.

My son Liam is 13 now; after we started realizing we had problems with the food and we started making changes, a couple of months later, I was taking Liam to the Ear, Nose and Throat Doctor (ENT). He had fluid on his ears for as long as I could remember. He had two sets of tubes and he had his adenoids removed.

The ear infections stopped around a year and half, but he still had speech issues because he couldn't hear properly. The tubes helped only for a couple months, nothing to get excited about. I took him back to ENT. The resident was young and she looked into his ears and says "Oh he has fluid on his ears; looks like we're going to need to put the tubes back in again." I said, "No we're not" and she stepped away and looked kind taken aback by my response. I said, "Were going to find out why he keeps getting fluid on his ear," and she looked at me like I had two heads. She stammered a bit and said, "Well I'm going to have to have the doctor come in." I said, "Yes, that would be good." The doctor came in and looked in his ears and said, "So, I hear that you don't want to do the tubes again." "No," I said. "I want to find out why this keeps happening because I want to stop it." She looks in his nose, literally 10 seconds, both nostrils and says "He has allergies, you might want to take him to an allergist." I looked at her and asked, "So, how come we didn't suggest that before the last $4,000 surgery?" She didn't have an answer for me. She showed me inside his nostrils; it was all purple and swollen, and she told me that's a clear sign that he's got allergy issues. He didn't have a runny nose, runny eyes or any of that. He simply had fluid on his ear.

I took him to an acupuncturist, not an allergist and she said he has issues with gluten, corn and dairy. We had already cut out the gluten and corn, so I just stopped buying milk and cheese. It threw my husband a little bit because he loves cheese. We keep a little in the house for him to eat, but other than that we tend to stay away from dairy. However, we do goats milk and he loves goat cheese now. It took only about a month or so and it cleared up. The fluid in his ear kept getting better. I put him through speech therapy. We had to clear candida out of his system. The sugar cravings in that kid were unbelievable.

Sugar is more addicting than cocaine (not to mention it is sprayed with glyphosate, just before harvest, just like the wheat and cereal grains). When I read that, I figured out why it wasn't so easy for him to give up the sweets and the treats, especially when he's surrounded by it at school.

For my son the other big thing was behavior. He was my outburst kid, very high energy and was all over the place. He never thought before he acted. I can't tell you how much stuff the kid broke. We always joked that when he took over my husband's construction team that he would be in charge of demolition. Over time, with a fair amount of work and lots of probiotics and some other supplements, he's become a normally energized child. He's a boy and they have a lot of energy, but now he's like the average boy. He doesn't have any health issues; he doesn't get sick anymore. So for him, getting that GMO processed crap out of his diet made a huge difference.

What Were They Thinking?

If they would have just left the food alone, I think it would have been fine. For example, look at dairy; many cultures in the world don't even drink milk. It was decided that everyone should drink milk, so they industrialized the production of milk. We take a cow that's supposed to eat grass and feed it GMO corn and soy. Now the cow is sick, so they give it antibiotics and all of that transfers into the milk - the illness and the GMOs transfer into the milk. The (glyphosate) chemicals they use on genetically modified crops, transfer into the milk and all of that goes into our kids and adults too.

The idea was that we needed to industrialize and grow mono-crops, like corn, as a primary source of starch. Then genetically modify it so it's resistant to bugs, so they could get higher yields and higher production, but it didn't really work. Now we have super weeds to deal with. They started modifying our crops in ways nobody understands, not even the scientists doing it. They don't understand how it affects your body. They've genetically modified corn to produce the low-grade insecticide, called Bt corn that can actually implant itself in your gut and produce a low-grade insecticide. There's evidence and research to support this. So you have potentially an element in your gut that comes from genetically modified corn, producing your insecticide that is constantly traveling through your blood stream with unknown consequences.

You can only imagine if you drank Roundup or OFF or RAID, you're going to get very sick. Well, we're doing it over long periods of time. So we're getting it through the milk we drink, through the meat we eat and we're getting it through the grains. Of course, there are the neonicotinoids, which is what they believe are killing the bees. Plenty of these chemicals have been linked to cancer, infertility and many other illnesses, that are being consumed on a daily basis.

We're surrounded by corn, soybean and potato fields here, and while I was driving on the highway the other day, my car got sprayed by the crop duster that was spraying the field next to the highway. It's in the water supply. We have a Monsanto and a Pioneer plant about 10 minutes from us and the town that they're in; the water supply is entirely contaminated. They're both seed sorting facilities here. They grow the seeds around here and then sort them and bag them.

If I look at the primary reasons we were getting sick from what we were eating, we can look at wheat as one example; biblical wheat and wheat itself is an heirloom crop. It is very nutrient dense, high in B vitamins. The oils are beneficial and even the starch has a little bit of benefit as well.

We got smarter than nature and decided we could do it better, genetically modified it and sprayed it with lots of chemicals. This started in the 80s and if you track the illnesses from then until now, it's an exponential rise. We're eating more of it. We're surrounded by it. I don't know how we aren't being impacted by it.

The Light Bulb Moment

Once I knew there was this limitation in modern medicine, regarding chronic illness, there was a light bulb moment sitting there in the ENT with my son, that they don't know why and if they do, they aren't telling anybody and that I wasn't going to get my answers there.

I was working full time, coaching soccer and being a mom. I had to do my research in very spare moments. I started changing our diet and adding a few supplements here and there. I started reading about detox, and I tried it. I tried this and I tried that, and putting together the pieces was very difficult. I knew that the job I was doing was not what my life's mission was going to be. I didn't know what it was and I remember reading an article in a clean eating magazine, I picked up to get some recipe ideas. The article was about people that had changed careers in the middle of their life and I was 39 at the time. There was a woman in the article named Andrea Beaman (IIN graduate), and she had been on that show *CHOP*, where they compete in one of those competition cooking shows. I remember her because I thought all her recipes sounded really interesting. I *Googled* her, got on her website and sent her an email. I said to her, "I want to want to do what you do. I want to be a health coach. What does it mean to be a health coach? Where did you learn how to do it"?

I happened to go to the Green Festival in Chicago and I came around the corner and here was a booth for CNHP—Certified Natural Health Professionals and they had all of these classes on natural health and I thought to myself, "Cool, they can teach me!" I found out that they were partnered with Trinity Health, and their naturopathic doctor program. I said to myself, "Whoa, what is that?" I had no idea. I never even heard of it. I looked into the program and signed up for the eight-day intensive. I figured that would be my bellwether to see if it was the right path for me. If I got energized by it, I would sign up for the full MD program; if not, I'd find a different way. I called my husband right away. I said, "I'm doing this … I don't know how were going to pay for it but I'm doing it." He was so wonderful and supportive; he said, "We'll figure it out." I started school while I was still working full time.

The thing for me was that I didn't want people to have to put it all together the way I did it. Some people don't want to spend the money to come to see somebody like me. I understand, but you have to spend the money to get the knowledge and the expertise. I can't even tell you how many people come to me that have been struggling for a long time. They don't understand it; they can't put it together, and their doctor doesn't know what to tell them. We put together a program that works for them. I don't force anything; I don't say, "You must do." But people who come and see me have to want to do the work. The reward is huge, absolutely huge. I look back to the age of 37, where I could barely get out of the chair every single day and look at me today. I am 99 percent headache free. I'm hiking with my kids. I'm biking with my kids. I'm spending time with them doing physical activities that benefit all of us. These are things, I've never done before. And my son, well he doesn't sneeze 75 times a day. He was a typical moody teenager and had adrenal fatigue with some major spells, but he's doing much better. His growth has normalized. Not a moody teen anymore, of course, everybody has their rough days, but no big deal. So we've gotten through those issues.

The beautiful thing about developing education around a healthy lifestyle is when something pops up at home, I can find an answer for it. I've developed a knowledge base of experience at home, through my education and from working with other very knowledgeable experts in the field.

My youngest son's hearing is really quite remarkable now, giving where he came from. He was only hearing about 40 percent, according to the hearing tests they had given him. Now he's hearing between 87 and 93 percent. He does so well in school anyway, and now his hearing isn't all hampered like it was.

Roughly 80 percent of health is diet. I think most of our improvements were the result of changing the food we ate. You got to clean the diet up because you can't outrun a bad diet, so yes, we saw huge improvements from cleaning out our diet.

I can really tell the difference in my boys and in myself when we eat junk, were not supposed to have. We suffer for at least two days. The diet absolutely must get cleaned up.

How I Do It

I would put our diet about 85-90 percent organic. We are a busy family, so once in a while we do eat out, but we are very selective about where we eat. I grow a lot of our food in the summer, hit the farmers markets, and I'm a member of my local CSA (Community Supported Agriculture).

Meijer's is a grocery store chain based out of Grand Rapids, Michigan that is doing a brilliant job of bringing in a lot of organics and they even have their own organic label. Certain things I can't get locally from the farmers market or I can't make myself, I aim for their organics. I've also got a Costco membership because they have a lot of organic fruits and vegetables. In the winter time, when I'm making smoothies and really want to keep our vegetables up, I can go there and it's inexpensive. Costco usually has organic chicken, sometimes organic beef and bison. Natural is not the same thing as organic. The natural label means nothing and can be GMO.

You do have to read your labels, which is getting to be more of a problem because country of origin is getting pulled off labels. I always look for organic grass-fed meats. They do have quite a few pre-packaged meals which I do very few of, like Amy's. I do some of their organics. Those are about the only pre-packaged meals I buy. We have a couple local health food stores where I buy a few specialty items that I can't find anywhere else.

We have four people in our household (two teenage boys and hard-working husband), plus our dog who also has an excellent diet, grain free, with mostly salmon. I would estimate that I spend about $700-800 a month on food. I spend about $125 week between Meijer's and the health food store, which is really not very much because food is getting stupid expensive! In August, we buy a half a beef which costs me a little over $5 a pound, and I put that in the big freezer. We eat that until it runs out, and then we get another one. I take coolers with me when I go pick up the meat. I almost never buy meat at the store or even at the health food store, because it's so expensive there. A pound of hamburger can sometimes cost as much as $8 at one of those stores. If you find a local farmer that raises beef, then it's going to be $5-6 a pound. We are a big family, and I have three big eating boys you know; so when I make meals, like tacos, I have to use two pounds of beef - the rest, I can pull together out of my garden.

You can grow a lot in pots. It's really much easier than you can imagine, growing your own greens and beans. You don't have to go hog wild ... just grow some of the basics you need. [Also] CSAs are becoming more prominent, where you can get a box of produce every week from a farmer. I pay for it in the spring, and we get 18-weeks of fresh vegetables. I go to pick up my box every Wednesday. It's fun and part of the adventure is all about – *What's in the box this week?* It's all local; it's all fresh ... it's all from farmers I know. When I walk up to get my veggies at Meijer's, nobody knows who I am, but when I go pick up my CSA box they all know my name; it's "Hey Julianna, how have you been; how are the kids?" You develop relationships; some of these farmers I get food from, I know their whole family. The place I get beef, I know most the people that work there and I go to their events. I take the kids to the farms so they can see the farming methods and where their food comes from. It really just becomes part of the adventure. Those become outings for us, instead of going someplace expensive.

We've really cut back on going to the movies. Instead of going and spending $70 for a movie, we'll put it toward really good food, go home have a BBQ on the patio, invite some friends over and have a really good time. We've set up our lifestyle a bit differently now, enjoying family time and less of the external kinds of things in life. It gives us much more enjoyment than the other stuff ever did.

As I've gotten more knowledgeable, I've become more of an activist, mostly online. I connect a lot with moms online and in groups like Moms Across America, because mothers make most of the food decisions in the household, not all cases, but generally that's the case. It was me that started digging for the answers, and it's me that say's okay the milk's gone. We are social creatures and having that fellowship is important. We need that network of people. If you have mom guilt, because you used to feed your kids fruit loops or whatever, you have a whole group of moms to help you navigate that and find the answers you need.

At first I was hesitant, because I never saw myself as an activist, but I figured out that this is how this movement works. We are advocating for our children. It is me sitting down, talking to other moms and other women for the most part. Sharing of information drives thought processes and then change happens. Those connections drive the movement. It's probably not going to change from the government level.

There's too much influence there and too much money being made. It's only going to change at the grass roots level. Look at Women's Suffrage, for example, women didn't get the right to vote because Congress said women should have the right to vote. It's because two women said we should have the right to vote, and we're going to do everything we can to make that happen. They rallied more women, fought hard for it and it was all at a grass root level, and we got the right to vote. Given the powers that be, that would have never happened if women wouldn't have stood up and said, 'This is what's right, and this is what is going to happen!' That's really what it's going to take for this tide to turn. It's going to take that ground swell and grass root movement to say 'no, absolutely not, I don't care what they say or what they do, I won't bow down to it and I won't feed it to my kids!'

I know when I cut genetically modified food from my family's diet, we got better. And when I cut out gluten, we got better. That's all the evidence I need. I don't need a test. I don't need a doctor to confirm it. I know when I cut red dye out of my son's diet, he stopped bouncing off the walls. A mother knows. You have to experience it for yourself, and you can't give up. I tell people, this won't be a two or three-week thing. It's not a pill you can take. You can't cut out gluten and all of your problems are solved. You can't cut out GMOs and all of your problems are solved. It's going to take a commitment.

Teach What You Know

I've taught classes on organic gardening and fertilizer and how to brew your own compost tea. I also teach people how to do a medicine cabinet makeover and what I call "living with" classes, where I teach them how to live without processed foods and live with high nutrient dense foods.

I was approached by a woman at one of my classes recently. She said to me, "So, you say your kids don't eat at McDonalds anymore; how did you get your kids to stop eating it?" I said, "Yes that's right. We don't eat fast food anymore … in fact, my kids think it's gross." I hesitated for a moment, because normally, I would have a soft answer like, "You have to talk to your kids about it." But I've found that talking doesn't work when there's such a strong craving for it. I looked at her and said, "Maybe I'm a mean mom, but I figure I'm driving the car and it's my wallet, and I'm not going to feed them something that is going to make them sick. So, I just stopped going. There was a little bit of protest at first. I just explained the reasons why. They were young and didn't fully understand it. They just knew Mom was not going to McDonalds. Now we don't do any fast food and we don't miss it at all."

The key is, you have to be the CEO of your household because you're the big decision maker. If the decision is, this is not good for my kids, then it doesn't come into the house. Pepsi is a great example. My whole family was addicted to Pepsi. It's not good for us. I stopped buying it.

When we decided to go dairy free for Liam, I just stopped buying milk. People would say to me, where you get your calcium. Of course there's calcium in spinach and other leafy greens, almonds, sesame seeds and the calcium in these foods is more absorbable too. We refer to that as bioavailability.

Calcium comes from grass. Cows that are providing dairy milk aren't eating grass. The calcium in the milk is lab created, and we know that's not the right formulation for the body. It might work invitro, but it doesn't work in the body the same way.

Bag the Lunch?

Thinking back, I had on my red cape with a giant "N" on my shirt for nutrition. I was going to change the world. I was going to tell everybody about GMOs and sugar. Their eyes were going to be opened, and everything was going to be great. There were two efforts that I undertook; school lunch was at the top of my list. I sat down with the principal of my kid's elementary school. That was an eye opener for me. I realized that she had very little control. I encouraged her to discontinue snack carts and consider less sugar for parties and such. She said she has parents who get mad if they can't bring cupcakes for their kid's birthday. Her hands were pretty much tied.

I then went to the food service director at the school; I had another individual with me. We were going to start a program, a campaign, to educate people; then we were going to take it to the school board. The director told me he has a $1.41 to spend on each meal that's it. How do you do that? They also have to provide free breakfast for the kids in the morning. From his perspective, he's hog-tied by the rules that govern him in the government food program.

There are two places where schools have to change. We have to change the federal level in terms of what we value, and we should put more value in nutrients over calories and allow schools to be a little creative and maybe have a little more money to spend, and we've got to educate the parents. Even if we manage to change the schools, the parents are blind to it. They don't know why the food isn't good for their kids. They don't know why vitamin A, vitamin D and C are better for them than calories and carbohydrates. There will be a bunch of uproar and backlash because there will be parents that say, "well my kids really like pizza and chicken nuggets." We got to get through all that. It's a lot of effort and a big undertaking.

When we started out, I told my kids I'm not paying for school lunch anymore. "We're going to pack lunches from now on." We went through a laundry list of things they liked and didn't like. My youngest likes salami, so I buy uncured salami with no nitrates. He takes trail mix with raisins and nuts; he likes that. If he wants a treat I'll make it myself using clean ingredients, like coconut flour and stuff like that. If I send him a drink, besides water, I make sure I get him organic juice boxes. There are some good ones out there and the pricing, I think, is competitive; mostly he drinks water. We have a non-traditional way of eating in my household. Sometimes it can be a struggle but we've found ways to manage it. I buy two loaves of gluten free bread a month. When they're gone, they're gone, that's it. It's expensive and they don't need it.

Check out the Paleo recipes. There's a ton of them out there; you don't have to have food allergies or be gluten free to enjoy the benefits of it. They have a huge variety of amazing, grain free, dairy free recipes. You can find cookie recipes made with almond butter and sweetened with coconut sugar. Say they need a treat for a birthday party that you feel good about with clean ingredients; the kids don't know the difference.

You Don't Know, What You Don't Know

There are certain books that I suggest everyone read and movies they should watch. Educating yourself is an important step ... watch movies like, *Genetic Roulette, Food Inc., The Future of Food, King Corn, Forks Over Knives, Food Matters, Fed Up, Bought and Doctored.* They are all great documentary films that will give you the background and context you need to solidify the why.

• •

Note: Often these movies are made available online to watch for free. You can *Google* the name of the movie, followed by the words "watch for free." Be sure that you are watching from a trusted site. *Netflix* carries many of these titles as well.

. . . .

Armed with knowledge, we are much more effective and we can stay much more on course. Keep learning, that's the real secret to success here. Empowering yourself with the truth here is absolutely essential.

Communication is another important factor when you make changes in your child's diet. Let their teachers know; let the cafeteria people know, and let family and friends know. Make sure they know what you are doing so they can support your efforts. It comes down to what's best for your kid. You're in charge and you have the ultimate say in the matter. You get to say, no, that's not for my kid. Often I feel like the government and the schools are dictating everything, saying we're the experts. This is disempowering people and making them fearful of change or making determinations and acting outside of the accepted norm. "My doctor is going to yell at me because I'm not feeding my child milk," for example. We have to empower ourselves and take our own responsibility and teach our children in this way as well. In doing so, we can stand up taller with that really big accomplishment.

I know that the changes that I made with my kids will affect their lives forever in a positive manner. I know that because I was strong, I educated myself and stood up for them. Because I did that, they don't have health issues and they are going to live longer, healthier lives. I'm the mom - that's my job and I feel like we've given that up, handed it over to people that don't even know our name and don't know anything about us. Then they force us into a one size fits all food system and one size fits all medical system. We are all different.

People ask me, "Why do you spend so much money on food"? I answer, "Because I'm not spending it at the doctors." I have a choice to make; do I spend it on doctors or do I spend it on really good food? "Well can't you just give your kids McDonalds once in while?" "No, I can't, because I know the damage that it does, and I'm not willing to do that to them anymore!" If I have to spend an extra hour preparing food for the day, then so be it, because their health is so much more important than a bag of crap from McDonalds.

Go, Go, Go

The real key here is preparation; if your kid is going to a party then you make something for them to take, that works for them and that keeps them out of trouble, if you will. When we go to family functions, I basically just bring a whole meal for my family because I have no idea what's going to be there. I prepare a main dish, a vegetable and a dessert, something sweet. We eat our food and they eat theirs. It's really not a big deal. When we go on vacation or on road trips we take a cooler and snacks. I always take food for the kids when we go on outings. It's essential to go prepared. You never know what's going to happen. We also go shopping when we get to our out of town destination. I take my nutria-bullet with me because I have a smoothie every morning. I always do my homework ahead of time to see where I can shop or if there are any local clean-food options in the area.

I know that I'm doing something right because I've lost 70 plus pounds and I'm training to run a marathon. That would have never happened before. My family is so much healthier now so it's all worth it.

Diana

Diana Reeves is a powerful example of what one strong, courageous woman can accomplish. She's a powerhouse in the *cleanfood* movement, who deserves a world of gratitude and appreciation for her hard work and commitment to the cause.

The Motivation

We lost our first child to cancer when he was just two years old; he was diagnosed with a tumor in his brain. This was many years ago in 1987. The tumor was inoperable at the time with modern surgical techniques. It was a deep-seated tumor in his brain. The doctors said he was born with it. I couldn't understand how a baby could be born with cancer in his brain. That was something I really struggled with. I asked myself many, many times, "what did I do, what did I do?" At the time, I didn't have an answer.

We had a two year battle and he went through every treatment under the sun. We went to the Mayo Clinic and did everything humanly possible, but we lost him. He wasn't quite five; he was still four and a half when we lost him. He is my special angel; he sits on my shoulder and he helps me do what I do.

It was very early in my first trimester of my pregnancy, I had just found out I was pregnant and I was in the yard with my husband, and there were weeds. Everyone sprayed Roundup in those days, and I even read the bottle very carefully. It said non-toxic to humans and it said biodegradable, because it said that back then. I said, to myself, 'if it's safe then okay, why not?' This was about a week after I had a positive pregnancy test, and while I was spraying the nozzle on the bottle exploded and the Roundup went all over my hands. I just stood there staring at them and saying to myself, "it better be right, because if anything happens to this child, I'm going to know why," and I tucked that away, because I never had cause to dig it out. It never came up during my thought process around what did I do, what did do, because the bottle said non-toxic and biodegradable.

Then last summer, I was fortunate enough to meet two well-known scientists, one of them was actually on the Séralini study team. I asked him what type of cancer did they find in the group of rats in the Séralini study that were fed environmental levels of glyphosate/Roundup in their drinking water. He told me it was only one type of cancer, rhabdomyosarcoma and that's what my son had. My son's cancer was very, very rare.

Rhabdomyosarcoma is cancer of the connective tissue and there's hardly any connective tissue in the brain, so doctors looked for a primary sight elsewhere in his body and there was none. They said what he had was so rare there were only 37 other diagnosed cases in the history of modern medicine.

Both of the scientists I met told me, "don't beat yourself up, there could be other factors, one never knows how certain chemicals come together and what the specific cause of something like this might be."

I do know more now. I have a genetic defect in my body, called the MTHFR mutation. I got my tests results back a couple months ago. This mutation inhibits the body's ability to detox itself.

In my heart I know when you expose an embryo, during critical stages of development to a carcinogen, it becomes a very real problem. I do believe, I honestly and truly believe this is what caused my son to develop a tumor in his brain. Having found this out much later, I had already started my battle on the GMO road. It just gives me strength and drives me harder to force this broken system that we have to change to protect children, so no one else goes through this. These are very, very real toxins with real risks.

I have since had three children; my oldest was born prior to losing my son. We actually found out I was pregnant with him, and a week later we found my son's brain tumor. The doctors said they didn't know why it happened. You always wonder if there was some kind of genetic breakdown and if it might happen again, so I went through all of these extra layers of ultrasounds with my second son. When he was 15 months old, I had a CAT Scan done to make sure there was nothing wrong with his brain and that there were no tumors in there. It can make you a little bit crazy having children after that. I am so glad we did. My oldest is going to be 28 this month. I've also got two girls. My middle daughter is turning 26 in November and my youngest is 21. She's going to be a senior in college.

Four out of five members of my family have health problems. We have an autoimmune disease. My son is the only one so far that doesn't. We all have celiac and all of us girls have Hashimoto's Autoimmune Disease and Hypothyroidism.

We've identified the triggers, so we're able to live in a healthy state. We avoid gluten because it triggers celiac disease. It also triggers the Hashimoto's Autoimmune Disease. We avoid dairy as well; it also triggers the Hashimoto's. I've confirmed that with blood tests, checking antibodies before and after exposure to dairy. We avoid soy. There's a number of reasons to avoid soy, most of it is genetically engineered. It also has a depressant effect on the thyroid, so that's not a good thing for us. We avoid gluten, dairy, soy and GMOs. Personally, I had to go carefully through the elimination diet (Read more about the elimination diet in Chapter 8—"GMO Detoxification") to figure out why I had chronic fatigue for over a year even though my diet was clean.

I wasn't eating 100 percent organic, but I was avoiding all GMO foods. I still felt like I couldn't get out of the chair during the day. I had horrible fatigue. One of my friends said, "check your vitamins; see if there are GMOs in your vitamins." I poo-pooed it, saying "I couldn't possibly be that sensitive, that's ridiculous." I finally called the companies that I was buying vitamins from, and it turns out that two of my vitamins were sourced with genetically modified ingredients. One of them had traces of GMO soy and I switched them out with something equivalent from companies that do not use genetically engineered corn or soy. Gradually, within a 3-week period my chronic fatigue lifted. I got my energy level back and life is good again.

I can't help but wonder how many people out there aren't feeling well and how many of them would feel better if they were able to do what I did, which is one of the reasons we need to know what we're eating. It's not a matter of "right to know." The "Right to Know" message is dead. It is a very weak message. If you listen to what Albert Einstein said, the definition of insanity is doing the same thing over and over again and expecting a different result. There have been four ballot measures that have used the 'Right to Know' message. That message is very easily countered by carefully crafted industry propaganda.

When you tell someone they have a right to know, then industry comes along and says it will cost you though. It's going to cost you $500 extra a year for food. They say maybe it's not that important and they back off. Industry is very, very smart. In developing these arguments they know how to manipulate. But when you tell people they *need to know* what they're eating, because they truly do and they can either pay the grocer or pay the doctor and the pharmacist. Then they do stop and think and they do listen, and they understand the importance of label because, we truly do need to know what we're eating. With a label we have the ability to trace and hold accountable and hold liable; without a label there is no traceability, so there's no accountability, and therefore, no liability and that's the way the agrochemical industry likes it. So this is a matter of needing to know what we are eating.

Something's Changed

In the 1990s, I woke up to GMOs, surprisingly, in a mainstream newspaper that was bragging about the wonderful things they were doing to our food and I remember sitting there thinking, they're engineering these foods so they can be sprayed with herbicide, this is a bad idea. This was something I had to keep on my radar because, in my mind, it would create health risks in the general population and the fact that it wasn't labeled; it was just showing up in the food supply, made me think "we need to keep an eye on trends with illnesses."

I sent an email to everyone I knew. The subject line said "Yes, you're eating it and no it hasn't been proven safe." I went on a little diatribe to raise awareness. Nobody responded to my email, not one person. Generally, people tend to think it's too inconvenient, or they're not sick yet, so they don't care.

You have to wonder, if 30 percent of the population have this MFTHR genetic mutation, that I have, and at least one of my children also has, if we're the ones getting sick. Someone needs to look into that.

Diana illustrates the importance of daily probiotics to help repair digestive issues and maintain gut health.

You need to know that even products that are "Non-GMO Project Verified" can still be sprayed with Roundup prior to harvest, as you read in Chapter 3—"Principles of Poison." I'm not saying don't buy those products, just be sure you do your homework to confirm that glyphosate is not being sprayed on the Non-GMO products you choose to purchase and feed your children. If there is a product that I really want, I will email or call the company to ask questions about their ingredients, processes and even what they feed their farm animals. Often they are happy to talk with me. If they aren't that's a big red flag. Diana told me more about her experiences:

I started cleaning out the family diet of GMOs about 7-8 years ago, after I discovered that I had celiac. We eat as organically, as possible and avoid traces of gluten, dairy and soy to manage my symptoms. Eating out in restaurants is something I'm just unable to do. I can't get trust someone else with my life and my health. I'm so sensitive to GMOs that I bought organic food for my puppy with trace amounts of barley, which still has gluten; then I even served it with plastic gloves and then still got sick.

. . . .

Note: this goes to show you that people respond differently to various things. Your child might be sensitive to foods that you may not even notice they are having difficulty with. Allergy testing is a very important tool, even if you suspect nothing is wrong.

. . . .

GMO FREE USA

In 2011 and 2012, I was part of a team in Connecticut, working to pass legislation for mandatory labeling of genetically engineered foods. The bill, in 2012, looked like it was going to pass. There was wide-spread bi-partisan support, and it was actually eviscerated at the last moment by the governor.

There was speculation as to what happened behind the scenes. We never found out, but it was speculated that it was a direct threat from Monsanto if legislation passed, because they did threaten to sue the State of Vermont. Perhaps it was trickle-down effect from the threat in Vermont. Our legislators weren't able to do their jobs because of corporate bullying.

I was one of over a million people that signed a petition to the FDA, telling them we needed mandatory GMO labeling. They put it in the trash. I said, "there has to be a better way," and so I woke up energized and decided we need to take back control of our food with a big boycott of a big food company and force them to change. The power is in the hands of the people. If we don't buy it, then they can't sell it and they'll stop making it.

I set off to find 5000 people, so I had enough voices to make them heard and make some noise and we started the boycott of Kellogg's; we'll stick with it until they remove GMO ingredients from their products. GMO FREE USA was born of necessity.

Note: Diana's story continues in Chapter 10—"The GMO-Free Movement,"—GMO-Free Unsung Heroes.

Amanyah

I started working on my health coaching certifications in 2010 and got initiated with something called the "90-Day Renewal Program," where they go deeply into the physiological functions and how your emotions and even your spirit, your daily activity, what you eat and the pollutants in the environment, and how it's all tied together. It's was really great; and I got a lot of insight.

I did the David Wolfe, raw certification course that was really comprehensive on raw food and plants in their inherent form before they're changed. There's so many, typically, more nutrients in raw food. Some foods you have to heat to a certain temperature to activate certain nutrients or deactivate natural toxicity that might be in the plant or to bring out more nutritional components. I learned a lot about those aspects of food. It was really wonderful.

I did the Body Mind Nutrition certification, which was two really comprehensive certifications that also went really deep into the physiological aspects, including how to program your body, how it works and what it requires in all physiological aspects. When you take all of these components under the holistic paradigm, you get results that count. I also did a sports nutrition program and studied the fitness models and got a cleansing certification, so I could teach others the ideal way to detox their body. All this education is part of my daily life and my family's as well.

When I work with clients we talk about the toxicity in foods, and we address those right away, so those foods (including GMOs) aren't part of the equation for too long. You can't get results if you don't know what you're eating and if you don't know what you're eating, you are probably eating GMOs, so we address that pretty quickly and get that out of the way.

I went through six certification programs and I'm still active with the colleges. Oh' and I did the Master Herbology course when I was 16, so

I've been at it a long time. My family has been organic since I was 15. I grew up researching anything and everything that we put on and inside our bodies. With that experience in conjunction with the education that I took, there's a lot to pull from.

Give the Body What It Needs

There are a lot of key components that need to be considered to properly execute a successful detox: you could turn up everything in the body, and then potentially can't eliminate it. Mineral replacement and nutrient dense foods play a key role. The very initial steps of my program, include certain components like adding Pink Himalayan Salt to your drinking water. It lowers the surface tension and activates dormant enzyme potential.

When we start giving the body what it needs, things like drinking more water, drinking good water, putting healthy salt on your food, all of it becomes a really comprehensive approach that initiates detoxification right there. Then you go GMO-Free and the body starts to get at what's been going on.

I notice people come to me and they're sort of sedated when they've been so subjected to toxicity and they come to a point where they are looking to get healthier. Often they are in a space where they are so inundated by it all that they are kind of in a fog and their attention span isn't so strong. It's very commendable when they are seeking help. People are really busy and distracted, so I really try to hone in with people so they become associated with the importance of going GMO-Free and organic where you can. It can get out of proportion with all of the media promoting these toxic foods. People tend to get confused because it's on TV and they can justify it.

At first, it's really about helping people get out of that fog and get them inspired to shift everything around. It's the initial steps that usually get it all going. It's really a beautiful thing. I see a lot of digestive issues in clients too. It's a typical problem, because most people haven't been providing the proper daily environment for their gut. Probiotics and balancing the gut bacteria is absolutely part of the equation that I address in the initial steps.

Mother of Inspiration

The most pivotal change I've ever seen was in my own mother. We'd always had a healthier approach to life. We didn't eat white bread, for example. We didn't realize that the eight-grain bread we were buying had high fructose corn syrup. Our approach was better than average, but we didn't realize the food had changed.

My mom, after getting married and having two more children, started accumulating all this weight. She didn't know what the deal was because it was never like that before. Initially, she took the Master Herbalist course; the same one I took. I followed in her footsteps there. They talk about your physiology and how you're made to function, how processed food and chemicals affect the body and basically it sludges everything up. Being the kind of person that she was, she believed we're responsible for what we know, and she took the initiative to change over the household to organic, almost immediately. She lost in excess of 200 pounds with no particular diet, except going from non-organic to organic -that's it. She just got rid of the chemicals and all the junk. All of that weight just came off effortlessly, in maybe, three years total, for the whole 200 pounds, but some pretty significant weight just started dropping off that first year, year and a half. It was a consistent momentum.

We've seen the same thing happen in other people too. People that get off the processed food and start eating a cleaner diet, they lose 160 lbs for example, and it just comes off with no problem. I've seen in many people that I've had a close association with. There are so many stories like that because the body says, "Hey, now I can function and the sludge is gone," and you're not putting that in continually. When you're actually putting real nutrition in the body, the body knows how to utilize it.

My mom also had Type 2 diabetes and that went away, along with carpel tunnel in her wrist which was calcification. It protruded about a ½ inch off her wrist and that too went away. With people in general who lose a lot of weight, because the toxicity isn't being fed anymore, they become a lot more clear and in tune with their own spirit and who they are, as opposed to being oblivious.

I was pretty young when all of that was initiated, but I can remember at 14 years old just feeling yucky. I would eat canned food or whatever we had at the moment. But then when we were eating organic, I didn't feel bad anymore. After having been really consistently clean, I remember trying to drink Nestle Cocoa and it made me feel horrible. I rarely strayed, because I was devoutly organic, but when I did, the toxicity was very pronounced. It was something I was desensitized to before switching to a clean diet. It was a good experience because I could really tell the difference.

Find the Balance

If you eat a lot of packaged food, then a good place to start is to change them over for organic ones. From there, you will take the bar higher and higher. I suggest you just start adding in new things. For example, if you eat cookies or mayonnaise or whatever, change those over to the organic versions. They will likely be available in the nutrition section of your local store. Your family will start feeling considerably better, just from doing that. Some stores disperse their organics among the other food items. I would recommend that you add a variety of organic fruits, vegetables, and even superfoods to keep stepping up your diet and improving your approach.

Something you should note, you're supposed to be healthy, so what is healthy should be appealing to you, but when a person is accustomed to eating synthetic food and junk food, sensitivity diminishes and you become desensitized, and that's why you're craving that food in the first place.

From what I understand, it takes two weeks for the palate to change. If you're accustomed to eating something, you're always looking for that, but if you start eating differently, in about two weeks your body will start craving what you're eating, rather than what you were eating before. Ultimately, if you're desensitized and you start eating healthy, you're going to become sensitive again and you'll actually crave foods that are good for you. The palate absolutely does change. It's not too hard. You just have to get the process started and be confident in knowing that you're not going to be craving the same foods you did before, and right now you're being desensitized to your food, and being desensitized to it is not in your benefit.

The Organic Compass

If it's organic it doesn't have GMOs in it. All of the junk, the herbicides and pesticides, don't go in there. We went straight to organic, so GMOs were never an issue and we just bypassed all that. I was taught that if it wasn't organic than we just expect that it contains all that. Organic food is really the purest form of food; it's what we were given in the beginning. It's what our grandparents ate.

Our food chain has absolutely changed, not just the GMOs, although it's the most significant one. With all the chemical pesticides and herbicides, just being GMO-Free isn't really enough, because all of the criteria isn't there like if it was organic which doesn't have any of that. Obviously, GMO-Free is a better choice, if that's all you can do, then you can aim to get cleaner and cleaner over time. As you know better, you can do better. That's how the process works.

I don't shop in most aisles of the store. I shop at a couple different stores. I love nutrition stores; they are one of my favorite places in the world, but generally, I shop at Fred Meyer. They have a nutrition section where I can find organics. Safeway has organic produce and then other options mixed in through the rest of the store. I also read labels. I want to know where the food is coming from.

We eat more of a whole foods diet, with fresh fruits and vegetables, with certain base grains and what have you. The boxed foods on the shelves are just riddled with chemicals and additives. They don't have the nutrients that your body needs to function. I buy a lot of fresh foods, living foods. Like I said, if you buy a lot of boxed foods, begin to switch over to the organic options. People say, just stick to the outer regions of the store, but there's more to it than that because there's plenty of GMO foods to be found in those outer isles as well. Know what you're getting and stick with organic, whenever possible. As far as making it affordable, co-ops are wonderful; farmers' markets really help and then we grow some of our own food to fill in the gaps.

I always encourage people to grow some of their own food, don't be defeated, it's really easy to do. Do what you can do and it really pays off. Obviously it's also important to consider your water source. It might be good to filter it. It really comes down to this: whatever is the healthiest choice use that one.

What's the Secret?

There's nothing that can't be overcome: you will learn to be resourceful. It's a unique lifestyle, but it shouldn't be. We are not radical for wanting to eat clean food. We are honoring what we know to be good. What they are doing to change the food; now that is radical.

Be prepared: if you anticipate going somewhere, take what you need. Prepare your kids and teach them the ingenuity to survive. Take the initiative and the responsibility to teach your children how to care for themselves. It's very empowering, and you will find amazing support for this lifestyle.

Engage in your purpose and contribute to the whole: for the benefit of yourself and your children, take responsibility for what you know; don't compromise and you will make healthier choices and so will they.

Everyone you care for can only be cared for in proportion to how you take care of yourself: you will become more effective and better able to function in your role. The foundation will be built and will take on the momentum you need, as you move forward.

Maureen

"Vermont was Green, before it was cool to be Green." I love that bumper sticker! It's true because it never has been large scale. It's always been about small family farms. Vermont was part of the food movement here before, I think, it hit most other places and the term "Localvore," I believe was coined here.

Of course, there's plenty of people that still eat at McDonalds and think the whole GMO conversation is crazy. When I first started looking at organics it was probably 2007, it's when I started clueing into environmental risks and the big picture. When I started to look there were already plenty of people here already doing it. I was quickly surrounded by people who get it, and I always had friends that were organic farmers and people that do their own organic gardens; that's how they feed their kids. It's been very much a big part of the culture of how I've raised my kids, so I've never had to deal with the feeling of having to be alone with it.

Vermont was the first state to enact a labeling law and the fact that they have Bernie Sanders—he has certainly stood up to Wall Street politics, even calling Monsanto out for its toxic practices. He speaks up for citizen's rights and believes that parents should have a right to know what they're feeding their children and since that topic is the one that is nearest and dearest to my heart, he has earned my vote.

Organic foods are readily abundant around here, and so I've found it is really different for me and my clients than for other coaches in areas where options aren't so readily available. It was really eye opening to me that other places weren't like Vermont, although the industry is booming.

The "Ripple Effect"

Author confession: I'm a little envious of Maureen in the sense that she also studied at the Institute for Integrative Nutrition (IIN), except she graduated three years before me in 2009, attending the program live in New York. As the largest, nutrition school in the world, the IIN network of health coaches spans the entire globe. We share a mission to change the world through what's known as the "ripple effect," using a holistic approach and nutrient dense food combined with the principles of common sense to empower you to heal yourself. All you have to do is begin where you are to re-establish your relationship with food. What could be better than that? Self-healing with real nutrition is about giving the body what it needs in order to facilitate health. That is the over-all defining concept that allows us to uproot the source of our dis-ease. Maureen told me about her experience:

When I was at IIN in 2009, I was part of a student group that was working really hard to bring GMO awareness to the student body. Ingrid Alvared started it. She's really a dynamo on this topic. It's something she's really passionate about. We made up T-Shirts and we're stationed at all the doors passing out information. This was when they were live in New York.

I remember we had to do it all on our own time, so it was something we had to organize and we held meetings after classes. We found ourselves having to explain what GMOs were to the other health coaches. It wasn't well known back then, and it really wasn't something that was covered in the curriculum. Today, of course, things have changed some.

One Sick Pup

I have three boys, my oldest is 19, then 17, and the youngest is 16. With regard to health and nutrition, I was very mainstream. I did what I knew.

I remember, my dog got really sick. I took her to the vet and they put her on medications, but her situation kept getting worse. She started having a problem with her paw. They did surgery and stitched it up but then when they took the stitches out it hadn't healed at all. Not a single collection of cells had reattached to each other. It still looked just like the moment they cut her open. They wanted to treat her paw, and she started to move and I put my hand on her to hold her still. I was barely using any pressure on her, but when I slid my hand away, I could see that not only did all of her hair, but her skin came off in the shape of my handprint. It was absolutely horrifying. I didn't understand what was going on. I was barely holding her! The vet told me she didn't have any connective tissue left. That's why she wasn't healing. He told me I had to put her down. I told him I needed time to go home and talk to my husband; I couldn't just put her down like this, so I took her home.

A friend suggested I take her to a holistic vet, two hours away and I took her in. They pulled her off all of her medications and the food she was on. They gave me a little cookbook, and I made all of her food, organic whole foods. Not even my kids were eating organic food yet, but the vet insisted it be organic, so I did. They also gave me some herbs and did some acupuncture and took some labs and they sent us home for the weekend.

The doctor was shocked when I told him that she was doing better than she had in two years. She was actually running and playing in the yard with our kids over the weekend, and she hadn't done that in years. Her paw was healing, and her back started scabbing over. He told me that he didn't think she would still be alive after seeing her labs. She had no thyroid function left and pretty much everything that could be wrong with a dog was wrong with her. She was literally on the brink of death.

We put her on a wholefood, organic diet and her life just turned around. She was 11 when that happened, and she lived another year and a half after that, but her quality of life was much better than the previous year and a half.

A Bad Batch?

I started looking at the food. That was about the same time my son needed to be hospitalized for what looked like measles, and we were quarantined after an MMR [measles, mumps, rubella] vaccine. They were concerned that he had gotten a bad batch of the vaccine. They wouldn't allow him to be hospitalized. He was actually seen in the parking lot, because they didn't want him to contaminate the pediatric ward. He was very, very sick and he had to have blood draws every few days at the health department, because they wouldn't see him in the pediatrician's office. The tests kept coming back inconclusive for measles. There was some portion of the blood that looked like measles, but it wasn't a direct match.

By day 10, he had a fever of 105 and was slipping in and out of consciousness. I called the pediatrician and said, "I think we're losing my son, we have to do something." This great guy was filling in, and thankfully, he admitted him to the hospital. When we were trying to figure out what it was, I asked the doctors if the vaccine was the problem, because I had overheard the doctors before saying something about the vaccine being bad. They were like "No, no, no…" They just did not want to have that conversation.

The nurses were talking about it being Kawasaki disease, but there wasn't a test that they could run for it. I asked them what it was. They said some doctors say that it's impossible, but it seems to go along with kids that have been exposed to carpet cleaners, and he could have some sort of chemical sensitivity.

When I was dealing with my son's health issues and all those unanswered questions, I felt like I needed to go forward on the assumption that he was chemically sensitive. I got rid of all our traditional cleaning products and replaced them with Seventh Generation, which is a local Vermont company. I was buying them from a health food store and started noticing all the different foods there. It really began a process for us.

Then my second son was born and he also had a bad MMR reaction. He would react violently to any dairy, whatsoever, after he got that shot. He had no reaction at all before the shot. Afterwards, he had open bleeding wounds. It was bad.

When I started looking for non-dairy things, I had friends that were part of an organic buy-in coop, and I started to buy a lot of food from them. That was in 1999. My third son was born in 2000. By the time I got pregnant with him I knew so much more. It happens that way you start looking, and you just keep learning more and more. Right from the beginning, everything in his life was organic. By that time, his brothers were too, but they didn't start out that way. It was also about trying to avoid the artificial dyes, herbicides and pesticides. The dyes affected my oldest son tremendously. It was a night and day difference for him. I could just see that my kids were really reactive to food and depending on how I fed them we would just see this radically different result. From the start we could see that our third son was a much healthier baby. He never had any issues of any kind. He was just totally healthy, in fact, he only recently had his first medication of his whole life.

The Gut-Brain Imbalance

Around 2007, I had an episode that felt like I had been shot in the head with a gun, I actually put my hands up and expected to see blood. I was in the hospital getting prepped for surgery, and they thought that I had an aneurysm. I was in my gown getting all ready for my operation, they ran the scan, and the doctor came back they didn't find anything, so they sent me home.

I didn't have an aneurism but I still wasn't well. I couldn't walk without assistance. My speech would come and go. There was definitely something seriously wrong. It started a whole long series of seeing different specialists and getting a variety of neurological exams done. Some were over 10 hours long and always coming to the conclusion that there was nothing wrong with me, yet I couldn't speak when I wanted to speak and four different times I was rushed to the hospital after I fell on the ground and I couldn't get up, talk or anything.

Something was wrong with me, but they couldn't figure it out. They were looking in my head, and they weren't seeing anything abnormal, so they would tell me, there was nothing wrong with me. This went on for about three months. We had to hire live-in help to take care of me, and I had three little kids at the time. This went on until I went to see this MD that several friends had recommended to me. She's also an osteopath and hands-on healer. She did an osteopathic treatment on me and instantly I was able to stand on my own for the first time in three months! She ran a bunch of tests to look at my gut function. At the time, I was having trouble speaking, and I thought to myself, I must have done a really bad job at describing my issue because she's looking at my stomach. Why is she doing that? It's my head.

Well of course, she knew exactly what she was doing, and the tests came back that I had a serious gluten sensitivity that I wasn't aware of an auto-immune disease going on, systemic candida, a parasite, a black mold exposure in the house and some other things too. We dealt with the whole thing with additional dietary changes and few lifestyle changes too, I really started noticing the difference when I started dealing with my gut health. I saw that doctor in October and I couldn't walk, by January I was training to run a half-marathon coming up in May. In less than a year I ended up being in the best shape of my life. I was doing wildly better than I was before all this had happened.

Aside from being organic and GMO-Free, it's also about figuring out what is toxic in the body, because everybody is different; then you begin addressing gut imbalances in order to increase the body's immunity. Afterwards you just need to get the nutrients that are needed, back into the body, in order to regenerate health.

It was, I think, two years later that I decided to go to IIN because my doctor was so impressed with my results, she wanted to refer people to me, but I felt uncomfortable without any training. So I decided to go to IIN, so I could start helping people. When I was in school and heard Mark Hyman talk. I think it's his *Ultra Mind Solution*, where he talks about ADHD and Autism Spectrum Disorder. It's an amazing book if you haven't read it. He's talking about our whole society with our kids and all of the chronic issues and autism going on and then with older generations too, we've had incredible increases in Alzheimer's and dementia. He says we're giving it all different labels, but it's all the same thing.

Our brain is tied to our gut and as soon as I heard that I knew that I could probably help my kids more than what I've helped them. Of course, we had huge improvements when we went organic, but they were at this level where I was still seeing them struggle. At that point, I took all three of my kids to our doctor and had them thoroughly tested for any dietary issues or sensitivities and with those results, made the necessary changes. I literally cleaned out the house of any traces of gluten and dairy, any sugar that wasn't raw honey or pure maple syrup and no additive of any kind, no carrageenan, I mean nothing, except for whole foods. I cleaned out everything within the course of a weekend, made those changes, and in less than a week, it was like I had a totally different son. Teachers were just shocked. His performance at school was just like night and day; the difference was amazing!

When it was me making the changes, I didn't feel it was right to make everybody change for me, but when it was our kids, it needed to be our whole family. We weren't going to buy wheat bread just so my husband could eat it. We were all in this together. With all the additional dietary changes, we saw miraculous improvements like socially, academically, wanting to participate. He became engaged, excited and funny, whereas before he just seemed kind of bored. We always knew he was super smart, but now he was really participating and engaged like we've never seen.

· ·

Note: Going GMO-Free or even fully organic isn't a cure-all. Years of damage, gut flora imbalance and decreased immunity have likely taken their toll with several potential sources coming into play; toxic buildup and nutrient deficiencies combined with your average GMO-Roundup based diet are bound to make bodies more vulnerable to all sorts of ailments. Foods with high nutrient density will offer more restorative outcomes in the body, thus allowing other issues to surface and become more straightforward to identify. In this way, you will get to the root causes of your child's suffering, knowing that you have addressed any gut issues through dietary cleanup and of course quality probiotics and/or fermented foods. Regardless of your child's condition, dietary cleanup is the best place to start.

. . . .

Genetic Testing

We took the kids to Mark Hyman's office and had $10,000 worth of genetic testing done on each kid. We had everything under the sun tested. We identified mutations that we all share. There was all kinds of stuff that they identified. We ended up with a two-inch thick book of everything we looked at.

. . . .

Note: Dr. Hyman teaches a class for the Institute for Integrative Nutrition (IIN). He is a medical magician, referred to, somewhat in jest, as the "Resort Doctor," he says, because he's often been the doctor of last resort. Even other doctors have been known to seek him out when they run out of options.

. . . .

Mark Hyman says we can have this genetic predisposition, but what's in your environment determines whether or not that gets turned on or turned off. [And] if we take a look at what GMOs have done to our health …. I didn't have issues, until a little over a decade ago. None of this stuff ever showed itself. I never had any health issues in my life and neither did my family.

Misplaced Trust

At some points, it felt like every time I turned over a stone there was something new; I had several moments of *Oh my God*, I can't believe this is happening, but for me the real revelation, and the thing that was hardest for me mentally to wrap my brain around, was that our government agencies were not looking out for our health. Why even have the FDA or the USDA? Why have the CDC? Why do any of those organizations even exist, if it's not to scrutinize our food and our drugs? That's what I thought they were doing.

We live in a sue happy culture; we joke that McDonalds coffee has to have the warning because it's hot. I feel like the average person thinks, if there was something wrong with it they would have been sued. We all go around thinking, perhaps it's not healthy food, but there's really nothing wrong with it. That was initially my opinion of junk food, not that it was harmful, it just wasn't helpful. It was beyond my wildest imagination, that there could be anything seriously wrong with the food, because I truly thought that the FDA and USDA were doing their jobs. We just have this underlying trust that it would not be on that grocery store shelf if it weren't safe. If it were carcinogenic, an endocrine disrupter or something that causes leaky gut, you would think it would not be allowed on consumer shelves, and I think people really believe that. Most people just cannot fathom that those agencies, that are seemly there to protect us, are not protecting us. So for me, by the time I found out about the GMOs, I had already wrapped my brain around the fact that that was true. It wasn't that big of a stretch, because I was already clued into the money trail behind it. It's all part of the food education.

The best way to get people to change is to let them get a taste of it themselves, and not spend too much of their time circling it around in their head, because it can make you crazy. Getting out there, sharing recipes is the best way to educate people, because that's really the bottom line isn't it? How does the food taste? If you give people delicious food that makes them feel good then it's a win-win situation.

Make it an Upgrade

If you are transitioning to whole foods-based diet, then there are so many sources of amazing recipes out there. You can *Google* foods—I do it all the time. If I go to the farmer's market and see something I haven't seen before. I'll *Google* recipes for it. Making it adventurous and more of a playful thing, keeping variety and tasting new things is essential. It needs to feel like a positive change, like an upgrade. It can't feel like we're suffering and we can't have all this other food. It definitely needs to be about what you can have, not what you can't have.

For any parents wanting to make that shift, the best tip is to find a couple recipes that you know, cook them and share them. Get connected with people you know. Connect with groups online. If you also need to go gluten free, there are a ton of resources online, follow some of the amazing blogs.

I think getting the kids involved, pulling out the cookbooks and getting everyone in the kitchen that is the best recipe for success. The real secret is that you can make almost any recipe organic. If you have older kids you can show them the GMO documentaries. As much as they roll their eyes, I see my kids being appalled at some of the things they see other kids eat. Not that my kids don't sometimes eat what I consider junk food, because they do and they will, but they have a real awareness about the quality of the food. They go to a school where the food awareness and the organic factor is very, very high. It's a very big deal. The kids aren't even supposed to bring junk food in their packs from home. It's part of their culture. Sometimes things come up and I don't get a lot of lead time, so I want to make sure we always have something special on hand for them to take.

At the beginning of the year when you have to fill out all the forms, always include all allergies and health risks. This isn't like a side note to somebody. Every teacher needs to get a copy of the list of flagged kids. I make sure it's on there, no artificial ingredients or colors under any circumstances and it's been totally accepted. This is a medical issue for my child; it doesn't mean he's going to drop dead, it's not that serious, but it is an issue nonetheless.

If you start seeing more than a few food allergies then you are not dealing with food allergies, but leaky gut and digestive disorder needs to be addressed. We learned this from Dr. Hyman at IIN. This is a bigger issue than just allergies. When you are reactive to everything in your environment then you've got a much bigger problem. GMOs have been so tied to food allergies. Why is it, people can't handle their food anymore? When we were growing up this was not an issue. You didn't see kids suffering from allergies, autism or ADHD and rarely from asthma. I had never met anybody with a food allergy in my life.

Every family is going to handle this differently, and not everyone in the family will be motivated to clean up their diet. I didn't always have everyone on board with what I was doing, but I really wanted to give it a shot and just see.

Honestly, to know what I knew and not try to help them, felt like it would be neglect. I can't know that I'm potentially harming their brains and their bodies, impacting their physical health and entire future and not try, at least, to do something about it. Thankfully, almost as soon as we did it, we saw such radical, amazing shifts, making it so easy for the whole family to buy into because it was so obvious.

I understand that it's going to be more difficult for some than others. You could have an access barrier; you could have a price barrier and then even family barriers. The important thing is to do what you can, as much as you can. No matter what the change is, whether you are going organic, GMO-Free, gluten free…no matter what the change is, it may feel daunting and really challenging initially, but whatever you can use to help it feel less so, will be helpful. For example, if you don't already own a crockpot, get one. It saves a lot of time. Then get yourself one or more slow cooker recipe books. Stephanie O'dea has a whole series of wonderful cookbooks based on crock pot recipes. During vacations, crock pots are a huge help. We bring our own food every where, so I always pack it and I love going out to play with the kids all day and by the time we get back, dinner is done. It makes for a really hassle-free vacation. So that's my tip.

The Best Food Ever

I'm so picky about the meat my family eats. Even if it's local, it has to be free-range, grass-fed, because if it just says "Natural" on the package, it is highly probable that it was corn fed. Cows cannot digest corn to begin with. It clogs up their insides and a lot of times gives them cancer.

In Vermont, it's just not an issue to find lots of organic options. I live in a small rural town, and I have to drive 20-30 minutes to do the bulk of my shopping, but we have a plethora of organic and GMO-Free options and even restaurants where I'm able to take my family out to dine.

When I made the big change with our diet, I promised them that it would be better than it was before. I didn't want them to feel cheated, like the quality of the food took a hit, so I really went to extended lengths to make the meals delicious and exciting. I really went way out of my way to keep it creative. I didn't want to make just two great meals a week, and the rest be passable. Every single night I really went above and beyond cooking them delicious home cooked meals that they loved. I said "if we're going to do this, it's going to be done right, and we were eating really, really good food." My kids were like, "Wow mom; this is the best food we've ever eaten!"

If you're going to make these changes with your kids, you want them to buy into it. You have to make it easy for them to buy into it. I made sure that the kids had treats when they came home from school. Usually, they would come home and just graze and I didn't have much to do with it, but I started to really make an effort to make sure they had something good to eat.

It's important to learn how to cook from scratch and buy in bulk, and that is really the key to dietary clean up. There are probably a lot of things in your diet that have no business being there, and your body doesn't even recognize it as food. The synthetic food movement has tricked us all into thinking we are eating real food. Often, It's not even close to a food-like substance with all its chemicals and additives. Growing bodies need real sources of nutrients and minerals. Enriched is not recognizable nutrition to the developing human body. We are getting sicker and sicker as a nation of overweight, chronically-diseased zombies that have lost the ability to think and respond intelligently to the world around us. Why? It's the gut-brain connection and all that it implies.

It comes down to how much nutrition you can buy for your dollar in order to feed it your kids. That's the way we need to start looking at it. It's important to get really basic and forgo the packaged stuff as much as possible because that's not where the nutrition is. Your kids just want to eat good food. They don't care where it comes from, just how it tastes. There's no arguing with the fact that real food tastes better. Combine that with how much better it is for your health, brain function and immune system and you've got yourself a winning combination of wellness factors, even your doctor can't even oppose.

Amber

I met Amber last year through Mom's Across America, along with Jennifer, whom you met earlier. We became fast friends and enjoyed a weekend camping trip with our kids on Camano Island, North of Seattle, Washington. We attended herbal healing classes, during the day, with some of the most skilled and knowledgable herbalists in the Northwest. By moonlight we enjoyed campfires, roasted homemade marshmallows, exchanged recipes and discussed the trials and tribulations of suffering children and sleepless nights. We talked about navigating the contaminated food supply, compared war stories and survival techniques and held organic potlucks with fabulous food. I felt a sense of camaraderie with these mama bears and their children that I hadn't experienced in a long, long time. That summer we formed a valuable lifelong bond.

With that, please meet this spectacular go-getter Amber King; a real GMO-Free activist out there on the frontlines for her kids, your kids and mine.

Our Story

I live in Seattle; I grew up in Southeast Alaska and Western Washington. I've worked in a wide variety of areas, mostly in the fishing and food service industries. I also worked for one of the first vegan meat companies on the West Coast, an organic CSA and I was a food auditor for a major grocery chain. I attended culinary school and worked in fine dining at several hotels and restaurants. I even worked at a winery in Washington, and did food service for Head Start and elderly care. I've worked in the food industry from "root to fruit." I've really run the gamut in things over the years. I did some non-profit management and also worked for public health a while.

After culinary school, I did an internship in Chicago. I realized pretty quickly then that I didn't like the fast-paced lifestyle that came along with fine dining. I needed more family time with my girls, so I came back to Washington and within a week, I found myself on a 1940's wooden scow filleting fish in Bristol Bay.

At the end of the fishing season I ended up getting seriously burned in a camping incident that left me unable to use my hands for quite some time. The skin on my face and hands was so damaged; I couldn't go back to the kitchen or do any cooking for quite a while. To open the oven for eight months was horribly painful. I couldn't have any heat near my skin. I have two girls; they are ten and five now. In 2006, when my first daughter was about a year old, we bought a house. Within a short period I got really sick. Six months later, I was diagnosed with an autoimmune condition called Sarcoidosis.

We'll get back to that in a moment.

A Real Food Connection

I became a vegan when I was 13, and was on my own by 16, and then I began eating little bits of meat again, mostly game meat. This was in Alaska. It was just too difficult to find food that was healthy. You got to think when you live in Alaska, your food comes to you on a barge. From field to warehouse it's about a week on average, then it sits on a barge for another one-to-two weeks before it even gets to the grocery store. That means that it only lasts a day or two in the fridge. So when you live in Alaska your shopping daily for food. Your broccoli has rotted within 2 days of buying it. I was having trouble getting enough protein on a vegan diet, so I went back to eating small bits of meat because meat is plentiful there and, of course, there's lots of seafood.

I learned about GMOs first in culinary school in 1997, so I kind of had an inkling about how that was going to work. I could see the opportunities there for them, so I always had it on my radar.

When I worked in the wineries I was in the hot fields, in grape fields and the apple orchards, I learned a lot about the agriculture business and how it works. It was a bad year for apples that year, and so they let everything fall to the ground and rot because they couldn't make enough profit on it. That's when I learned that all of the apple juice was coming from China.

I've always had my hands in the food industry, so like I said the GMOs were on my radar, but it wasn't until I got sick that I really had to clamp down on the toxins in my body. Like I said, I got an autoimmune condition called Sarcoidosis. It's a multi-symptom granulose disorder. You can compare it to tuberculosis of the body. You can get ten people in a room with it and they'll all have different stories. They'll be similar, but not the same.

I thought I was pretty healthy. I bought natural cleaners and I was about 50 percent organic, I would say. I was pregnant the year before that, and I wanted to make sure I was eating right so I did lots and lots of research and did the best I could.

Back then the trends weren't like they are now. They're really catching on. Stores didn't carry a lot of organics and in Alaska, where I lived, we had one tiny health food store in town. They had a deli and I ate lunch there as often as I could afford to.

When I was pregnant I cleaned out my house and cabinets of anything with questionable ingredients. I learned about natural birth versus hospital birth. I also learned that I had to advocate for my health in a whole different manner.

We don't eat beef or pork, only fish and organic poultry. My 10-year old has gone vegetarian in the last six months. Trying to find GMO-Free and soy-free meat alternatives is really, really difficult. It's the same thing with people trying to go gluten free, GMO-Free, organic options are almost non-existent. I don't see that as a choice because I believe the gluten intolerances are being caused by the GMOs.

Food has to be the top priority in the budget. Unfortunately, many people haven't been taught the importance of what they eat and they put food at the bottom. I can't go to work if I'm sick or my kids are sick; if they're sick they don't go to school. I'm paying for daycare that I'm not using and it all goes down from there. I try to inspire others to make food a priority because we really need to. It can be overwhelming when you start talking about making all these different changes. Often, we don't start focusing on it until we really need to, until somebody gets sick and we're forced to pay attention.

Early Learning Curve

When my second daughter was born her respiratory system didn't transition well from womb to world. She had a lot of trouble breathing at birth, so we were medevacked to Anchorage, where she spent two weeks in the NICU. They said she had something called PPHN, which is Pulmonary Hypertension of a Newborn. I think although they were helpful, it was a result of some of those interventions that she's very sensitive to things. Her skin is really sensitive. She gets a rash around her mouth if she eats GMOs—"GMO mouth," which tells me it's a toxic reaction to the chemicals.

My older daughter gets severe anxiety; I can always tell if she's been eating something she's not supposed to or she's found sugar, candy or red food dye somewhere. I can spot it a mile away. It can be hard to tell your kids no. You want them to have meaningful experiences, for example, try making an organic gingerbread house, it's going to cost you $900 and two weeks of research.

The more information you have to access the easier it is to make those decisions. Starting young and giving them a good foundation is key. This is how we're going to make things different. You can influence your children to make better choices. They are bombarding our children with their marketing and propaganda, both on TV and in the school room. These big corporations have influenced science and they've really influenced higher education, and now they're going after early education and getting to them young. They've been investing in our kids to bring them to the dark side for a long time. As parents, we're really outspent and outnumbered.

We need to give them opportunities to create meaningful connections with their food, teach them about how their bodies work and about science and make it fun. It's up to us to teach them how to feed themselves the kind of food that will nourish themselves, so they can live healthy lives. Children need to learn how to cook and with the demise of the middle class, families don't have the time to spend with the kids to teach them that.

My girls go to grocery store with me and they know what to look for. If it doesn't have a USDA certified organic label and they can't read the ingredients, they know it isn't coming in the cart. They need to know what it all means. Teach them about worm bin composting. Our school, back in Alaska started a composting project. We got a giant school garden going and the older children would harvest the crops and sell them at fundraisers to go on week-long camping adventures. The kindergarteners plant potatoes in the Spring and when they came back to school in the Fall as first graders, they would harvest. It really takes parents getting involved and becoming a force in the school.

The Navigational Pull

Amber offers some helpful insights about how to make your transition easier:

- **Connect with your neighbors, friends and family**: however you can make it happen. Perhaps you can have a potluck at your house. Offer to go in on food orders from local organic farmers, whether it's a CSA box that you split with them or a buying club, some of them have a $300 minimum. The biggest money saver is buying in bulk.

- **Find ways to get healthy food cheaply into your home**: if it's in a box or plastic container, you are paying for that box and that container, whether it's organic or not. The more you can get bulk food and store it safely in glass, the more healthy you will be and your children will be. It does take time prepping, cooking and changing the way you live, but the advantages far outweigh the time and cost involved.

- **Pressure cookers are great**.

- **Get a bread maker**.

- **Make healthy meals in bulk for much less than buying it in a grocery store**.

- **Grow your own food**: it is hard; it is work, but there's so much reward in it. I've continued even when I've lived in places where I had to grow in flower pots on my deck, but I've always had fresh herbs and fresh greens. In the winter time in Alaska, I did organic sprouts. You just have to push wherever you can to make that commitment.

- **Pay attention to your body**: it is an important component.

- **Learn how to use herbs**: cook with them often.

Also, It's really important to learn about science. There's a war on science happening. It's the science of nature versus the science of industry, that is at odds with nature. It's being played on this large scale, political and global platform, tied to our economy. We should all dedicate a little time to that, understanding what they're trying to do and what is happening with it, so you can make those educated choices for yourself and for your family. It can be daunting but very, very empowering at the same time.

It helps to stay positive and focus on the things we can do, rather than all the things we can't do. It's important not to give up hope, not to give up trying. Keep pushing and do whatever you can do. For me, that means teaching my family how to cook and how to keep making better choices, as well as, how to store things properly and make things from scratch. I think it could mean you have a generator for when the power goes out and a small garden, or perhaps you have two chickens in your yard. Maybe you hold community meetings, trying to change local laws. Every effort counts.

I always try to involve those other people. This isn't a solo mission. We need other people involved. *You grow the carrots this year; I'll grow the broccoli. You have room for chickens and I don't, so I'll trade you this or that.*

We have to get back to some of the ways this country was founded and how we got our freedom to begin with, which was through agriculture. It was through small farms. It was through seeds. George Washington, Thomas Jefferson, Benjamin Franklin, they were farmers. They had farms and they considered agriculture the path to gaining freedom from the control of the oligarchy. That's where we're at now, over two hundred years later and we have to take small steps to get it back.

The Best You Can Afford

At the beginning of 2015 I was in a situation where I had to be on Food

Stamps, and I had $500 a month to spend every month which, for us, was a huge luxury. Right now, I only have $50 a week to feed a family of three. That's not by choice, but I'm a single mom and so that's what I can afford and that's what I make due with. The bulk of it goes to my food box every week. I still get organic food delivery from the CSA company I used to work for. Every Monday I get a package on my doorstep with my produce for the week. Then the rest, I just supplement what's not in there. Our meat protein, I probably only buy once a month. We eat a lot of vegetarian meals. I have to live within my means, so it can be done. You can live organic on that budget.

A couple of years ago, I was getting WIC up in Alaska and they only allow you to get the cheapest of the cheap products, which are of course GMO. I tried to advocate for them to make some changes to the policies to allow some healthier options. I told them that I can't feed that stuff to my child; it would make her sick. They just didn't understand that. Honestly, when I was on Food Stamps that was about the most I've ever been able to spend, except for when I was working 70 hours a week in Alaska, I spent around $700 a month, but the prices there demand it. A gallon of organic milk is $10 up there.

The new goal I have is to advocate for glyphosate allergy testing. If we could prove that our kids are allergic to glyphosate, the USDA would have to provide organic meals to those children in the free lunch program that test positive for glyphosate allergy. The USDA School Lunch Program Policy says that they have to accommodate those children who have food allergies.

An Activist Perspective

I get really mad at injustice and I feel like GMOs are one of the world's worst injustices. I know how the food industry works in this country. It's such a sad travesty to our planet and our people. I had to get out there and tell everybody I know about it. I constantly talk about it and beat that drum. People get sick of it; stop following me on *Facebook*. I just don't give up on it. I find that friends and family eventually start to come around. Then they start beating that drum. It takes time and persistence for change to happen.

Food is a very powerful part of our life. We don't give it the time and attention that it deserves. Our connection with food is so much more than people think it is. It's so involved in our family lives, our emotions, our bonding experiences; they are often centered around food.

I became a certified lactation consultant, so I could talk to moms about what they're feeding their families and how they're doing it. I used every opportunity I could to get in front of people to talk about it. I also started selling products for a great company, called NYR Organics out of the UK. Their line of personal beauty products is very high quality, GMO-Free and organic. There's nothing else like it on the shelves. It's a great lead-in to talk to people about what their using and what they're feeding their kids.

I've always been out there talking to people about food, finding ways to have those conversations about what they're eating, why they're eating this or buying that. But as this health and food crisis has hit the country, several organizations, like Moms Across America starting jumping on the bandwagon.

NYR Organics linked me up with Moms Across America, who were marching in 4th of July parades all over America to spread the word about GMOs. Some of us got together, in Juno, and handed out samples of GMO-Free candy and samples of some of our organic lotions. That really got me started with Moms Across America.

I also helped with the Washington Labeling Initiative. Unfortunately the legislation failed, except in Vermont and Connecticut. I got involved and started doing everything I could to spread awareness. Afterward, I started participating in events like World Food Day and March Against Monsanto. There were a couple of years where it was just me and maybe two or three other people, holding up signs standing on the capitol steps.

In addition, I use to do a lot of childcare advocacy for mothers and children, so that played a part in it. I was part of a National Organization of Women's group up in Alaska that taught women how to provide meaningful testimony and how to track a bill through the legislature. We taught that process to mothers and childcare providers and how to navigate that political realm, which can be really daunting for regular moms that just care about their kids. People shouldn't just assume that they have to participate from home and not get out there and speak. It's important to give people a voice in their government policy. I lived in Oregon for a bit and started Moms Across Cascadia for people in the Northwest, sort of a spin-off of Moms Across America. I wanted to have a place so I could connect with families and get more information out there.

We were way outspent in the labeling campaign. People were so disappointed that the vote was so close and we lost. When you spread the lie that labeling will cost more, it scares people. It's a fear based tactic and it works. After we lost the vote I didn't want people to lose hope and I wanted to spread more information. I started doing social media for Moms Across America. We are a group of mothers mounting national campaigns.

I was inspired to go to Washington D.C., last summer during World Food Day. I had it on my radar for a year, and I was committed, come hell or high water, I was going. I did a *Go-Fund Me* and got the funding to go. I ended up being the volunteer coordinator for the event. I connected with all the people across the country that were going, coordinated where we were meeting and stuff like that.

We attended 37 meetings with congressional staffers, while we were there - dividing them among 30 of us, I think. Having never been to the East Coast or Washington D.C., it was really a whirlwind, with all the coming and going and different faces we met with. We just got out there and tried to speak to as many people as we could. Of course, you never speak to the actual congressman; you always speak to staffers. We targeted the DARK Act. If they were on the Senate Agriculture Committee or the Health Committee, we wanted to talk to them.

Senator Mike Pompeo's DARK Act made its way through the House, and was added to a budget bill as a rider, tying it to the federal operating funds of the government. It's all about wheeling and dealing with all the money tied in. If you can sneak something into something, that has to pass, to keep things operating, you have a much easier chance of getting it through. It's really sneaky.

Our take away, was just getting the opportunity to tell our stories. We had lots of information to present to them, lots of science and lots of data. We showed them the studies, but I think what really made a difference was the personal interaction and telling our stories about how this has really impacted our lives. We told stories about family members getting sick, our kids getting sick and then getting better after they change their diet.

Families are seeing illnesses that have never run in their family. Something is happening here. These are real people. This shouldn't be happening.

One in three babies is not being carried to full term. That number is enormous! What is going on? People are not hearing this story. It's heartbreaking what families are going through. So when we started talking about our stories and the real impact of it all, that is what made the most difference, I think. When we were kids, we heard of maybe one person in our town that got cancer. Now that number is one in three.

Previously, Zen Honeycutt went to D.C. to testify on behalf of Moms Across America, and they essentially blocked the meeting. In a sly move, a bunch of students were paid to attend the meeting and fill up the room. Even though Zen showed up several hours early to testify, she still couldn't get in and was unable to testify, because all of these other people were paid to obstruct the process. This is the kind of tactics being used. They will stop at nothing to keep this information from getting out. We're up against such a big animal, but we're so committed to not letting them win. It's so frustrating and maddening at times. The bottom line is the health of our families and the health of this country. The health of our children is worth everything. That's what matters here, and so we're not going to stop.

The Real Victories

The vote in Vermont was a big victory; that's why they've tried so hard to push through this DARK Act. It passed, they couldn't fumble the election, and they're scared for it to take hold. When that goes into effect, if they want to sell products in Vermont with GMOs, it will have to say 'contains GMOs' on the label.

(Little did we know during this interview that the DARK Act would be passed, overshadowing the Vermont law.)

The FDA decision to pull Enlist Duo was a step in the right direction. Revoking their certification was a huge victory, although we know that there will be several more lined up behind it. The EPA, FDA and USDA really have some major problems that need to be addressed, so the little victories we'll take but it's far from a real win on the matter.

The real victory here, what I tell people every day that are upset and have lost hope, is this, *we vote every day for GMO labeling. We vote every day for more organic options, every time a bar code crosses a scanner. And that by far is the most powerful vote we have and will continue to have.*

I've really seen the uptick in the market of organic products. New businesses are focusing on it. We've had a 50 percent increase in the growth of organic produce sales just here in Northwest. The growth has been dramatic as people have become more aware.

I worked for a local CSA here in Washington State that also delivers to Alaska. I was the Alaska sales representative. I can tell you it's so empowering to help somebody in Dutch Harbor or Kodiak working on some remote river in the middle of Alaska. Yes, it's very expensive because of shipping, but we can get you a box of organic produce. That is a huge win, because the reality is there are so many places in this country where it's not available.

I know the way this country is operating and the way the grocery stores chains work. There are many food deserts in large cities and different areas where it is very difficult to get nutritious, healthy food that will make you better.

Actions of Accountability

Our children don't have a voice in this, along with the elderly in our care. They aren't buying the food and they are at the mercy of those who are. Some universities require students to purchase a food card as part of their tuition now. Essentially binding them to the GMO processed options in the school cafeteria. They are being forced into something that is likely making them sick. It's forcing illness.

With a lot more voices aimed at overthrowing the Monsanto dictatorship, along with their monopolies controlling our food and sick-care system, the time has come to hold them accountable. We just have to get louder and stronger and work together more. When we organize and get the information out there, we have more impact. Personally, I'm working hard to try to get the information out in my own community.

Whole Foods just moved in and now my favorite little health food store, independently owned, is being driven out of business. It's sad and just awful to me. We've got to work on that. We've got to support these businesses and the makers, trying to do things right. If you understand the business model of these large companies, they aren't what they're cracked up to be. In this movement, I want to be the one throwing the ball; I don't want to be constantly reacting, and right now we're just all reacting to what is happening. There has to be that tipping point where we're throwing the ball. That's what I envision and intend to see in my lifetime. These little wins are starting to mean so much more than the awful losses. Things are beginning to really turn around.

Sophiah

Sophiah is a fabulous young woman that I first met and admired right away, just before her 15th birthday. She agreed to talk to me about what she remembers about her early GMO-Free transition:

In 2002, I was around four or five years old when we went organic. I've been organic about 14 years, and I'm almost 18. I really don't know any different. For me, it's just not an option to eat any other way. If I go out or to see a friend, I eat before I leave, or I take food with me and share. It's really not a big deal.

The food I eat is fabulous and so delicious! There are so many great recipes that you can make yourself. People can call me vegetable muncher if they want to. I don't care. They have no idea what that even means. This food is clean and healthy and it won't add to your waistline, the way that other food will. I like to cook; it's a big thing with me. I like to make people happy and I like to feed them. It all just goes together because food makes people happy and if you feed them healthy food, it makes them happier. I do a lot of baking; I make pies and pastries in large quantities. They go fast around here.

My mom was a large woman for a long time, about 300 pounds at 6'2" tall. I remember she was having a really hard time and her health was really bad. I remember after we made the changes she started getting thinner and thinner. She got a lot happier and had so much more energy. She lost over 200 lbs and that's what I really remember.

It has just been my life and I really couldn't tell you the difference. I have tried foods that weren't organic, regrettably, I always pay a high price. It makes me sick. My body rejects it pretty quick. I know there is definitely a difference, so I won't be doing that again.

Friendly Advice

Just give them the information and let them try the food. That's the big push here. Don't be afraid of trying new foods and making the changes. There's always alternatives to the foods you love, but you'll feel so much better afterward. You'll be eating real food that tastes so much better. You will feel the difference.

You might be afraid of giving up that donut or that cup of Jo or that pizza, but you'll find cleaner versions that are going to be so much better and will taste better. After you do this for a while, your taste buds come back to life and say "oh my goodness, real food, halleluiah, thank you!!" They want the real deal and so that's really the good push.

The food wasn't intended to messed with. You don't change the genetics. It's wrong what they have done to the food. They don't know how it affects your body. This is a way to slowly kill somebody. Mother Nature has a code, and you can't mess with that. It's horrifying and disgusting to think about it. You would think that people would have the wherewithal to know that's just so wrong. You can't mix up mother nature and expect it to be okay.

CHAPTER 6

....

GMO-Free Doctors

Why does the United States pay about 2 ½ times more for health care than most nations, yet still has the worst outcomes? According to the Peterson-Kaiser Health System Tracker the Total National Health Expenditures in 1960 for each person was $146, including hospitals, clinics and prescription drugs. In 1980, just 20 years later, the same care increases to an incredible $1000 per person. By the year 2000, we see it jump to over $4500, and in 2008, it rolls up to $7500. And, looking back at just hospital care in 1990, the total cost was around 250 billion dollars for that year. Comparing it to national expenditures for hospitals in 2014, the cost rose to over 971 billion dollars. Why are Americans getting so sick? [1]

Although there have not been any *official* GMO lab tests done on humans, we can, indeed, look upon these dark days as little rats in experiments.

Today many doctors and practitioners avoid genetically engineered foods and are advising their patients to do the same. Are they onto something?

American Academy of Environmental Medicine (AAEM)

The American Academy of Environmental Medicine is a team of global physicians that specialize in Environmental Medicine. "The AAEM provides research and education in the recognition, treatment and prevention of illnesses induced by exposures to biological and chemical agents encountered in air, food and water." [2]

Originally, the AAEM started calling for a moratorium on GMOs in 2009, after a comprehensive review of existing research and feeding study outcomes. Dr. Robin Bernhoft, the former president of AAEM, says that the Academy, "recommends that all physicians should prescribe non-genetically modified food for all patients and that we should educate all of our patients on the potential health dangers, and known health dangers of GMO food." [3]

Dr. Bernhoft appears with Jeffrey Smith in his film *Genetic Roulette*. He says that the public thinks that genetic engineering is a precise science; though that misconception is not at all accurate. It's more like, "microscopic shooting from the hip," Bernhoft notes. [4]

"Real Medicine, Real Health" is an article by Dr. Arden Anderson, exposing the suppressive efforts in the scientific community to conceal work by doctors and researchers that oppose genetic reorganization of our nutrition. [5] He says that they are using viruses to turn on new genes during the cloning process. Smith says this process of gene insertion plus cloning, "creates massive collateral damage. This can lead to hundreds or thousands of mutations up and down the DNA strand, and hundreds of thousands of genes that can potentially change their levels of expression," cautions Smith. [4] Smith worries that numerous side effects have the potential to occur from this type of haphazard methodology and that it could plausibly destroy our planet without any recourse for her inhabitants.

The AAEM has asked physicians to advise all of their patients to avoid GM foods:

... several animal studies indicate serious health risks associated with GM food consumption including infertility, immune dysregulation, accelerated aging, dysregulation of genes associated with cholesterol synthesis, insulin regulation, cell signaling, and protein formation, and changes in the liver, kidney, spleen and gastrointestinal system. [2]

Dr. Anderson implicates the foreign gene sequences in our food supply that are not found anywhere in nature. He says that our immune system, with its hypersensitive electromagnetic logic, doesn't recognize it as food and so the body attacks. I would just add that, clearly, the body is smart enough to know the difference even when the mouth is fooled. [6]

Earlier we explained that inflammatory responses can occur in your body, when it is being bombarded by what it sees as foreign invaders. This can lead to chronic health conditions that may indicate impending disease.

Physicians of Fortitude
Emily Lindner

Dr. Emily Lindner is a doctor of internal medicine. She says increasingly she is seeing patients suffering from digestive issues, allergies, impaired immune functioning, bloating, irritable bowel syndrome, colitis, leaky gut, autoimmune disease, neurological disorders and a whole host of diseases, that are getting better for her patients in a matter of days and weeks, following the prescription of a GMO-Free diet. [6]

Vitality Magazine, one of Canada's largest publications on natural health, spoke with Dr. Lindner about her observations:

I tell my patients to avoid genetically modified foods because in my experience, with those foods there is more allergies and asthma, as well as digestive issues such as gas, bloating, irritable bowel, colitis, and leaky gut...and what emanates from that...is everything. Lots of arthritis problems, autoimmune diseases, anxiety... neurological problems; anything that comes from an inspired immune system response.[3]

She says that recovery time varies depending on the person and the symptoms they experience. Linder describes what she notices when she changes her patients from a GMO diet to a GMO-Free diet:

I see results instantaneously in people who have foggy thinking and people who have gut symptoms like bloating, gas, irritation. In terms of allergies, it might take two to five days. In terms of depression, it starts to lift almost instantaneously. It takes from a day, to certainly within two weeks.[3, 6]

The doctor also appears in the documentary film *Genetic Roulette* illustrating her clinical experience with GMOs and allergies:

In most of my patients, because they have some sort of immune or inflammatory response to the GMO foods, I have to take them off the non-GMO foods that are related. So I have to take them off of all corn. I have to take them off of all grains...once the immune system has been inspired to have a response, they react to GMO and non-GMO.

Dr. Lindner says that most people tend to see full results in about four to six weeks, adding that elimination of GMOs from the diet is the most critical component. She uses some telling examples; one patient, a trial consultant named LaDonna C., was taking six pills a day to manage painful cramps and constant diarrhea from irritable bowel syndrome. Ladonna recalls, "My doctor told me I would be on this forever..." But then she saw Dr. Lindner and, "The first thing she did was take me off GMO....within two months, I didn't need the medication any longer." [3]

John Boyles

Ohio Allergist Dr. John Boyles explains, "I used to test for soy allergies all the time, but now that soy is genetically engineered, it is so dangerous that I tell people never to eat it."

The good doctor condemns GMOs:

> This exchange of DNA between the species is totally against nature. We simply don't know what it will produce. We don't know if it is safe, and it has not yet been proven to be safe. We do not fully understand how gene splicing works within a single species. We certainly can't predict how it will work when attempting to combine more than one species...by altering genes, scientists are creating a separate allergy to foods that did not exist in patients before. By changing or altering the structure of the plant, GMOs can cause separate reactions from the same food. You owe it to yourself and your family to make healthier food choices. Any allergic person can benefit from a diet with increased organic foods. Control what you can...steer clear of GMO foods. [6]

Boyles says his patients with allergies have to stay away from GMO foods, because they react to them and they'll tell you that. [4]

Richard Lacey

Dr. Richard Lacey is a food safety expert and author. Previously, he served on a UK government advisory panel on food relating to human and animal health. In an article "Doctors Against GMOs," Joel Edwards reveals that Dr. Lacey started raising the red flag with officials in 1989, condemning the practice of feeding cattle meat products from other animals, predicting the epidemic of mad cow disease before it every occurred. [6]

Dr. Lacey has written five books on food safety, even publishing one with Cambridge University Press, including a detailed examination of the evidence surrounding GE food:

It is my considered judgment that employing the process of recombinant DNA technology (genetic engineering) in producing new plant varieties entails a set of risks to the health of the consumer that are not ordinarily presented by traditional breeding techniques... [and] that food products derived from such genetically engineered organisms are not generally recognized as safe on the basis of scientific procedures within the community of experts qualified to assess their safety...recombinant DNA technology is an inherently risky method for producing new foods...part due to the complexity and interdependency of the parts of a living system, including its DNA. Wedging foreign genetic material in an essentially random manner into an organism's genome necessarily causes some degree of disruption, and the disruption could be multi-faceted... the disruptive influence could well result in... unexpected toxins or allergens or in the degradation of nutritional value... and our understanding of them is still quite deficient — it is impossible to predict what specific problems could result .... [and] I am not aware of any study in the peer-reviewed scientific literature that establishes the safety of even one specific genetically engineered food let alone...these foods as a general class...the only way to base the claims about the safety...is to establish each one to be safe through standard scientific procedures, not through assumptions that reflect more wishful thinking than hard fact. [6]

Ronald Weiss

Internist Dr. Ronald Weiss sold his thriving medical practice in New Jersey after 25 years and bought organic farm so he could treat patients with food instead of drugs. [7] "Fruits and vegetables contain nutrients that prevent inflammation, which is believed to be cause of many chronic diseases," says Weiss, a 52-year-old assistant professor at the Rutgers New Jersey Medical School in Newark. [8]

Dr. Weiss advises his patients about the best way to overcome disease:

> Plant-based whole foods are the most powerful disease- modifying tools available to practitioners — more powerful than any drugs or surgeries...I am talking about treating and preventing chronic disease — the heart attacks, the strokes, the cardiovascular disease, the cancers ... the illnesses that are taking our economy and our nation down... I am not saying if you fall down and break your ankle, I can fix it by putting a salve of mugwort on it. You need someone to fix your fracture. [9]

Weiss set out to establish Ethos Health as community-supported agriculture project, which "offers individuals direct access to its 'living medicines'...the nutrient dense and delicious fruits and vegetables Ethos conscientiously grows to prevent and reverse chronic illness." [7]

Michelle Perro

Dr. Michelle Perro is a prominent integrative pediatrician in California at the Institute for Health and Healing. She is genuinely concerned about the health hazards of eating GMOs.

She works diligently with her young patients and parents to establish cleaner eating habits in order to rebuild a state of health and wellness.

She presented to an audience in New Zealand in May 2015.

She says, "were having such a problem with food allergies in California that right now; it's a state law in California that schools have to stock EpiPens." She explains that one in two children in the US has a chronic disease now and nearly six million children have allergies. Dr. Perro refers to CDC reports from 1997-2011, illustrating a 50 percent increase in children's food allergies. [10]

She says our children are suffering more than ever from

digestive disorders, along with one or more of following chronic health issues that she sees walk through her door every day: [10]

- Immunological dysfunction
- Respiratory dysfunction
- Fertility problems
- Neurological disorders
- Endocrine diseases

In addition, Perro sadly recounts the high number of kids that have come into her clinic with asthma, food and environmental allergies, chronic ear infections and sinus infections. She complains about the huge rise in kids with ADD and autism … *"1 in 50 kids right now. Back when I was a resident, it was 1 in 10,000."* [10]

Dr. Perro says she sees a lot of little ones with abdominal pain and things like acid reflux, bloating, gassy tummies, constipation, diarrhea, obesity, immune dysfunction, failure to thrive. Inflammatory bowel diseases (IBS) like Crohn's are frequent. She even diagnosed an 18-month-old toddler with ulcerative colitis, which the doctor says was previously unheard of in a child so young. [10]

I would note, she indicates early on in her presentation that her practice is located in an upper class neighborhood, so these children are not kids living in poverty. These are upper income families suffering ill-effects from what she and many doctors believe could very well be their GMO-glyphosate filled diet.

Perro defines the seriousness of leaky gut syndrome that allows food to pass through into the blood-stream without being properly broken down first. The immune system attacks the body thinking the food is a foreign invader [8]. This provides further confirmation about what we discussed earlier in relation to the gut-brain connection, allergies and the intensity, in which the body responds to these synthetic food-like substances, unrecognizable as real nutrition in the body.

Like many scientists and practitioners, Dr. Perro also expresses deep concern about the hazards inherent problems of using glyphosate in farming, and the health effects on consumers, especially our children, when it acts as a chelator, binding to the essential minerals our body needs for hundreds of different functions. [10]

The good doctor makes a prime example with Zinc, something she says we need for around 250 reactions in the brain, along with magnesium for another 200 functions. The blood tests she runs on patients are showing up with significantly low zinc and magnesium levels. This is highly concerning considering the disturbance this can cause in the health and development of our children. She and other doctors note that glyphosate inhibits Cytochrome p450, which is the main detoxification system in your liver, and it also inhibits our vitamin D. This is problematic because it can easily lead right into a hormone dysfunction in our children and in us adults. [10]

Earlier we discussed that glyphosate is a toxic herbicide that kills the beneficial bacteria in the body. This is something Dr. Perro drives home, noting the significance of the relationship between the rise in celiac disease and the introduction of farming practices spraying glyphosate on non-tolerant crops to dry them out, prior to the harvest. [10]

Perro illustrates with study outcomes, showing high toxicity levels in Dr. Judy Carmen's pigs that were fed GMO food. As a result, the animals developed significant amounts of intestinal inflammation, according to Dr. Carmen's reports. Dr. Perro says this is something she's noticed among many of her own patients with high toxicity levels. [10]

We know that chronic inflammation is a precursor to most of our chronic diseases, if not all of them. Inflammation is a warning sign from the body telling you something isn't right. We are seeing an abnormally high amount of gut inflammation in our young kids and that is not a normal state of being human, so we must ask ourselves why.

Dr. Perro says a toxicologist she knows suggested that she might be able help these kids with an amino acid called glycine, which comes in a powder. She reports that some of the kids that were particularly toxic got better. [10]

At this point, let us recall, in Chapter 2, Dr. Samsel and Seneff's latest discovery with, "Glyphosate V..." and how "it provides a strong case for the possibility that glyphosate, acting as a non-coding amino acid analogue of glycine, can get into proteins by mistake during protein synthesis." Might this be the reason that glycine supplementation helped some of the more toxic cases recover?

Dr. Michelle Perro prescribes an organic diet to her patients, she says. She is pleased with the positive health outcomes she sees in her young patients after they make the recommended changes. Parents continue to report significant improvements in the health and well-being of their children following dietary cleanup of GMO foods. [10]

Dr. Perro adamantly opposes any detectable levels of GMOs and glyphosate in baby formula and food products. In her article, "GMOs in Baby Formula? A pediatrician provides answers," *Dr. Perro* encourages parents to read labels and make better choices for the health of their babies:

> There are several formulas to choose from, and there are certain "musts" that I do insist upon. One "must" choose an organic preparation. Because of the toxic effects of herbicides, particularly glyphosate (due to its prolific usage) as well as organophosphates and genetically engineered foods, formula that is not organic is not an option for infant feeding...[and] can have lifelong detrimental health impacts for children. Those ingredients include GMOs, glyphosate and other pesticides and herbicides...the Roundup formula eliminates beneficial bacteria found in our intestines. Beneficial bacteria play a key role in many important functions in the body, particularly immune function. The depletion...allows pathologic bacteria—which is at the root of many serious chronic diseases—to take up residence in our intestines.... [11]

Dr. Perro further cautions,

there is an alarming rate of childhood disorders on the rise in the US including: allergies, autoimmunity, neurological disorders (autism and ADHD), growth failure, endocrine disruption, etc. There are modifications to the immune function that can take place prenatally and early in life which may lead to the above disorders ("developmental immunotoxicity"). Increased exposure to environmental toxins during those sensitive times may contribute to the health conditions noted above. In animal studies where animals were fed GMOs, there were profound changes in the animal's intestines as well as immune function...[11]

Bayshore Pediatrics

Bayshore Pediatrics in New Jersey recommends parents feed their children organic. On their website they educate parents about GMOs and encourage them to vote with their dollars:

The really frightening thing is that food labels are not required to list whether ingredients are GMO. So avoiding these ingredients can be a challenge. Organic foods cannot be GMO so sticking with these products where possible is a good way to limit your family's exposure. [12]

Carla Nelson

Dr. Carla Nelson, a pediatrician working in Hawaii, reports that she and other doctors have seen a rise in birth defects and illnesses in patients, that she and the other doctors suspect are the result of the high rate of pesticide being sprayed on GMO corn fields. She condemns the fact that it has been the major cash crop on four of the six main islands over the past three years. Local residents complain that the wind carries the spray particles in the air even on days they aren't spraying. It causes stinging eyes, headaches and vomiting in the town's people.

Nelson says there's an American Academy of Pediatrics' report called, "Pesticide Exposure in Children," where they found, "an association between pesticides and adverse birth outcomes, including physical birth defects."[13]

The story reports that the local schools have been evacuated twice; numerous children have been sent to the hospital because of pesticide drift. Nelson wants doctors to start receiving prior notice of the spraying. She says, "It's hard to treat a child when you don't know which chemical he's been exposed to." Middle school teacher Howard Hurst says, "Your eyes and lungs hurt, you feel dizzy and nauseous. It's awful. Here 10% of the students get special-ed services, but the state average is 6.3%. It's hard to think the pesticides don't play a role." [13]

A PubMed study from 2011 showed:

> [An] estimated 43% of US children (32 million) had at least 1 of 20 chronic health conditions being assessed, increasing to 54.1% when overweight, obesity, or being at risk for developmental delays were included; 19.2% (14.2 million) had conditions resulting in a special health care need. [14]

Let's look the following evidence to determine if it would benefit our children if we applied the precautionary principle, along with some common sense, to improve health outcomes that may be declining as a direct result of our dependency on the GMO food system.

Bellwether Babies

The Centers for Disease Control (CDC) has identified an unhealthy dose of reality, in regards to the offspring of Monsanto's generations. Autism rates continue to skyrocket, as parents and providers seek out new ways to manage the challenging disorder.

A CDC report, published in 2003, in *The Journal of the American Medical Association,* surveyed incidents of autism among children ages 3 to 10, in metropolitan areas of Atlanta, Georgia. The report period began in 1996, and was the first-time researchers began to track and report autism rates in the US. That first year, 987 children with autism or related disorders were identified, showing 3.4 cases of ASD per 1,000 children. [15]

Fast forward to a 2012 CDC report, looking at just 8-year-olds in selected areas - 1 in 68 children was identified with an autism related diagnosis. This is according to estimates from the CDC's Autism and Developmental Disabilities Monitoring (ADDM) Network. [16]

Identified Prevalence of Autism Spectrum Disorder ADDM Network 2000-2012 Combining Data from All Sites				
Surveillance Year	Birth Year	Number of ADDM Sites Reporting	Prevalence per 1,000 Children (Range)	This is about 1 in X Children...
2000	1992	6	6.7 (4.5-9.9)	1 in 150
2002	1994	14	6.6 (3.3-10.6)	1 in 150
2004	1996	8	8.0 (4.6-9.8)	1 in 125
2006	1998	11	9.0 (4.2-12.1)	1 in 110
2008	2000	14	11.3 (4.8-21.2)	1 in 88
2010	2002	11	14.7 (5.7-21.9)	1 in 68
2012	2004	11	14.6 (8.2-24.6)	1 in 68

CDC's 2015 *National Health Statistics Reports* show 1 in 45 children surveyed, ages 3-17, was identified with ASD. In this study, it was the first time that survey responders were asked to self-identify (only) one child, per household, with an ASD diagnosis from a medical doctor. The report stems from a 2014 National Health Interview Survey, demonstrating clear-cut indicators that our children, are indeed, drowning in a quagmire of autism related symptoms. Meanwhile, ASD service provider waitlists are still brimming in cities across the country.

We can only conclude that the *principles of poison* appear to leave little doubt as to fault line of this rising epidemic, underlying the contention that they, themselves, are fully aware of the detriments of the GMO food supply and the pockets they serve.

Infant Mortality Rates

How does a rich country like America end up with a higher infant mortality rate than Cuba, Taiwan and Israel? We lose about six babies per 1,000 live births here, whereas South Korean infants, and even those in Slovenia, are about twice as likely to survive. Why is our infant mortality rate higher than 27 other affluent countries? According to the Center for Disease Control (CDC), Spanish infants were twice as likely to celebrate their first birthday in 2010, than their American counterparts. Japanese babies were three times as likely to survive birth than children born here in the US. [18]

Perhaps Americans spend more on health care than any country on the planet, but if we look at our 2013 infant mortality rate in just one state of the union, you would never guess it. For instance, in Mississippi parents saw more infant deaths (per capita) than those in some third world countries, such as Sri Lanka. [18, 19]

Is this the inevitable outcome of GMOs and their toxic companions found all throughout our environment and food supply for, at least, the past two decades? Farmers who had no intention of growing GMOs are finding them in their fields. Parents who had no intention of buying GMOs are finding them on their plates. Doctors and scientists all over the world are reporting concerning outcomes in the health of patients and lab subjects, who are consuming these "contaminated" products on a daily basis. [20]

Meanwhile, for a food or substance to be categorized by the FDA as "generally recognized as safe" (GRAS) it must be the dominant theme of an extensive number of peer-reviewed and published studies (or the equivalent of) and secondly, there must be overwhelming consensus among our scientific communities that the product is indeed, no-doubt, safe. Scientists say that GMO foods have never passed either of these standards. [21]

CHAPTER 7

....

GMO-Free Tips, Tricks & Tools

In "GMO-Free Testimony" we tilled a lot of rich soil, and I hope you were able to glean some practical ideas that are relevant for you. I want to be sure that we don't lose track of what's important while you are transitioning into your new way of life, and that is your child, your family and how this impacts them and you; because at the end of the day if I leave you lost and confused in the GMO jungle, I'm not doing you any favors.

The best way to begin to facilitate your transition is to start at the dinner table with a mental and perhaps physical accounting of what is important to you and your family, with regard to the nutritional options available in your kitchen. Are you are a vegetarian or a Class A carnivore? Is your family into traditional American Cuisine or cultural foods or a little of everything? It doesn't matter what kind of "food-style" you've been engrossed in, the patterns of a healthy diet begin in how you feel about your food. In essence, it boils down to your relationship with food.

For the Love of Food

Examining how you feel and respond to food is a vital part of changing the habits that are not benefiting you or your family. Our emotional connection to the food we eat runs deeply into all aspects of our daily lives, whether we realize it or not.

Your childhood was peppered with examples of how you manage your relationship with food as an adult. Take the child, for example, let's call her Rita. Rita is growing up in a household consumed with being and becoming fat. Perhaps her mother doesn't accept herself and is verbally judgmental or even downright self-abusive in response to her negative self-image and lack of self-control in response to food. Maybe Rita's mom lives in the binge-guilt cycle where she fills up on garbage, and then she feels guilty, so she goes into starvation mode to make up for it.

The emotional reflections of ourselves shine through the eyes of our children who mirror the best and worst parts of ourselves.

What is Rita learning from her mother about self-worth and her relationship with food? What if Rita begins to repeat the patterns of her mother in ways that engage her in eating habits that destroy her health and sense of self-worth like so many generations of boys and girls in the world? The negative role her mother plays, however unintentional, will become the basis from which she establishes her overall relationship with food.

I can't overstate the importance of respecting the role of the gut-brain connection in relationship with what you eat. It goes a long way in establishing your mental and emotional state of being. Remember how the gut-brain connection works and the importance of maintaining it? The chemicals and toxins rampant in the food supply have taken their toll on our physical and psychological state, and they have to be addressed to resolve what could be a mental dysfunction simply resulting from damage to this delicate system. It's highly possible to reverse this damage in noticeable ways, and once you've taken the steps to do so you will likely find a world of difference in how you and your children act, feel and think.

Taking advantage of everything the *cleanfood* lifestyle has to offer will allow you to successfully overcome any mental challenges the rocky road-blocks presented in the past. You will see how you can navigate those sticky situations through which these lifestyle patterns have kept your mind and body confused, burdened and likely exposed to high levels of toxins.

Don't fret if you can't imagine how you're going to pull this off now. Let the overwhelming feelings motivate you to commit to finding your way through the cloudy haze of uncertainty, so we can replace it with confidence and lofty amounts of opportunity to transform this entire SAD (Standard American Diet) paradigm from where you sit. The awkwardness will pass and so will the disorientation of it all.

I recall at this point in my journey I was terrified. I think I was literally afraid of food. I never said that out loud to anybody, much less myself. Imagine discovering your child has over 60 food allergies to navigate around. I often thought, "This is ridiculous - how can I be afraid of the very thing that was designed to keep us alive?"

Food is a glorious, beautiful experience. It's not just some irrelevant sidebar, like it has become in so many of our lives. It's sustenance, it's life, it's the very essence of who we are as human beings. This relationship is so intimate that we can't go on living without it. So don't you think that we should have a little more respect for our food and for whence it came?

In this chapter, we will go over the details of how you can personally manage to find resources in your local area and on vacation that are committed to providing you with sustainable, organic and GMO-Free options at a price you can live with. Here's where we really take off, and discover new ways of feeding the family well while maintaining within our grocery budget. Combining the practical advice and tips from the GMO-Free families in Chapter 5 with my some of my own experience, I aim to provide you a livable reference section to help guide you through the maze and haze with righteous certainty my friend!

I cannot overstate the importance of appealing to the comfort level and taste buds of your little ones during the course of this transition.

Humans need real living foods not dead, chemicalized, man-made non-foods that offer growing bodies nothing, least of all the love of a mother who just wants to please her kids. Appeasing them with (GMO) sugar and additives does nothing but short term and long-term damage to their health, brain and behavior (according to the studies in Chapter 2) and once you kick them to the curb for your new cleaner, greener alternatives you will begin to see what all of the rave is about. Nobody expects you to change everything overnight. That's too much for most people to fathom, although after the real evidence has been presented those that can, often do.

You don't have to stop eating the foods you love or start eating foods you hate. There isn't anything that you can make with your recipe that I can't make organic. What is important to consider is the nutritional content of the food we feed our kids, and to realize that it is a direct investment in their future. Think of it as a savings account, banking on the health and future of your child, because it is just that. We all want to give our kids their best chance in life. Their best opportunity is a clean, healthy diet to nourish the development of a macrocosm of bodily functions for a lifetime, ensuring longevity and cognitive functioning well into old age. The *SAD* GMO diet of Americans has come to collect, and the price of our health and that of our children is the toll of us all. We bought their crap, and now they just want to sell us more crap. It is high time that we take back our food system and demand high quality, real food.

Quality Protein

Good quality protein is key for the body's functions, and there are many different avenues to get there, including your plant-based proteins which are highly essential to growing bodies. Meanwhile, for you carnivores, let's talk about where you can get your meat.

Where's the Grass-fed Beef?

So how do we define high quality grass-fed beef? One key consideration that has a huge bearing on the quality is whether or not the cattle have been raised on pasture, as opposed to a feedlot in what is known as a Confined Animal Feeding Operation (CAFO).

Joey Jones started *GrassfedNetwork.com* and has been largely involved in the grass-fed beef market, he says, for over 17 years. He and his wife started one of the first organic co-ops in Houston, Texas. Now he teaches livestock producers how to improve the way they raise their grass pastured animals.[1]

The "Natural" label means nothing in terms of GMOs, pesticides or even the conditions in which animals are raised. Producers get away with it, because the regulations are vague and allow ample room for interpretation. The bottom line is ranchers typically raise calves on pasture grass for "some amount" of undisclosed time period, so those producers can get away with calling their beef grass-fed, when it's really not. [1] 100 percent grass-fed beef is what you're shopping for.

Jones emphasizes the key to a truly grass-fed product is all in the finishing. As you too will discover, in regards to taste, texture and fat content, the very best beef really is both grass-fed and grass-finished:

> It is true that all animals are fed grass at some point unless they're dairy animals...but almost all beef animals are going to be on grass at some point in their life. It definitely is the grass-finished product that you're after. And the difference is big. [1]

"What You Need to Know About Grass-fed Beef" details an insightful interview with Jones by Dr. Joseph Mercola. Jones talks about a test he performed with one of his livestock clients with their cattle. He says they were raised and then finished for two different grass-fed meat buyers. One of the organizations, he explains, accepted dried distiller grains with solubles (called DDGs) used as a supplement in the animals. DDGs are made from corn that has been processed to remove the starches. Without the starch, Jones says, it technically qualifies as a grass feed supplement. The second buyer didn't allow DDG use. The one group of the animals got about two pounds of DDG a day and the other group got only grass. [1]

Jones illustrates the differences he observed in the quality of the two meats:

> When we processed those animals and sold them, we took a meat sample from both groups. In that three- month period... [the DDG-fed] group had no health benefits left whatsoever in the meat. The group that didn't get those DDGs still had all the health benefits that we expect from a grass-finished product...many times the health benefits reside in the fat more than the meat itself...[1]

Grass-foraged/finished beef has been proven to contain higher levels of something called conjugated linoleic acid (CLA) which is highly beneficially in disease prevention, according to several recent human and animal studies. Surprising lab results show that as little as .5 percent of CLA in the daily diet could reduce tumors by over 50 percent. Grain-fed beef has been shown to contain less of the other healthy fats too. [1, 3, 4,]

We need to maintain the balance of essential fatty acids in our daily diet with a good ratio of both omega-3 to omega-6 to keep our body is a good state of wellness. Processed foods and vegetable oils can ultimately lead to dramatic increases in your omega-6 fatty acids over the omega-3s. When they're in check omega-3s work to alter the brain chemicals that correlate with your mood and behavior. They also monitor over 100 genes in your body that are involved in the transmission of information between brain cells. Omega-3s work to alleviate the chronic inflammation that leads us to things like heart disease, Alzheimer's, cancer and dementia. Omega-6 fatty-acids, on the other hand, can promote inflammation putting us at a higher risk for all kinds of diseases. [2]

The Union of Concerned Scientists reports their analysis shows grass-fed steak has nearly double the omega-3s as your standard grain-fed steak. Another study published in the *Nutrition Journal* confirms those numbers, proving that grass-fed beef is far superior to its grain-fed counterparts, no question about it. [3. 4. 5]

Joey Jones says, "some of the grass-fed beef in the US is coming from Brazil, Mexico, Nicaragua and Uruguay, although most of it is actually being imported from Australia and New Zealand." The main reason, he points out, they are importing the grass-fed beef is because it's cheaper in those countries to finish animals on grass than it is here in the United States. The market for US beef has been grain driven, so few ranchers have opted for grass-fed operations.[1] As with all other commodities, when the demand for real grass-fed beef is realized, the market will respond and expand to accommodate the need. Currently, only about 3 percent of our beef cattle are coming from grass pastures, but the beef sales for grass-fed animals has increased around 20 percent over the past 6 years, Jones says.

The trend toward greener, cleaner eating will continue as more and more people demand it. And they certainly are.

How do I Know it's Quality Beef?

If you don't have access to local ranchers, try looking for grass-fed beef at your local grocery store. They very well might be selling certified USDA organic beef and chicken. Although producers no longer have to include the country of origin, some producers are stamping it voluntarily.

Now there is a point where Jones and I begin to diverge a little in our philosophies. Being that he is involved with American producers, it is his job to recommend that you stay within our grassy beef borders. Of course, I always choose local above national and imported meat options, where available, but he stresses the importance of being certain that you are buying a US-based product, because you don't know their methods and philosophies. While I agree with this angle whole-heartedly, he did mention that only 3 percent of American producers are committed to providing grass-fed products. If I'm *unable* to get my hands on a quality grass-fed and finished meat from the US during my grocery store visit, I am not above purchasing it from places like Brazil or Australia, as they are more likely to have raised and finished the animal on pasture alone, without any grain supplements added at the end, as Jones says himself.

I won't buy any meat without a country of origin indicated on the label. I personally will not buy food from China as a general rule (unless I do my homework thoroughly on the producer), due to the amount of environmental pollution plaguing many of the country's waterways and natural resources.

Jones advises that we call the producers to find out what their standards and protocols are. I've called and emailed many companies to find out about their processes and ingredients. Often the number appears on the packaging and if it doesn't, then *Google* is a great resource to find contact information. He also says that we should think of our grass-fed beef like a seasonal product, because there's a season for raising and a season for harvesting and most producers follow that seasonal pattern. This makes perfect sense to me as a consumer; I try to stick with this pattern as well, as economics allow, because when I'm unable to, I pay a higher price later. Undoubtedly, I will end up paying more for organic beef, pound-for-pound, if I miss my window of opportunity to get my beef from a local rancher. I typically fill up my freezer in the Fall, as economics allow. The processing season will depend on your farmer and where you live.

Organic or Grass-fed?

USDA organic is fine, but we can't take it as a total guarantee that the meat has been grass-fed and grass finished. In fact, the organic label costs so much to establish and maintain that ranchers a lot of times will opt to raise their beef cattle using high-quality methods that provide superior beef, without an organic label. Jones says in his mind, "a truly grass-fed, grass-finished product is superior to organic." [1]

Whenever possible, I always choose the local option, and I take every opportunity to get to know my rancher, so I can be assured that I'm buying the best beef for my family at the most economical price for my wallet. If I'm convinced that my producer is as passionate about *cleanfood* as I am, then I'm perfectly willing to forgo the extra cost of a certified product. I suggest that you don't take anyone's word for it, until your confident that you've asked all the right questions. It gets easier with experience.

You recall in the testimonials that we discussed the importance of knowing where your food comes from. We talked about the value of visiting local farms and ranches in the area, whenever possible. Most small farms and ranches will welcome you and your family and show you around. They want customers that are knowledgeable and engaged in what they're doing. The ones that have something to hide, are those you do not want feeding your family.

Jones shares a handful of helpful questions for you to cover with your beef producer, so you can get a clear indication of the practices they use with their animals. He makes a really good point; see if the farm is clean and well-run, but don't expect a sterile environment. It is a farm after all. [1]

Some valuable questions I ask and Jones suggests:

1. What do you feed your animals? Is it organic or non-GMO? (Remember: Alfalfa can be GMO and glyphosates are sprayed on some grasses prior to harvest.)

2. Are the animals fed any grains, hay, corn, soy or DDG supplements? If so, are they organic? Either way, I would walk away if they feed any of these, besides the organic (or at least GMO/pesticide-free) hay. The bulk of the diet should be grass. They are cows afterall. Cows eat grass, period.

3. Do you use any antibiotics or vaccinate the animals? If so, when and why? You're educated about antibiotics now, with regard to what they do to the gut bacteria, so you can you use your own judgment there. I suggest you do your homework when it comes to ingredients in vaccinations for animals and your kids. I will stop there.

4. Are the animals given any hormones? If so, goodbye.

5. Are the animals in a large pasture or confined? Confined feed lots make for unhappy cows and a new European study in *Science Daily* proves happy cows have more nutrition.

6. At what age is the animal being finished? The ideal for optimal fat content and taste, Jones notes, is around 20-24-months, but it's fine to go as long as 30 months, he says many producers do. [1]

I've noticed that a lot of small farmers like to name the animal because they love them; they treat them like part of the family. Obviously, it's not necessary for them to have named your cow. My point is, the more they care about the welfare of that cow, the better they will feed you and your family.

Jones offers some great advice in order to find a higher-quality meat, "You're looking for a shorter and wider animal, instead of a tall and leggy animal," he says. [1]

Good, Clean, Local

Good resources will make all the difference in your world. Here is a boatload of *cleanfood* resources offering you a wide selection of quality local meat and produce. It would be well worth your time to check out a few of these website links below. (Thanks Dr. Mercola; I wish I had found these long before.) You can follow the links to find various descriptions under an assortment of farms and ranches in your state. They provide an overview of their practices and philosophies, as well as the products they have to offer. The descriptions really allow you to get to know a little about the people you're dealing with, so you don't have to start from scratch trying to find local producers.

GMO-Free Online Tools

organicstorelocator.com—Locate your area organic stores

organic.org/storefinder—More search options for your area

pickyourown.org—Find local U-pick farms

eatwild.com—US, Canadian and International Farms & Ranches, featuring over 1,400 pasture-based farms and ranches with state-by-state search options. Find local grass-fed beef and dairy. This website is always being updated with new options. [1,7]

localharvest.org—Connects people looking for good whole food with the farmers who produce it. [1,8]

ams.usda.gov/local-food directories/farmersmarkets— Find your local farmer's markets.

eatwellguide.org/info- Curated directory of over 25,000 hand-picked restaurants, farms, markets and other sources of local, sustainable food throughout the US. [1,10]

grassfedexchange.com—Coordinated effort for grass-fed producers and buyers [1, 11]

greenpeople.org/btc/buyingguide.cfm—The *Green People Directory* has lists of local health food stores, organic food and your green products.

foodroutes.org—*The Food Routes Network* is working to rebuild local community-based food systems. As of April 2016, the site was still in the development stages, but promises to be a fabulous information, communication and tracking tool for producers and buyers alike.

coopdirectory.org—Find local food co-ops with this handy online directory of information of natural food co-ops.

wewantorganicfood.com/directory –More search options for organic food across the nation. Includes a very comprehensive directory of directories and information on certification and organic trade associations.

**whatsonmyfood.org** –*What's on My Food?* This is a great resource! It is very user friendly, letting you choose from a wide variety of produce to find out the chemical content of your conventional foods vs. organic. This site is provided by the Pesticide Action Network (PAN). They cross-referenced toxicology data from the EPA and others with the USDA's Pesticide Data Program (PDP). This tool allows you to see the pesticide residue levels in a wide selection of foods, that you can choose from, on their list. The site lets you access toxicological information for most of the pesticides tested by the USDA. They also include the chemical combinations and associated risk factors.

Long-term Suggestions

Here is a list of items that you might consider purchasing when you have the funds.

Consider Buying:

- Big freezer for extra freezer space
- Good blender/food processor (I love my Vitamix!)
- Canning jars/lids (Ball makes BPA free lids)
- Glass containers for left-overs and food storage
- Hand mill to grind your own flour
- Spice/coffee grinder to grind herbs
- Quality non-toxic cookware [19] (cast iron, glass)
- Gardening supplies
- Heirloom seeds, plants and trees (if you have space)

Consider Ditching:

For an added bonus you might eliminate a few or all of these unncessary hazards.

- Plastic containers, dishes and flatware [20, 21] (often BPA)
- Aluminum pots and pans [22]
- Teflon coated pots and pans [23]
- Microwave [24]

How do I Get Food?

- Community Supported Agriculture (CSA)
- Buy-in groups
- Farmer's market
- Buy bulk
- Shop around
- Avoid stores without organics
- Find local and organic restaurants
- Buy produce weekly
- Grow a garden
- Hunt/fish or find someone who does
- Buy a half/quarter grass-fed/finished beef
- Be a bargain shopper
- Minimize lunch meat—high cost/low nutrition
- Buy whole foods—low cost/high nutrition
- Keep it local

Important note:
You can tell GMO produce apart from organic by the PLU Number that appears on the sticker: [24]

- Four-digit number means the produce is conventionally grown
- Five-digit number beginning with 9 means it's organic

- Five-digit number beginning with 8 means it's GMO

Go Social—Make Friends

Take it from me, don't try to go it alone. The more support you have in this new lifestyle, the more successful you will be in every aspect of it.

- Talk to your farmers—ask questions
- Call the company
- Find local organic growers, not necessarily certified yet
- Encourage local restaurants to add organic menu options
- Meet others who get it
- Introduce your children to other organic families
- Talk to family, friends and neighbors
- Talk to teachers and school staff
- Have potlucks
- Visit food fairs and farms

How Do I Get My Kid to Eat Healthy Food?

- Explain why—so they understand
- Ask questions—what do you like, what don't you like?
- Offer options (two at most when their small)
- Check in—feelings and physical update
- Be flexible where you can
- Make adjustments and changes as needed
- Lace food with nutrition—compact nutrition at every meal
- Try new foods and encourage the same
- Take food on the go—don't buy for convenience
- Have snacks ready—it will save money

- Keep a healthy snack tray—it will save time and a lot of whining
- Make homemade yogurt—freeze
- Add infused water
- Pinterest—when stuck in a rut
- Lazy Susan—give them access to healthy nuts, seeds, fruit and veggies
- Freeze leftover cakes, cupcakes and muffins—be party ready
- Cook meals ahead and freeze—great for emergencies and long, busy days
- Fermented foods—happy tummies—happy eaters
- Encourage a bite or two—taste buds change
- Crowd out bad food with so much good—no room for garbage
- Find recipes for family favorites—so easy to find online!
- Cook foods in new ways—keep trying different ideas and methods.
- Find what works for you
- Skip it if they don't like it—it's not worth the fight
- Set clear expectations
- Give them your best—they deserve it and so do you
- Make a "I Can't Live Without It" list –find GMO-Free alternatives
- Cook it from scratch (almost all recipes are online)
- Encourage fresh raw vegetables—whole food is the best food
- Get input from other GMO-Free parents
- Include smoothies—lots of compact nutrition
- Set good examples—show them how to eat healthy
- Ask do you like it, what would make it better?
- Don't like it—don't say it out loud (adults and siblings)
- Keep it simple
- Make it an upgrade—feed them better than ever

Honor the Body:

- Listen to it
- Trust it
- Encourage mind-body relationships
- Respect the gut-brain connection
- Watch for allergies and sensitivities
- Discontinue anything questionable

Learn About:

- Herbs and spices—compact nutrition, medicinal benefits
- Superfoods and whole foods—nutrient dense
- Chemicals and additives- *Google* the Chemical Safety Data Sheets for any household chemicals
- Ingredients—what is it, where does it come from?
- New food and chemical studies
- Vitamins, minerals and nutritional needs for growing bodies
- Vaccine chemical additives—mercury, aluminum (ASK Dr. for and *read* the vaccine insert for all vaccines.) http://vaxtruth.org/2011/08/vaccine-ingredients/

Remember:

- Garbage in = garbage out
- Healthy doesn't mean yucky
- Cook with Love
- Taste buds change
- You're the parent
- Question everything
- Organic = GMO-Free
- GMO-Free ≠ organic (not necessarily)

- The US President doesn't eat GMOs—(why should your child?)
- Review products—be mindful when products change producers and/or ingredients
- Ask for help
- Stand your ground
- Cook from scratch where possible
- Read labels and know your ingredients
- Minimize products with more than 5 or 6 ingredients, and be sure you can pronounce them and know what they do in little bodies. Can't say it? Don't eat it.
- Don't fall for fads—this lifestyle doesn't have to be expensive.

Most of all Remember:
It's a Process Not an Event!

CHAPTER 8

....

GMO Detoxification

"Plant-based whole foods are the most powerful disease-modifying tools available to the medical practitioner."
- Ron Weiss, M.D.

Mindset Matters

Food can be your best friend or your worst enemy. It can be a slow ride or a rapid crash. You've known folks, maybe yourself, that have relied on food to manage emotions, stuffing their face, rather than speaking up and addressing the situation at hand. Fear and anxiety can affect how we eat, as well as pain, happiness, boredom, depression, or any other emotional justification we can put our hungry little fingers on.

Perhaps you have experienced times in your life where you had little control over impulsive binges or the last cookie on the plate. This is not anything, except normal. This is how the human animal was designed. Forage and feed was a matter of survival and primordially you are on the right track; only fill and fuel has taken on a whole different concept in terms of our health, and the recent changes in man's dietary choices.

Our children aren't much different from us. Those hungry little humans can be quite the munchie mouths, eating when they are not hungry, filling up on sugar and preservatives, looking to fill idle hours or perhaps a sad day. Other times, they're moving too quickly to slow down and eat something good for them.

It's important that we talk about food with our kids, teaching them how to experience the real joy surrounding a healthy, nutritious diet and mindful eating techniques that will influence what they put into their mouths and how it affects their health and moods. They are indeed what they eat. Empty calories and sugar do not do the developing brain or body any favors. Lacking attention to what we put in our bodies, will ultimately only pay off for our doctors and the pharmaceutical industry.

Try looking at food with a different perspective, devoting yourself to cleaning up your eating habits. This can benefit your family and your waistline, not to mention your ability to function on a daily basis. Do you need more sleep? Are you suffering the perils of digestive failure? Are you foggy thinking or feeling moody? So are your children. You might only need to look as far as the gut and perhaps your refrigerator to get to the root of the problem.

The central theme of mindful eating begins at the checkout counter and ends at your kitchen table. The secret is this; add so much of the good stuff, that you don't have room for the bad. That means if little tummies are full of good, nutritious food, it doesn't leave much room left over to put in all that bad stuff. My brilliant teacher and the owner of the Institute for Integrative Nutrition, Joshua Rosenthal calls this strategy "crowding out." It works.

I know it seems they always have room for sugar, true statement, although it comes back around to availability. You buy it. They eat it. Don't forget that sugar feeds the bad bacteria in the gut, making it a good place to grow candida. Removing offending foods and replacing them with healthier, GMO-Free, wholefood options will kick this deal into high-gear for your entire family.

The following is not a specified detoxification program. It simply shares a compilation of methods and techniques that I use with my own family. The purpose is to rid the body of a variety of chemical substances, toxins, GMOs and heavy metals. Do not begin use of any detoxification protocols

with your child before consulting a trusted licensed medical practitioner.

The author makes no specified guarantees or representation as to the effectiveness or results that will be experienced by either you or your child with regard to any of these methods. It's important to use your own judgment and observation skills when using any detox program.

Take note and respond with your common sense to any signs of discomfort or unintended reactions to these or any detoxification methods. Discontinue use if you or your child are feeling uncomfortable with any of the results. There are many valuable, natural detoxification options that you can incorporate gently with your child, these are simply just a few of them. I encourage you to do your homework and further research these and other simple, natural detoxification methods, while avoiding overpriced store bought products that promise results. There are a ton of food and herbal options that you can incorporate into your diet that will super boost immunity and the body's ability to cleanse itself. Again, it is important to find out what works for you and your child.

With that said, this is not your mama's detox program. We need to take this slow and steady with little bodies, while going in with a gentle, yummy approach to reducing the overall toxic load.

Western medicine seems to completely disregard the significance of detoxification in the wellness plans for their patients. The body's ability to cleanse itself is instrumental in maintaining a disease-free life.

When you overlook the signs and symptoms your body is trying to tell you that's when disease jumps in to help communicate the dire message. The body is trying to make us aware that it is having difficulty getting rid of toxins and other waste burdens, and it needs our help to do that. Rather than ignoring these malfunctions that are hindering our natural self-healing mechanisms, we need to truly address the root causes of these problems in order to get the body functioning on its own again. When things are left to climax under the chemical strains of daily exposures, this weighs down and essentially affects everything we do and everything we are. As these systems become impaired their regulatory abilities cease to function as designed, and that is when cancer heeds the call.

Detoxification is the central theme for maintaining our regulatory mechanisms in order to prevent disorder and disease. With a little effort we can assure proper functioning of the liver, kidneys, colon, lungs, skin and lymph system, which are all intricately involved in keeping the body clean and in well working order. [1,2]

My goal as a parent of a sensitive child is to always seek out the most gentle and thorough options for my money. I look at all of my herbal and nutritional choices first. Will they do the job, or do I need to compliment them with supplements to assist the process? Pharmaceutical answers are considered as a very last resort in my family; obviously it depends on the potential outcome of their treatment vs. the reliability of my own.

I'm confident in my healthcare judgment. You should be confident in yours. The more you educate yourself about all of your different options the more certain you will become that you are making the best possible choices for your child. You don't have to choose the pharmaceutical quick-fix when you know they often bring a whole new set of problems.

A Cleaning System

Detoxification involves several important organs working together to regulate the whole individual. Staying mindful of their needs will help keep the body thriving and running well, to assure longevity for yourself and for your youngster.

Liver

The liver is dedicated to maintaining digestion, breakdown and conversion of nutrients, storing of nutrients, breakdown of toxins, hormonal precursors and regulation, destroying invaders and overall functioning.

As your major detoxification center the liver works hard to remove harmful substances that you consume, extracts waste materials from your blood, and it deactivates toxins so they can be eliminated by the body. Unwanted viruses, cancer cells, fungi and bacteria are destroyed by powerful and very special cells in your liver called Kuepfer's cells. They permit filtering and eradication of harmful attackers. There are countless things you can do to enhance proper functioning of these important processes, along with your liver and therefore many other wellness factors. Stay tuned. [1, 2, 3]

Kidneys

Our kidneys work overtime to protect us from all sorts of various harmful substances, medications and chemical influences in our lives. Toxins get filtered out of the blood and flushed out into our urine for convenient disposal. Some harmful substances can do a lot of damage to the kidneys and clog the filtering processes, hindering removal of toxic elements in the body. [1, 2]

The kidneys are an important organ for managing fluid balance at the cellular level and within the blood vessels. They are an important center for blood pressure.

Intestines

Digestion starts in the mouth, continues in the stomach and heads to the intestinal tract, connecting with a microcosm of competing organisms vying for the nutritional content of your last meal.

Complex food molecules get converted to simpler forms that our cells are able to recognize and absorb. Nutrients like amino acids, fats, minerals, vitamins and sugars enter through intestinal membranes via capillaries; then are transported to the liver for purification and redistribution into the blood stream.

Unwanted chemicals, toxins, drugs, heavy metals and even

your excess sex hormones are quickly purged and dissolved by the liver, turning them to bile to be excreted in the stool. [1]

The colon is in charge of the last stage of elimination. With the help of special micro flora it breaks down any leftover useful substances, such as fiber, transporting it to the liver for decontamination. The intestinal mucous membranes absorb nutrients for use and remove contaminates from the body. When these filters are healthy and working properly they expel unwanted materials like heavy metals and pesticides from the blood stream. Anything left over gets turned into fecal matter and flushed. [1]

When these vital processes get delayed or impaired digested food cannot be discarded properly and begins to ferment. It will putrefy the gut, turning good bacteria into bad, as micro flora mutates into aggressive microorganisms that emit other toxic substances into the body to fight the invasion. This can become a vicious cycle with damaging outcomes for adults and children alike.[1]

Lymph System

The lymph system is also a very important part of detoxification and defense. Lymph fluid runs its course through your lymphatic vessels, circulating throughout the entire body at any given time. Lymph is formed from the extra cellular fluid that protects each of your cells. This system is pressurized and runs best with frequent movement and activity to keep it free flowing. [1]

This fluid detoxifies cellular waste to be carried away by the bloodstream and eliminated. The lymphatic gland groups purify the body and produce white blood cells for defense. During invasions white blood cells increase rapidly, gaining intensity to match the aggressor. The lymph nodes that are closest to the site of infection are the first to swell in response.

When lymph nodes get clogged the body looks for any alternative routes to remove the garbage. If none are available, it begins to make a lot of extra mucous, signaling that there is a problem. Another alternative is to send toxins out the skin. That's why we get acne and other skin issues. When lymph gets trapped and is unable to be released, lactic acid begins to form and store up in the body causing inflammation. [1, 4]

Remember, inflammation is part of your normal repair process, but if it gets out of control it can be a precursor to disease. It is the alarm system warning you that your body is fighting something.

Lungs

During normal air and blood circulation toxins are transported into the lungs and released through exhalation of carbon dioxide gas. Phlegm also plays a major cleansing role; it is produced and released by our mucous membranes to keep our lungs clean. This sticky substance collects and traps unwanted invaders to be expelled from the body by any means available. [1]

Skin

Your skin is the largest organ of the body, taking in toxic exposures unfiltered like a giant sponge, sending them straight into the currents of your bloodstream. Rashes can signal a toxic discharge of some sort. The skin works to maintain your temperature to keep you comfortable. Its amazing sensory abilities play an important part in toxic filtering and elimination using the sweat glands for release.

These organs can get mucked up with daily exposure to all sorts of environmental toxins. Minimizing the damage, starts with assessing those toxic load factors in your life and in the body. This can help you determine how and where you need to focus your efforts.

Toxic Load

Your toxic load is essentially the accumulated toxins that are burdening your body's organs at any given time. Toxins enter and attack from a variety of sources like the environment and your food. These toxins are also stored in fat cells which become a toxin, in and of themselves, as they emit excess estrogen. Your consumption habits are the worst offenders of this whole process.[1]

Little bodies, and big ones too, are having more difficulty these days ridding themselves of these pollutants, heavy metals and pesticides due to their extensive overuse all around us—all the time in homes and industry in nearly every community. Inevitably they lurk in the air we breathe, the water we drink and the food we eat. These contaminants are well known for causing developmental issues and delays in children and fetuses, along with disease and disorders in people and wildlife. Removing them as efficiently and naturally as possible from our bodies, our homes and our children is in the best interest of our health and that of our little people.

Knowing isn't half the battle; action is required here in full force, but gently of course. What I mean is, it will take continuous and ongoing efforts on your part and on their part, as well, to remain essentially toxin free because the world around us is full of it. What we need to do is re-program the body to do its job again. The key here is to remove the gunk, free up the systems and recapture the vibrant ability to cleanse ourselves naturally. Assuring proper methylation is the door that fits this key.

We can help to maximize the body's ability to function and restore itself by promoting good methylation. This will allow our children to overcome the damage from these past encounters to welcome in the age of wellness.

Methylation

Methylation is the cornerstone of the body's ability to detoxify itself. It involves combinations of methyl groups. Think of them as communities of little workers, inside your cells, that essentially determine the essence of who you are. Methyl groups pass important signals back and forth as the central function of methylation. They decide everything from how you look to how you act and what you become; they form your genetic expression [6].

The entirety of this system depends on the very accuracy of the methyl communities and their ability to deliver and execute their orders accurately, so that genes are turned on and off, as needed, throughout the entire 67 billion miles of genetic pathways that make up your human genome [5]. That's a lot of responsibility on these little guys, being in charge of human functioning to such a grave extent (some pun fun).

Methylation is hindered by deficiencies in folic acid (Folate-B9) and/or in vitamin B12. Folate (folic acid) comes from a variety of green vegetables and the B12 comes mainly in animal proteins. Vegans need to supplement this important nutrient. When methylation breaks down the pathways become impaired and messages can get really fouled up. We start to see autoimmune and neurological diseases like autism, ADHD, chronic fatigue, dementia, anxiety, depression, lupus, multiple sclerosis, seizure disorders, etc., etc., etc. [6]

When your methyl groups are happy and methylation runs smoothly the less desired genes are quickly shut down and turned off, while more favored genes are turned on and reproduced. This is essentially the order of communication between your nervous system and your immune system, as methylation acts as the master of detoxification. [6]The troops are mobilized and threats are averted as the attackers are destroyed. Toxins become water-soluble during proper detox so the body can eliminate them more effectively. [7] Your hormone functioning also relies on proper methylation, as it controls histamine to minimize allergic reactions and things like asthma. [6]

Poor methylation will also disrupt nerve performance that can lead to such issues as muscle twitching, numbness, weakness, seizures, fatigue, memory, vision and even hearing loss. The Autism Spectrum Disorders (ASD) generally have very poor nerve functioning as well. Methylation imbalances have been implicated in anxiety, depression, bipolar disorder, insomnia, OCD, Parkinson's, schizophrenia, and will most certainly affect your concentration and focus. [6]

The overall growth & development of your child relies on the quality of these methylation processes, even commanding cell repair for healing. This cellular regeneration becomes compromised as toxins, pathogens and pollution work to interfere with the body's production of these vital methyl groups and the messages they carry. [6]

How can you ensure that your child's methylation processes are well functioning and detoxification is going smoothly? There are so many beneficial actions you can take to clean out your little munchkin. Besides consuming GMO-Free and organic, as much as possible, here are some additional considerations.

Eat Whole Foods

Whole fruits and vegetables will give little bodies the right balance of vitamins and nutrients so they can naturally detoxify themselves. Whole foods contain those crucial phytochemicals to help remove yucky buildup and toxins from the liver and kidneys so that they can function at their best. [6]

Eat the Clean 15

The Environmental Working Group (EWG) releases a yearly list of the fruits and vegetables with the lowest levels of pesticide residues. To be honest, I amended the most recent list for your GMO-Free ease—removing corn, papaya, and pineapple (soon to market). I relocated them to the "Dirty Dozen" list (now the "Dirty 15"?) because of GMO concerns (sorry Environmental Working Group.) Now what's left on your *cleanfood* plate is, avocados, cabbage, sweet peas (frozen), onions, asparagus, mango, kiwi, eggplant, grapefruit, cantaloupe, cauliflower and sweet potatoes. These contain the lowest pesticide residues of any food crops. The EWG ran pesticide tests of 48 most common produce items. The results are listed at *ewg.org*. This list will help you determine which fruits and vegetables you want to be buying organic versus ones you can likely trust for minimal exposure. [8]

Eat Grass-fed Meat

The poultry, pork, beef and fish sold in your typical grocery store and in restaurants is likely being raised on corn and soy products, with standards that inherently cause a buildup of toxins in the meat. Grass-fed beef, for example, is full of B vitamins to keep methylation running smoothly.

We know these commercial practices work against us by depleting the healthy fats from the meat. Consuming it can have a toxic effect, wreaking havoc on hormone production and our metabolism. [9]

Add Probiotics and Fermented Foods

Adding beneficial microorganisms to the body through consumption of fermented foods and quality supplements is vital to rebalancing internal detoxification. These little microbes live throughout the body in little ecosystems. They protect us from harmful invaders and control immunity while also managing the gut-brain connection.

These beneficial bacteria depend on us for a rich source of plant-based foods that should be readily available from our daily diet. This is where you really get ahead of the game. Probiotics work to repair the damage and restore gut function and boost immunity. Fermented foods are simple and inexpensive to make; plus they are a great way to get quality probiotics in the diet, naturally. [10]

Add Quality Coconut Oil to your Daily Diet

Earning its superfood status, this outstanding anti-inflammatory, coconut oil, contains a surplus of health benefits. It can be used safely at high temperatures without going rancid like other oil, including olive oil. Studies show this healthy fat kills off viruses, harmful bacteria and fungi, along with staph and candida. It also promotes digestion, weight loss and can increase liver function.

Coconut oil has many proven anti-cancer properties, and it has even been used to moderate seizures, because it increases ketones throughout the bloodstream. [11] It also works great as a skin moisturizer and even a non-toxic sunscreen for you and the kiddos, because it has a slight Sun Protection Factor (SPF) of around 4-5. So it's good for short jaunts.

We use coconut oil several times a day in my house. I might even suggest everyone incorporate it into a daily oil-pulling regimen for the entire household.

Add a Daily Oil Pulling Regimen

Oil pulling has been commonly used throughout Asia and India for over 3,000 years. It is an ancient Ayurvedic traditional treatment that is helpful in cleansing the body via the mouth. It also helps to reduce inflammation, kill infection and improve oral health. [12] I suggest you try it first, become comfortable, and then demonstrate it for your child. My youngest doesn't mind doing it at all. It's something that's easy and kind of fun. Begin by swishing about a ½-1 teaspoon of coconut oil in your mouth (sesame and olive oil can also be used). Ideally, you could get to a point where you are swishing 15 minutes, one to three times a day and more during periods of illness or infection.

. . . .

> **Note:** Be sure your child is old enough to understand the process. The oil is not to be swallowed, as it turns to a toxic, milky-like, foamy substance in the mouth. It must be discarded (spit) into the toilet, trash or outside where it will not be walked in and tracked about. Do not spit it into the sink. It is toxic and can clog your drain. Afterwards, rinse your mouth completely with warm water a couple times, and then brush your teeth well.

. . . .

My family uses oil pulling in between regular brushing. On occasion when someone has a toothache, I find that it really helps to minimize the pain and helps kill the infection. Stepping up the process to 3 times a day will prove beneficial if you are fighting issues elsewhere in the body and for prevention purposes. [12]

Buy BPA-Free Products and Canned Foods

You've probably seen the BPA-Free labels on baby bottles and other plastic kitchenware. Did you know it is in your canned food products too? Bisphenol-A (BPA) is an industrial chemical used to make hard plastics, and is also used to line food and beverage cans for preservation. BPA is made from what used to be used as a pharmaceutical replacement for the female hormone estrogen; until they figured out they could manipulate it into a hard plastic material. It has been linked to cancer and serious developmental damage in fetuses and young children.[13, 14]

In 2010, I stumbled across a website called *ourstolenfuture.org*, and I was shocked to discover the controversy behind the use of BPA. That same year, the National Toxicology Program reported that they had *"some concern for effects on the brain, behavior, and prostate gland in fetuses, infants, and children at current human exposures to bisphenol A."* [13, 14]

Glass jars, containers, cups and bowls are always preferred over plastic. If you must purchase canned food, look for producers that are committed to using BPA-Free containers. Some producers have stopped using it in their cans, like Trader Jo's and Eden Foods, except for their tomato-based products because of the high acidity. I only buy tomato products that come in glass, because they do not come in BPA-Free cans at all. You will want to run a search for BPA-Free producers.

When this chemical is used in food cans and plastic drink ware, it has been known to leach differing levels of synthetic estrogen hormones into the food and drinks of our little tykes (and big peeps too). BPA is used to make the large plastic jugs (#7) that you see on water cooler systems in doctors' offices or perhaps where you work.[13, 14] (See the science for yourself at *ourstolenfuture.org*).

Add Pure Drinking Water

Did you know that the water you drink becomes part of your bloodstream after 30 minutes? Clean water is essential, and the best water on the planet is filtered spring water which has been collected from a mountain. Natural spring water is free of most of the contaminants you usually get in tap water when harvested correctly. It is also a good source of essential minerals and maintains the body's pH levels in a way that promotes a state of alkalinity for your body. Freshly harvested spring water can be the purest, cleanest water available. Being that water is a big part of the body's detoxification process, it's important to encourage it rather than drinks of any other kind.[14]

Drink Lemon Juice in Filtered Water

There is good reason to drink lemon water. It's not just for fancy restaurants. It actually serves a valuable purpose, most people don't realize. A little lemon alkalizes the water and helps to maintain your body's pH in a healthy range—that is not too acidic and not too alkaline. Ideally, the body prefers a tidy 7.4 reading on that little color strip. I typically keep them around the house to check our levels and those of our drinking water.

I encourage my family to drink one cup of water before breakfast with one teaspoon of fresh squeezed lemon juice, *without adding sweetener, not even honey.*

Raw Organic Apple Cider Vinegar (ACV)

It seems odd that something so acidic would change your pH levels in the gut making them less acidic and more alkaline. My husband says you can remember it like this, "Acidic foods make you sweet, sweet foods make you acidic." Thanks Robert! That's a great tip! Besides lemon water, another great way to maintain our pH balance is to drink the following mixture: Begin with ¼-½ tablespoon of ACV to 2 ounces of water, or even organic apple juice (at first), 1-3 times per day. Once you've establish that, you can work up to a full tablespoon mixed with 2 ounces of water or the organic juice, if needed. Although, ACV is packed full of benefits it has a strong, very acidic taste that takes time to adjust to, and it will eat the enamel off your teeth, so don't drink it strait.

ACV is great for flushing out toxins and heavy metals like mercury from the body and brain. It's been used for centuries as a cure-all and it's not hard to see why. Cider has strong anti-viral, anti-bacterial and anti-fungal properties. The father of modern medicine, Hippocrates, prescribed ACV to his patients for all kinds of ailments. It has been used to alleviate symptoms of acid reflux, acne, allergies, arthritis, candida, chronic fatigue, gout, gum infection, high cholesterol, joint pain, rheumatism, sinus infection, sore throat and much more. (15)

Whenever one of my family members catches cold or begins to feel that tickle in the back of their throat, I pull out the ACV, and generally, it tends to knock out that bug before it has a chance to take hold. Usually by the next day it's pretty well gone. ACV reacts to many of the toxins in the body, converting them into less toxic substances so that they can be safely flushed out.

If you eat the standard Western diet it wreaks havoc on your insides, which are probably more acidic than they should be. You can test this using standard PH strips that you can get in most pharmacies. The exciting part is that, once you start maintaining your body in a more alkaline state, you literally cannot get sick. This is the real key to staying well and avoiding all sorts of chronic illness and dis-ease. [15]

Incorporate Regular Movement

Involving daily amounts of physical movement, you know exercise, increases your blood-flow, boosts serotonin and balances out those wacky-ass hormones. I don't need to convince you that regular movement has an entire semi-truck load of health benefits and makes a world of difference in the attitude; but did you know that it's also necessary for proper detoxification and metabolism? Your physical activity acts as a pump, cleaning the entire lymphatic system. That's important for the health of your whole body, and it keeps everything from becoming stagnant which will allow toxic buildup.

Glutathione

Another key performer in the body's natural detoxification activity is something called glutathione, which is often recognized as your "master antioxidant." Inside your cells, this little-known superhero comes to your rescue, day and night, with an invisible cloak of protection that neutralizes those harmful, free-radical attacks from environmental chemicals, pollutants and radiation. Glutathione enhances the immune system and cleanses your liver - making it an essential component of detoxification. [16]

Consider this, under the toxic strain of modern daily living low glutathione levels can shove us right into a full fledge, toxic overload situation, that can keep us, and especially little ones, sick and exhausted for a good amount of time. Glutathione recycles the antioxidants, including itself within all of your body's cells.

Glutathione is naturally composed, by the body, using three amino acids that must be present: cysteine, glutamate, and glycine. It can only be formed precisely from these amino acids when magnesium, potassium and sufficient energy are all available to work the cycle together. [16]

Again, I can't help but to think about how this ties in to the potential consequences of what Dr. Samsel and Seneff reveal in their study series "Glyphosate, pathways to modern diseases...I-V." Remember, "Glyphosate III..." focuses on glyphosate's chelation of manganese and the resulting health effects, including a compelling link to autism. And... "Glyphosate V..." that provides a substantial case for the possibility that glyphosate masquerades as an analogue of glycine, getting into our proteins by mistake. This feature alone, the researchers say, could easily explain the rise we are seeing in multiple modern conditions and diseases, such as autism, Alzheimer's, diabetes, obesity, rheumatoid arthritis, kidney failure and various cancers.

Could this be the pivotal smoking gun that connects the "roundup" of chronic disease, with the body's *inability* to detoxify itself, directly aligned with modern "advancements" in synthetic nutrition? In other words, are these the expected consequences of GMOs and their pesticide companions in bodies that do not recognize them as genuine nutritional components?

Glutamine

Your brain produces another amino acid called glutamine; this is your body's most common amino acid, made from glutamate. It turns into glutathione. This stuff is more precious than gold because it naturally flushes out those heavy metals, toxins and phytochemicals. Amazingly, it also stops and repairs genetic mutations caused by chemical elements and other biological threats. It keeps the nucleus from breaking down and being destroyed. This battle rages on every day within all the cells of your body. [16]

The great news is that real food sources can really help to replenish glutathione, either directly or through natural conversion. It is generally produced inside the body but is also found in raw meats, fruits and vegetables. Phytochemicals like sulforaphane in broccoli, Brussel sprouts, cabbage and cauliflower, along with the chlorophyll in greens, will all help bring glutathione levels back up in the body. Turmeric, cinnamon and cardamom also have compounds to restore those levels. Beets will boost enzymes, helping to facilitate this process as well. [16]

Studies have shown that oral supplements and some food sources of glutathione are not the best way to raise cellular levels, but they can even be absorbed into cells of the intestines to support digestive health and further the detoxification process. Note: there is also strong evidence that glutathione supplements may interfere with your body's own glutathione production, so you might find it best to stick with real food sources and let the body do what it knows. [16, 17] Some synthetic supplements can signal your systems to stop producing certain substances, so do your homework on the supplements that you choose for yourself and your children. [16, 17]

Researchers report that glutathione is destroyed by heat, pasteurization and processing. Only raw vegetables, raw fruit, raw eggs, raw unpasteurized milk and dairy, along with raw and rare-cooked meats are high in glutathione, although I never suggest feeding a child raw meat or raw eggs in order to increase their levels. [16, 17]

Breast milk studies show a remarkable 73-80 percent reduction rate in glutathione readings only after 2 hours of being frozen. Amounts decreased over 79 percent after refrigeration, and at room temperature the glutathione levels were dropped by as much as 73 percent, so you can recognize the importance of breast feeding from the source, rather than pumping and preserving. [17]

There is hard evidence that vitamin D increases intercellular production of glutathione. Raw whole foods, herbs and spices can properly support glutathione, using precursors that will help to recycle the oxidized (used) glutathione back into the usable form that the body needs.

Fever Reducers and Glutathione

Acetaminophen fever reducers, like Tylenol, are known to deplete levels of glutathione during a process of conversion the body uses to change the drug into something less toxic. This is so your kiddo doesn't end up with liver failure. In fact, you might be interested to find out acetaminophen is the second highest cause of liver failure in the United States. In the UK it's reported to be number one. Keep in mind that fever, all by itself, essentially isn't a threat. Whenever your child gets a fever it works to raise the glutathione levels in the body to facilitate the healing process. Administering a fever reducer is likely to slow the healing process, rather than hasten it.[18, 19]

Use your own motherly instincts to determine when it is appropriate to administer drugs to remedy discomfort.

To increase glutathione levels naturally, try to avoid:

Processed Foods

Processed foods typically contain a number of toxic synthetic chemicals, preservatives, MSG, dyes, "spices", "natural" and artificial flavors. These are *dead* foods that are synthetically made to taste good to get you and your kids addicted.

They are highly toxifying, unnatural non-foods, regardless of what they say on the box. (20, 21)

The "Dirty Dozen"

All of your fruits and vegetables should be eaten organic, if possible, to avoid pesticides. When it's not possible you have the "Dirty Dozen" list, created by the Environmental Working Group (EWG). Their analysis has determined that to minimize pesticide exposure we should avoid the following foods: apples, celery, cherry tomatoes, cucumbers, grapes, hot peppers, nectarines (imported), peaches, potatoes, spinach, strawberries and sweet bell peppers. This list focuses specifically on pesticides and is updated every year by the EWG. [22]

Toxic Cleaning and Personal Hygiene Products

Chemical ingredients like Sodium Lauryl Sulfate, Triclosan, Polysorbates and many others appear in these products. These toxins easily absorb into the skin, which soaks them up like a sponge, absorbing them directly into the blood stream. Cleaners and many personal products increase toxic your load factors considerably. Your local market has many safer, greener alternatives. [23]

Antibiotics

Antibiotics destroy healthy gut flora, impede detoxification, causing long-term immune dysfunction. Minimize exposure to foods treated with glyphosate and/or Roundup which act as antibiotics to destroy your good gut bacteria where most of the immune system resides.[24]

I incorporate recipes from all kinds of "food-styles," from the Weston Price diet to Paleo, vegan and even some raw food. It's really all about what works best for you, your family and your wallet. [26]

Barring any dietary restrictions, I try to avoid putting myself and my family into any sort of rigid dietary box, outside of organic and GMO-Free, because it makes good food easier to find when I keep my options open.

By eating organic you can limit your family's exposure to GMOs, toxins and pesticides. Outside of that there are many ways to maintain a clean healthy diet. The best thing to do is to experiment with different foods. Try incorporating foods from other cultures and seek out different dietary concepts to see what works best for you and your body, as well as your GMO-Free child.

Try Paleo, if you are a carnivore who suspects gluten issues, dairy allergies or the need to limit carbs. Check out *paleodiet.com* for a huge, delicious assortment of wheat free, gluten free and dairy free recipes. [25]

Weston A. Price Diet

Weston A. Price was a dentist that traveled the world examining different dietary habits of various cultures, prior to and following the processed food revolution. His dietary recommendations were written in 1920, and include some of the best and most straight-forward advice for healthy eating.

Weston A. Price discovered that our best fat-soluble activators, come in the form of vitamins A, D and K and are found in high amounts in traditional diets containing foods like eggs, meat, butter and some seafood. His approach includes,

- Eat foods that are natural, unprocessed and organic (and contain no sugar except for the occasional bit of honey or maple syrup). [26]

- Eat more foods that grow in your native environment, that are in season. Eat local as much as possible.
- Eat unpasteurized dairy products (such as raw milk) and fermented foods.
- Eat at least one-third of your food raw.
- Be sure to get enough healthy fats and omega-3s from animal sources and reduce omega-6 intake from vegetable oils. [26]

It is highly important to understand when your body is deficient in essential metals, it will start using toxic heavy metals as replacements in order to make up for the lack of those minerals. [27]

GAPS Diet

We've had good luck implementing portions of the following nutritional programs, based on my daughter's changing needs. Many parents have seen major improvements with food allergies, physical symptoms, communication skills, cognitive functioning and even learning abilities can really increase.

It's been quite a process, but I do believe it has been a strategic combination of our GMO-Free/organic diet, along with adaption of the relevant parts of the Gut and Psychology Syndrome (GAPS) Diet, that has really helped the situation with my daughter improve. GAPS is used as a natural alternative therapy for patients suffering from autism, ADHD/ADD, dyslexia, dyspraxia, depression and schizophrenia.[29]

Following her son's struggle with learning challenges, Dr. Natasha Campbell-McBride created this specialized approach to address the multitudes of digestive and immune disorders, learning disabilities, psychiatric and psychological disorders that are overwhelming our medical communities, our children and the parents who love them.

The purpose of the GAPS treatment, the doctor says, is to detoxify the body, removing toxic brain fog while allowing for proper development and cognitive functioning. She suggests we clean up and repair the digestive tract to reverse a major source of toxicity in the brain and body. [29]

About 90% of the poisons in your blood and brain are directly from your gut, says Dr. Campbell-McBride. Gut repair efforts tend to show significant drops in toxicity levels for the body. She knows, because her clinical outcomes display massive benefits in thousands of adults and children worldwide who have experienced meaningful recovery using these methods. [29]

GAPS protocols are separated into three segments they are: GAPS Diet, GAPS Supplementation and GAPS Detoxification. Each one specifically works to, "heal and seal the gut lining, rebalance the immune system, and restore the optimal bacterial ecosystem within the gastrointestinal tract," the doctor says. It restricts all forms of grains, commercial dairy, starchy vegetables and all of your processed and refined carbohydrates. She focuses on foods that are easily digestible and nutrient dense.

For children struggling to overcome the trials and tribulations of the standard Western diet, she recommends parents ease them into it, in stages, beginning with the Full GAPS Diet, which limits food intake to meat, fish, eggs, fermented foods, vegetables and bone broths. Skipping the Introduction Diet is also acceptable, she says, if your kid is only experiencing mild symptoms. However, with cases of severe allergies and digestive issues it might be best to start with the Introduction Diet, working your way through the different parts as suggested. [30]

She offers a comprehensive line of GAPS books, videos and even a cookbook to make the whole process easier to navigate.

I would note that I do not benefit financially from making any of these statements about GAPS or any other program or product I mention in this book. I have not thoroughly implemented the full program. Like everything else, I take what we need and leave the rest. You should do what you feel is best for your child and your situation.

In order to reap the highest level benefits, the doctor suggests that the GAPS Supplementation protocols be customized to fit the individual needs of the child (or adult). [31] Generally speaking, the doctor also encourages a quality commercial probiotic that will provide the most beneficial bacteria for gut repair and digestion. It includes supplements of essential fatty acids, cod liver oil, plus targeted digestive support that is central to the GAPS program.

A special detoxification protocol is used to flush out toxic chemicals and heavy metals that can damage young guts and developing minds, inhibiting colon and liver functioning. Detoxing these pathways is a key component of the GAPS approach. Her website, *gapsdiet.com,* has a ton of great information and recipes to help you "heal and seal the gut," and to repair the gastrointestinal system within. She offers a really easy way to determine allergies with her Food Sensitivity Test. She also highly recommends daily consumption of homemade bone broths. [29,30, 31]

We do a lot of bone broths at our house. You'll find the recipe in Chapter 9.

Elimination Diet

Allergy testing can be very expensive but for children suffering from food sensitivities and digestive disorders, following the elimination diet for a minimum of 2-3 weeks could be the most helpful and simple technique to identify offending foods. [32]

Some describe results as nothing short of a miracle, as they eliminate specific foods for a short period of time. Slowly, they reintroduce those foods one at a time with a close watch for potential reactions or return of any symptoms. Although it can be difficult, the more food restrictions you put in place during this time, the greater the outcomes will be and the more information you will gather. The most effective elimination diets will always exclude the greatest number of foods, allowing you to investigate and discover the biggest troublemakers for your child's digestion. It is the most efficient and effective way to determine where the issues lie.

Remove foods you suspect might be problematic like dairy, gluten, eggs, wheat, soy, sugar, nuts, beef, citrus, coffee, corn, dairy, fish, nightshades, pork, oats, palm and canola oils. GMOs, pesticides, processed foods and additives of all kinds should also be strictly avoided. [32]

Although they may feel like their missing out on a lot (only at first) the return of some of these foods, one at a time, after the elimination period, will most undoubtedly be a clear indicator of whether or not that particular food is a cause for discomfort. Once you remove all these foods and start providing only what the body essentially needs, it will undergo a total metabolic reset. This allows the body to rest, ease inflammation and restore proper digestive functioning. [32] It's kind of like hitting "control, alt, delete." It's the do-over the body needs to regain its ability to do its job.

You and/or your child may experience periods of withdrawals at any of these junctures, which can cause everything from moodiness, to cravings, headaches, stomach aches and even flu like symptoms and rashes may occur. Sometimes the exorcism of these toxins can cause adverse reactions, and things may get a little worse, before getting better. Anything that is cause for alarm should be stopped, and it bears repeating that you should contact a medical professional in the event of an emergency. [32]

Don't worry, this simplified plan still has plenty of tasty options like quinoa, chicken, turkey, fish, lamb, most fruits and vegetables. If it has been determined that coconut is not an issue, you can try coconut oil, coconut sugar and coconut milk for healthy alternatives to their counterparts. [32]

At *Precisionnutrition.com* there's a very useful table to help you determine which foods you might want to eliminate and which foods you might want to keep.

For the best results you will fully reintroduce each food, one at a time, eating the same quantities as before. Any sensitivity, large or small should be easy to spot, since the body has been free of it for this time period. Log any signs of discomfort.

Next, you will avoid that food again for a minimum of 3 days in order to recognize any delayed responses or subtle changes. If no symptoms are experienced or if only slight, you can try reintroducing it again. If another response is detected then you will want to eliminate this food for several months before reintroducing it. Food sensitivities tend to come and come go, so it doesn't necessarily mean your child will have to avoid any certain food for a lifetime. [32] Food allergies can be a little more tricky.

Lacto-fermented Foods

Fermented foods are nothing to fear when they are done correctly. They can be miracle workers for your health. They have been used in different cultures throughout the world, for thousands of years, to sustain wellness and maintain the gut.

You're familiar with fermented foods like cheese and pickles, but did you know that raw cultured vegetables are an important part of a well-balanced diet? Lacto-fermented foods allow the release of beneficial micro-organisms that are naturally present in the vegetables, and in the digestive tract, to break down sugar and starches and allow for proper digestion. [33]

Rounds of antibiotics and environmental toxins can upset the delicate balance of our gut flora, increasing the risk of overgrowth by a naturally occurring yeast, called candida that will inevitably cause additional health problems in your child's body, if not addressed. Raw fermented foods are equipped to manage candida, and put the balance back in our favor to boost digestive power and secure our level of wellness. The best health insurance against chronic illness is a well-balanced microbiome, as we discussed earlier.

Raw cultured vegetables improve immune functioning and have been shown to be an effective treatment for conditions such as allergies, colic, constipation, cystitis, diarrhea, digestive disorders, inflammation, ulcers, ulcerative colitis and even vaginal infections. [33]

Many physicians have written about the health benefits of these magnificiant foods. German Doctor Johannes Kuhl wrote several books on the subject of cancer including, *Cancer in Check*, where he offers ample evidence that regular consumption of raw cultured vegetables can prevent cancer. [33] In another book, *Healing with Whole Foods*, Paul Pitchford (one of my respected IIN instructors) discusses the benefits of cultured foods to promote better nutrient absorption from the diet. Besides restoration of healthy gut flora, cultured foods can also help:

- Break down food and improve digestibility,
- Enhance blood circulation,
- Balance acidity in the gut, restoring pH levels,
- Protect against chronic illnesses and cancer,
- Work as a disinfectant, killing bacterial infections and;
- Produce vitamin B12 that is essential to our blood-cell development and DNA performance. [33]

Cultured foods are hugely beneficial to any detox program, but they are especially important for children with chronic health and digestive issues due to ever increasing toxic load factors. [34.36]

As you can see, there are many facets to consider with any gentle detoxification program that you choose. I suggest taking it slow; after all it is a process and not an event. Be aware that your child may begin to show some detox symptoms that can include body aches, constipation, diarrhea, headaches, nausea, sinus congestion, sore throat, skin rashes, or even flu-like symptoms, because the cells in the body begin releasing stored up toxins and pathogens that need to come out. [35] It is important to maintain hydration during this time.

The body's pathways have been obstructed by toxic waste, and once they begin to move symptoms may arise as a result of dying pathogenic microorganisms that release toxins into the bloodstream. [35] Scale back on the process a little during periods of discomfort. Discontinue methods if anything arises that you feel is concerning and seek medical attention immediately. Use your best judgment and keen mama senses. You know your child best.

Eliminating the incoming toxins is really a critical component of any detoxification program. Take it slow and feed them well and they will respond, Mom and Dad (just watch and smile :)!

At times elimination diets are not enough. Sometimes the

body needs a little extra help with detoxification. That's where a qualified natural practitioner, such as a naturopath, can be an invaluable resource and a mom's best friend.

Toxic Load Reduction Quiz

Here's a quick analysis tool to help give you a general overview of the toxic burden, weighing on your child, from day-to-day exposure levels. [28] There are many, many factors that need to be considered. This quiz is not meant to be a diagnostic tool. Answer honestly, and then allow other family members to participate, if you wish. Add up the scores to see how you might step up your healthy options in order to better serve you and your child.

	Always 5	Mostly 4	Some-times 3	Never 0
I buy organic produce.				
I buy organic dairy.				
I eat grass-fed meat/organic poultry.				
I avoid grilling or eating burnt food.				
I drink quality filtered or spring water.				
I avoid prescription drugs where possible				
I avoid processed foods with more than 5 ingredients.				
I buy GMO-Free vitamins and supplements.				
I avoid cooking in a microwave.				
I avoid Teflon coated non-stick pans.				
I avoid plastic for food storage and BPA- lined canned foods.				
I avoid eating out at restaurants.				
I use green household cleaners in my home.				
I avoid standard bath and hygiene products.				
Pesticides/herbicides are not sprayed around my home, school and/or office.				
I avoid dry cleaning services.				
I avoid mercury dental fillings.				
Total				

75-85 Excellent!

You are really making a sincere effort to keep your toxicity low and maintain a healthy environment for your family. Way to make a difference!

64-74 Honorable efforts

You are clearly taking steps to decrease toxicity levels in your family and in your home. You are determined to make a difference. Keep up the good work!

53-73 Average efforts

You can see the benefits of reducing toxins from your food and environment. You are on the path of change and just need to step up your game a little to maintain a healthy, toxin-free environment for your family. It will make a difference.

42-52 Below average

You can do better. Taking action, right now, to reduce your family's toxic load will benefit them and you, immensely. There are so many measurable steps that you can take to cleanup your food and environment, and it will certainly help your family to live a more disease-free life.

0-41 Warning high toxic load!

Any, and all, efforts that you make to reduce the toxic load burden, right now, will be a huge benefit to your family. They are being bombarded with things like chemicals, pesticides, GMOs and heavy metals that are affecting their health and yours; although you may not know it yet. These and other toxic ingredients like parabens, phthalates, mercury, lead and organophosphates really have an impact on our health, especially for the little ones.

Some chemicals are endocrine disruptors, others impact the neurotransmitters, immune system, development and/or digestive functioning. The sooner you get on the road to change, the sooner you will begin to reverse the damage and reap the major health benefits of doing so. [28]

CHAPTER 9

····································

GMO-Free Recipes

When diet is wrong, medicine is of no use. When diet is correct, medicine is of no need.

—Ayurvedic Proverb

Here's the big secret to organic cooking. Are you ready? There is not one recipe, nor any dish that you can imagine, that you cannot make with organic ingredients. There is always a way; that is why this process will be much easier than you think it will be. You can take your favorite recipes and make them better. Make them organic and you will see how quickly your family adapts to this new healthy lifestyle.

Please assume that all of these recipes call for organic versions of each ingredient, if and when possible. However, the ingredients that I specify "organic" below in the recipes, should undoubtedly, be organic or at least GMO-Free to properly maintain your GMO-Free child. You can only do what you can do, but be sure to do what you can to maximize all of the benefits organic has to offer your family, as your economic standards will allow.

You don't want to overlook all of the fabulous recipes online. You can entirely recreate your favorite meals into healthier, even more delicious versions than they already are.

Let's start thinking outside of that GMO "SAD" food box and

begin to find the real pleasure in healthy living. Good luck and happy eating!

· ·

Helpful hint: Soak all raw grains, nuts and seeds for 12-24 hours before consuming to induce sprouting and minimize levels of phytic acid that block digestion, nutrient absorption and the live enzymes that help you break down your food.

· ·

Breakfast

Best Yummy Detox Smoothie

Kids just love this thick and creamy smoothie! It gives them a great start for the day and helps them get rid of all those toxins.

Ingredients:

1 cup cold home-made almond milk*

1 small handful of kale

1-2 pieces of fresh parsley

1 organic chilled green apple

1 frozen medium banana

2-3 pitted dates

½ avocado

Ice optional (made with purified water)

Optional ingredients: Frozen Berries Flax or Chia seeds

Serves: 2

* See recipe under "Alternatives & Replacements"

Directions:

Slice up banana and freeze it in pieces in an air-tight container overnight. Add ice to the recipe, if you missed this step. Combine all ingredients in the blender, mix well and serve immediately. Beneficial enzymes in the food begin to break down soon after blending. Smoothies should be consumed within 10 minutes to maintain nutritional integrity.

Berry Fruity Smoothie

Ingredients:

1 overripe frozen banana

1 cup blueberries

½ cup raspberries

½ cup romaine lettuce

½ cup spinach

½ avocado

½ cup filtered water

½ cup homemade almond* or organic coconut milk (carrageenan free)

Serves: 2

*   See recipe under "Alternatives & Replacements"

Directions:

Slice banana and freeze pieces in air-tight container overnight or add some ice to the recipe if you forget. Combine all ingredients in the blender, mix well and serve right away.

April's Good Morning Granola

Ingredients:

2 cups organic and or gluten free oats

½ cup mixed nuts and seeds (chia seeds, sesame seeds, pumpkin seeds, sunflower seeds all work well)

½ cup shredded coconut

4 tablespoons coconut oil

3 tablespoons organic butter

1 teaspoon cinnamon

¼ cup raw honey

¼ cup organic raw coconut sugar or agave

1 teaspoon of vanilla

Servings: 2-3

Directions:

Heat up 2 tablespoons of coconut oil in a frying pan over medium heat. Add oats and stir very frequently—cook 5-6 minutes, being watchful, since they tend to scorch easily.

Remove oats from pan and set aside. Lower burner temperature to medium low. Add the rest of the coconut oil, butter, honey, vanilla and coconut sugar (or agave) to the pan and stir constantly, until it bubbles. Stir in the oats, mix well and continue to cook on medium-low for 1-2 minutes. Put mixture into a large bowl and then add your nuts, dried fruit, seeds, shredded coconut, cinnamon and any other ingredients you like. Allow to cool. Store granola mix in a sealed container.

For some extra flavor try adding: dried cranberries, cherries, chocolate chips and/or almond butter.

*Helpful hint: This goes fast around my house. You might want to double the recipe. Enjoy!

Mama's Muesli

A healthy, satisfying good-to-go breakfast for work and school.

Ingredients:

½ cup organic rolled oats

¼ cup walnuts and/or almonds and seeds (flax, chia)

¼ cup of dried cranberries, cherries or dried fruit

1 teaspoon raw coconut

1 teaspoon raw local honey

1 teaspoon organic coconut sugar (optional)

½ cup dairy free milk (canned coconut milk tastes great!)

½ teaspoon of vanilla

Serves: 1

Directions:

Put all of the ingredients in a glass bowl and stir well. Seal with a lid and refrigerate a minimum of 2-hours, but overnight works fine too. Taste your muesli and adjust sweetener and other ingredients as needed.

Vanilla Coconut Pancakes

Ingredients:

1 cup coconut flour

½ cup organic coconut oil melted

3 medium organic eggs

½ cup organic applesauce

½ cup coconut milk (carrageenan free)

¼ cup raw honey

2 tablespoons organic coconut sugar

2 teaspoon vanilla

1 teaspoon baking soda (aluminum free)

extra organic coconut oil to fry with

Serves: 1-2 children

Directions:

Combine coconut flour, coconut oil, eggs, applesauce, milk, honey, vanilla, coconut sugar and baking soda in a bowl. Mix up ingredients well. Coat the frying pan with coconut oil. Pour pancake batter and cook on medium heat 2-3 minutes until both sides are thoroughly cooked.

Almond Corn Flakes

Ingredients:

2 cups (only organic) corn meal or corn flour

1 cup almond meal or almond flour*

3 tablespoons ground flax seed

3 tablespoons hulled hemp seeds

3 tablespoons chia seeds

3 tablespoons raw organic coconut sugar

1 teaspoon Pink Himalayan Salt

2 teaspoons vanilla

1 ½ cups purified water

Servings: 4 cups

* See recipe under "Alternatives & Replacements"

Directions:

Preheat the oven to 350 degrees. In a large mixing bowl, combine dry ingredients and mix well. Add vanilla and water to the mixture. Stir batter, until it is smooth and thin. Pour onto baking sheet, lined with chemical free parchment paper. Then spread your mixture out, until thin and even. Bake for about 50-55 minutes. Cut into small bite-sized pieces and store in a glass container with a lid.

Fancy Banana Nut Muffins

Ingredients:

3 eggs or egg replacements*

3 cups gluten free flour mixture* or almond flour*

¾ cup chopped nuts and seeds—walnuts, almonds, poppy and chia seeds are good options (don't cook flax seeds—unless ground).

2 teaspoons baking soda

¼ teaspoon Pink Himalayan Salt

½ cup of melted organic coconut oil

¼ cup organic apple juice

¼ of homemade almond milk*

Makes: 12- muffins

* See recipe under "Alternatives & Replacements"

Directions:

Preheat oven to 350 degrees. Then smash bananas in a large mixing bowl. Mix all wet ingredients in with it. Combine all dry ingredients in a second bowl and mix well. Add ingredients from the first bowl and stir briefly, just to combine. Do not overmix. Pour batter into well-oiled muffin tin, until ¾ full. Bake for 20-23 minutes. Then test with a toothpick, until clean.

Gluten Free Cinnamon Toast Crunch Cereal

Ingredients:

2 eggs or egg replacements*

¼ cup coconut oil

¼ cup organic applesauce

¼ cup organic whole milk or you can use coconut or homemade almond milk*

1 teaspoon cinnamon

2 teaspoons vanilla extract

¼ teaspoon baking powder

Plus: 2 tablespoons of coconut sugar + 1 ½ teaspoons of cinnamon for coating, mixed.

Makes: about 5 cups

* See recipe under "Alternatives & Replacements"

Directions:

Preheat oven to 350 degrees. Mix all of your dry ingredients together in a mixing bowl, then combine the wet ingredients and stir up well. Roll dough up into two balls, seal in a glass container and put in the refrigerator for one hour or until firm.

Sprinkle parchment paper with flour and add your dough. Cut the dough in half and set one part aside. Coat the rolling pin with flour. Roll out the dough into a thin layer. Transfer it to a (non-aluminum) baking sheet and brush with a light layer of water. Sprinkle on your cinnamon-sugar coating to taste, or just leave it off. Cut into squares. Bake for 12-15 minutes and turn over pieces and cook another 15-18 minutes or as needed.

Honey-Almond Pumpkin Bread

Ingredients:

1 ¾ cups almond flour*

½ teaspoon Pink Hima-
layan Salt

4 large eggs or egg
replacements*

1 ½ teaspoons baking
soda

2 tablespoons pumpkin
pie spice

1 tablespoon cinnamon

1 cup pre-cooked
pumpkin

2 tablespoons raw or-
ganic honey

½ cup of raw organic
coconut sugar

Makes: 2 small
loaves or 1 big loaf
or 12 muffins.

* See recipe under
"Alternatives &
Replacements"

Directions:

Mix together the dry ingredients in a large
mixing bowl. Add the rest of the ingredients and stir until completely blended or
use a hand mixer or blender if you like.
Scrape batter into well-greased pan(s) and
bake at 350° for 20-25 minutes for muffins.
Bake 35-45 minutes for small loaves and
45-55 minutes for a large loaf. Test your
bread with a toothpick or butter knife and
make sure it comes out clean. If not, put it
back in the oven for 5-7 minutes and check
again.

Happy Day Donuts

Ingredients:

3-½ cups organic non-bleached white or

whole wheat flour (sprouted wheat flour is preferred)

2 cups raw organic sugar or coconut sugar

1 teaspoon Pink Himalayan Salt

1 teaspoon nutmeg

5 tablespoon of coconut oil

4 organic eggs or (equal amount ground flax or soaked chia seeds)

2 level teaspoons of baking soda

2 cups of organic buttermilk or organic whole milk, or use a milk alternative mixed a 1 tablespoon of white vinegar

Directions:

Heat oil to 375 degrees. Combine baking soda and milk, Mix in sugar and nutmeg. Add the rest of the ingredients and mix well, until you have thick dough. Dust rolling pin with flour and use to roll out dough, until it's about 1/2 inch thick.

Use a donut cutter. Then deep-fry each one until it turns light golden brown. Flip over once, remove and then you can glaze them with butter and/ or sprinkle coconut sugar, or you can make a nice honey butter glaze for them.

Lunchbox

G.G.'s Potato Salad

Ingredients:

3 pounds organic russet potatoes

1 medium finely chopped onion

6 hardboiled organic eggs chopped small

½ cup small Kosher Dill Pickles, diced (no pickle juice)

2 cups organic mayonnaise (or to taste)

4 tablespoons organic yellow mustard

½ cup finely chopped organic green pepper

½ cup finely chopped organic celery

Add last: Salt and pepper to taste (both black and white, if you have it on hand) ½ teaspoon of dill seed, 1 tablespoon of turmeric and celery seed (optional) to taste.

Optional adds: Celery seeds, Chopped black olives, green onions or chives

Directions:

In a large pot, boil whole potatoes with the skins on, until you can stick a fork in the biggest one, easily. Let them cool at room temperature (Do not refrigerate), until you can safely remove skins (optional). Dice into small or medium size chunks. Add all ingredients in a large mixing bowl, except spices, and mix well without mashing potatoes. Add salt and pepper to taste, along with the other spices. Refrigerate a minimum of one hour before serving.

Note: G.G. says do not refrigerate the potatoes, prior to mixing; they will become sticky and will not absorb flavors. Also, do not add pickle juice to this recipe, G.G. says it changes the taste dramatically, and then you are just on your own!

Makes about: 4 pounds

Cheryl's Delicious Broccoli-Cranberry Salad

Ingredients:

3 heads fresh raw organic broccoli, chopped small

1 medium head of red cabbage, shredded

1 cup organic carrots, shredded

1 cup seedless organic grapes, chopped

½ cup of dried cranberries

¼ cup of organic celery, chopped

¼ cup of raw sunflower seeds

1 small red onion, chopped

¾ cup of organic mayonnaise

¼ cup of yellow mustard

1 teaspoon of Balsamic Vinegar

1 teaspoon of Pink Himalayan Salt

1 teaspoon of turmeric

1 teaspoon of pepper

Directions:

Combine all vegetables into large mixing bowl, mix in mayonnaise, mustard and spices. Mix well and refrigerate in air-tight container for a minimum of one hour and serve.

People Pleasing Pesto

Ingredients:

½ cup Brazil nuts, chopped (almonds or walnuts work too)

1 ½ cups of fresh basil leaves

½ cup fresh parsley

2 medium cloves of garlic

½ cup extra virgin olive oil

1 teaspoon of Raw apple cider vinegar

¼ cup of organic sharp cheddar cheese or parmesan cheese (optional)

Salt and pepper to taste

Directions:

Place nuts in food processer or blender. Blend until smooth. Add oil and pulse, until mixed. Then add remaining ingredients, and mix to desired consistency, being careful not to overmix.

Fermented Summer Salsa

Fermented foods are a great way to provide the body with the good microorganisms it needs to repair the gut and boost immunity.

Ingredients:

1 medium onion, finely chopped

2-3 pounds of tomatoes, diced

1 medium red pepper, diced

2-3 cloves of garlic, minced

½ cup of fresh cilantro

1 whole lemon juiced

2 tablespoons of Pink Himalayan Salt

2 tablespoons raw apple cider vinegar

Directions:

Mix all the ingredients together. Place the salsa in canning jars, pressing the mixture down to release excess liquid. Ideally the vegetables should be well submerged. Add more water as needed.

Sit the canning lid on top (do not put on ring) and put in an out of the way spot where it won't bumped. Let it stand and ferment for 2-3 days at room temperature. Screw on the ring and refrigerate. It will stay good for about 6 months.

Fruit leather

Ingredients:

2 cups organic mangoes (fresh or frozen)

3 cups of organic raspberries (fresh or frozen)

1 cup purified water

2 teaspoons organic lemon juice

4 tablespoons raw organic honey

Makes: 15-16 strips

Directions:

Preheat oven to 175 degrees. Stir all ingredients together into a pot and let simmer for 12 minutes, mix completely and pour into mesh strainer. Spread out the mixture into a thin layer on to chemical-free parchment paper and bake 7-8 hours. Remove from oven and let stand, Peel from paper and cut into strips.

Rosemary Flatbread (gluten free/vegan)

Ingredients:

1 ¼ cup sorghum flour

½ cup teff flour

2/3 cup arrowroot powder (or tapioca starch)

2 teaspoons chia seeds

¾ teaspoon baking soda

¾ teaspoon Pink Himalayan Salt

1 cup warm water

¼ cup extra-virgin olive oil

2 tablespoons raw honey

2 tablespoons raw apple cider vinegar

½ tablespoon minced rosemary

½ tablespoon minced thyme

1 tablespoon ground turmeric

½ teaspoon black pepper

1 tablespoon sesame seeds

Serves: 4-5

Directions:

Preheat oven to 375. Generously, grease a large baking sheet. Combine flour, arrowroot, chia seeds, baking soda, and salt in a mixing bowl and mix well. In a second bowl, combine your wet ingredients and mix. Add your herbs, spices and sesame seeds. Mix together. Then add dry ingredients and stir until mixture becomes a thick, sticky dough. Coat your hands in flour and put dough on baking sheet and press out evenly up to the edges. Poke several holes in the dough so it doesn't bubble up during baking. Bake for 25-30 minutes. Then cut into pieces.

Gluten Free Sandwich Bread

Ingredients:

3 cups of gluten free flour mix*

1 ½ cups warm organic milk or milk alternative

1 teaspoon of ground flax seeds

1 tablespoon of non-aluminum baking powder

¼ cup raw organic coconut sugar or raw organic honey

2 teaspoons of dry active yeast

1 teaspoon Pink Himalayan Salt

2 teaspoons of raw apple cider vinegar

1/3 cup of coconut oil

2 large organic eggs

Makes: 1 loaf

* See recipe under "Alternatives & Replacements"

Directions:

Oil and flour your bread pan well. Warm up your milk just slightly. Mix in sugar and then add the yeast. Let sit for a good 10-12 minutes. It should get fizzy. If not then your yeast is no good.

Mix all of your dry ingredients into a large mixing bowl. Then combine your wet ingredients in a second bowl and stir well. Combine the dry and wet ingredients, then mix them together thoroughly.

Pour your bread mixture into well-greased bread pan (glass is best) and place into a warm area and let it rise for 25-30 minutes. The dough should double in size, but not above the rim of the pan.

Meanwhile, preheat your oven to 375 degrees. Then bake your bread for about 35-45 minutes, until it appears golden brown.

Chicky's Corn Bread

Ingredients:

- 1 cup organic whole milk or coconut milk
- 1 tablespoon organic raw apple cider vinegar (Bragg's is great)
- 2 cups organic corn meal
- 1 teaspoon Pink Himalayan Salt (84 minerals)
- 2 tablespoons aluminum-free baking powder
- ¼ **cup** raw organic cane sugar or raw honey
- 2 tablespoons coconut oil
- ¼ **cup organic** applesauce

Directions:

Preheat oven to 425 degrees. Oil an 8x8 baking dish. Mix vinegar and milk in a mixing bowl, and set aside. In a separate bowl, combine dry ingredients and mix well. Then add the rest of the ingredients to the milk mixture, stir, and then combine with dry ingredients. Mix well and pour into baking dish. Bake for 25-28 minutes. Use a toothpick to check if it's done.

Dinner

Chicken Soup

Ingredients:

6 cups of home-made chicken bone broth (recipe below)

3-4 medium carrots peeled and shredded

2 celery ribs, diced

1 large onion, diced

1½-2 cups shredded chicken

1 whole package of spaghetti noodles or gluten free pasta or homemade noodles if you have the time.

Fresh herbs like rosemary, parsley thyme and/or oregano.

Directions:

Combine all ingredients into 10-quart cooking pot. Cover and cook on medium-low, until vegetables are tender. Uncover pot; then increase temperature to medium-high. Add noodles and cook, until pasta is the desired consistency. Salt and pepper to taste and serve.

Chicken Bone Broth

One of the most tasty and effective gut repair techniques I use is bone broth. It's really helpful to keep a homemade soup stock around the house. Bone broth has been used for centuries to aid the immune system and you can use almost any meat.

Broth is great to have because you can just pull it out, add some fresh organic herbs, veggies, pasta and/or beans; then *poof* you have a highly nutritious soup in minutes. Yay supermom!! My family loves the chicken soup I make from this broth. My husband brags about it all the time!

Here's a simple way to make your own. Start by roasting a whole organic chicken for dinner the night before you want to make your broth. Feed the family well, but be sure to save a good hunk of meat or two for your broth, along with all of the leftovers, even from the plates. Don't forget the giblets.

Ingredients:

Whole chicken left-overs—meat, bones, giblets, soft tissue

Pink Himalayan Salt to taste

Black pepper to taste

1 tablespoon turmeric

Purified water

One large pot—5-6 quarts

Directions:

Place all meat, bones, soft tissue and joint pieces (a ton of restorative properties), into a 10-quart cooking pot, along with the chicken grease from the pan. Add filtered water, filling pot to about ¾ full to start with. Then bring to a full boil. Lower heat to medium-low. Add salt, pepper, and turmeric. Cover and allow mixture to simmer on for 4-5 hours. Broth will become more concentrated. Watch that it doesn't fall past the ¼ line mark. Keep adding water, as needed, to maintain your broth at a desired consistency. Use your own judgment; when it starts to look and taste like broth to you, then it's ready. I like my broth more concentrated, so I tend to add less water at the end. Finally, use a stainless steel, fine-wire mesh to strain broth. Do your best to remove all meat and remaining soft tissues from the bones to use in soup (beneficial in gut repair). Beef bone broth can be made the very same way.

Note: Dr. Campbell-McBride (GAPS Diet) suggests that you pound on the thick bones, to release visible bone marrow, onto a solid wooden butcher block, while it's still warm.

Home-made pasta

Ingredients:

2 organic large eggs

2 cups of organic sprouted wheat flour or unbleached organic white flour

½ teaspoon Pink Himalayan Salt

2 tablespoons whole organic milk

Directions:

Mix eggs, salt and milk in a large bowl. Add flour slowly, while stirring; continue mixing until you have dough. Separate dough and roll into two balls. Use a rolling pin, dusted with flour, to roll out the dough into a thin layer. Let it sit for about 15 minutes and then cut into strips, dust with flour. Use pasta right away, or hang dry and store in an air-tight container for later. Cook pasta in hot water or soup for 6-8 minutes.

Garlic–Cauliflower Alfredo Sauce

Ingredients:

4 cloves minced garlic

1 tablespoon organic butter

3 cups raw cauliflower

¼ cup of raw cashews

1½ cups organic vegetable broth

¼ cup organic grated parmesan cheese

½ tablespoon coconut oil

½ teaspoon Pink Himalayan Salt

½ teaspoon black pepper

Serves: 4

Directions:

Add cauliflower to pot and cook for about 8-10 minutes, or until cauliflower is soft but not mushy. Drain, then add broth and bring to a boil.

Sauté garlic in butter on low. Cook for approximately 2 minutes. Transfer your cauliflower and broth mixture into the blender/Vitamix, then add butter/garlic mixture and the remaining ingredients and blend until smooth. Heat on low and serve over your favorite organic pasta.

Mama's Meat Loaf

Ingredients:

2 lbs. grass-fed hamburger

½ cup organic catsup

1 large onion, diced

3 organic eggs

1½ cups organic and or gluten free rolled oats

salt and pepper to taste

1 tablespoon turmeric

1 garlic clove minced

For extra flavor: add fresh herbs like, parsley, basil, thyme and/ or Rosemary.

Serves: 4-5

Directions:

Preheat oven to 350 degrees. Mix ingredients together, adding oats last. Add mixture to well-oiled 9x5 bread pan and bake 45 minutes or until the sides of the meatloaf separate from the pan.

Mexican Soup

Ingredients:

1 pound carrots, peeled and chopped

1 medium-sized onion, diced

1 red pepper, diced

2 cloves garlic, minced

2 tomatoes, chopped

1 teaspoons cumin

1 teaspoons coriander (I substituted 1 teaspoon fennel seeds)

1 teaspoons chili powder

1 teaspoon Pink Himalayan salt

1 pound grass-fed hamburger

3 cups beef bone broth or vegetable stock

2 cups cooked black beans

1 lime

Optional: Fresh oregano, thyme, cilantro and parsley may be added at the end for extra taste and nutrition.

Directions:

Add all ingredients to crock pot (except lime) in the morning and cook all day for a delicious meal whenever you are ready. Add a squeeze of fresh lime before serving.

Sweet Potato Love

Ingredients:

3 large sweet potatoes (not yams) peeled and cut in chunks

3 tablespoons raw honey

3 tablespoons coconut oil

1 teaspoon cinnamon

1 teaspoon nutmeg

1 teaspoon turmeric

Pink Himalayan Salt and pepper to taste.

Serves: 3

Directions:

Preheat oven to 400 degrees. Melt coconut oil in a saucepan. Put sweet potatoes into a well-oiled glass-baking dish, along with the other ingredients and pour on coconut oil. Bake for 35-40 minutes, cool and serve.

Steak Fajitas

Ingredients:

1 pound grass-fed steak or roast, thin-sliced

1 medium-sized red pepper, thin-sliced

1 medium-sized green pepper, thin-sliced

1 medium yellow onion, peeled and sliced

2 large cloves garlic, minced

2 teaspoons honey

2 teaspoons chili powder

1 teaspoons cumin

1 teaspoon parsley

2 tablespoons purified water

Pink Himalayan Salt and pepper to taste

Serves: 2

Directions:

Cook steak in frying pan until almost done, leaving it slightly pink. Add peppers and garlic. Cook on medium for about 2 minutes; then add remaining ingredients. Lower heat to medium-low, cover and cook for another 8-10 minutes and serve hot with warm tortillas and cooked black beans.

Alternatives and Replacements

Almond Milk (Made Easy)

Almond milk is a good source of protein, vitamin E and calcium, but most packaged almond milk contains synthetic vitamins the body can't absorb. Most have something called carrageenan, a thickening agent that has no nutritional value and is known to cause inflammation in the body.

Ingredients:

1¼ cups raw almonds

4 cups purified water

¼ teaspoon of Pink Himalayan salt

½ teaspoon cinnamon

1 tablespoon vanilla

White agave, honey or coconut sugar to taste

Note: you will need a nut milk bag or cheesecloth for this recipe. (cost about $3)

Directions:

Soak almonds in purified water for 12-24 hours to reduce phytic acid that inhibits digestion. Drain and rinse almonds. Add almonds with purified water into blender or Vitamix. Blend several minutes until smooth and creamy.

Pour mixture into cheesecloth or nut bag and squeeze contents into a large bowl, until pulp becomes dry and cakey, like wet flour. Pour batch into a canning jar and set aside. Repeat the process, several times, until you're comfortable that you got the most milk from the almonds. I tend to refill the blender, remix and re-squeeze the pulp three times. Milk gets thinner as you go, so mix batches together for consistency.

When finished, pour milk back into blender. Add your sweetener (try soaked dates), vanilla and cinnamon. Keep milk chilled in a sealed, glass jar. Use within 5-7 days. Empty the cheesecloth and set the dry contents aside. You can use the leftover pulp to make almond flour in your oven. Stay tuned for that recipe.

Almond Flour

If your GMO-Free child is also gluten free and without almond allergies, you will love this recipe. Almond flour is a great way to make yummy moist baked goods, pancakes and desserts. The nutritional value is nothing to cough at either. Almond flour has over 21 grams of protein per ½ cup, compared to the same amount of wheat, which has less than 10 grams of protein action. Almond flour has a super low (<1) glycemic index (GI), making it a perfect alternative to wheat flour, which registers a big fat 71 on the GI scale. The higher the number, the more the food raises your blood glucose levels. That messes with insulin balance in the body and can lead to hyperglycemia and even diabetes.

Finally almond flour has a whopping 10.4 grams of fiber (wheat = 2.4 g) and less carbs (19.44 g) than a banana or even unsweetened applesauce.

Directions:

Save your pulp after making almond milk (recipe above). Once you have your pulp in hand, set oven to the lowest temperature. Coat a glass baking dish with coconut oil or line with chemical-free parchment paper. Spread mixture into a thin even layer. Cook on low, until completely dry but not burnt, usually about 3-4 hours depending on the amount. Put mixture into blender. Blend until it looks like flour. Use it in place of wheat flour on a 1:1 basis.

Gluten Free Flour Mix

Ingredients:

4 cups oat flour

4 cups teff flour

4 cups tapioca flour

4 cups garbanzo flour

8 teaspoons of xanthium gum

Makes: 16 cups

Directions:

Combine ingredients into large mixing bowl and mix well. Store in airtight container. Glass is best. Use in various gluten free recipes.

High-protein Gluten Free Flour

Ingredients:

5 cups garbanzo bean flour

4 cups sorghum flour (med. weight)

4 cups tapioca (light starch)

4 tablespoons of ground flax seeds or whole chia seeds (to replace guar gum and xanthium gum)

Makes: 16 cups

Directions:

Combine ingredients, seal in glass container and use in various gluten free recipes.

Sweet Condensed Milk

Ingredients

1½ cups organic whole milk

½ cup organic brown sugar or organic raw sugar

3 tablespoons organic butter or coconut oil

1 teaspoon of vanilla

Makes: about 1 cup

Directions:

Combine milk and sugar in to a medium size pot, bring mixture to a boil and keep stirring. Reduce heat and cook on low for another 20 minutes or until desired thickness, stir in vanilla and butter and mix well.

Cover and refrigerate for at least 45 minutes, before using.

Ingredients

1 teaspoon chia seeds
or ground flax seeds

3 tablespoons purified
    water

Directions:

Mix chia or flax seeds (measure after grinding) with purified water. Stir, then chill for 15 minutes.

The mixture will set up and can be used as egg replacements. Use the same amount as you would if you were using an egg. Large eggs are about 3 ½ tablespoons. You can also use applesauce as a viable egg replacement.

CHAPTER 10

....

The GMO-Free Movement

Modern GMO Affairs

Congress is always seeking to extend the same failed policies as prior administrations. As they push for further expansions on "free trade," like the Trans-Pacific Partnership (TPP) and Transatlantic Trade and Investment Partnership (TTIP), combined with the hazards of the DARK Act, we find that it all conveniently comes together to further endorse Monsanto's genetic revolution.

NAFTA demolished our "American Dream," locking us into the chains of a broken system. It took our jobs, it took our sense of American pride in a product that was worth buying. Thanks to the Clinton's "free trade" and Walmart (Hillary's former client), we traded in quality made standards and invested our money in disposable, cheap plastic products that pollute our environment and fall apart in a week. Think it's not all connected? Think again.

The dangerous provisions of the new "free trade" agenda limit local government and state's abilities to apply restrictions on genetically modified organisms (GMOs) not only in America but all over the world; thus allowing a free global market of questionable food ingredients and setting the stage for even more dubious food technologies lurking on the horizon.

Under debate has been the US Farm Bill, which was designed with an increase in benefits and compensations for corporations and large-scale farms while essentially working against the plights of small farmers, businesses, consumers and our environment.

Clinton's original "free trade" tied us to this toxic big food scheme, dominated by shareholder pockets and corporate manipulation. Across the country and the world, we are opting out in order to restore healthier, local options ingrained in local economies, that work together to sustain, cultivate and bridge the vital connections between the farm and your kitchen table.

By voting with your dollars, you are sending a clear message of objection to this massive human experiment. This act of revolutionary defiance must be made by the American people to overrule and topple the perpetual GMO feeding trough, refusing to allow our children to become just another lab rat in their money making trap.

I think we can agree that evolution of our species must continue. The synthetic restructuring of our entire planet and its inhabitants is indeed a detriment to our existence. The keys to the entire planet have been offered up on a false altar of sacrificial egos in dirty backroom deals. There comes a time when accountability comes to call. That time is now.

Families are fed up trying to navigate the GMO food circus that could be making their kids sick. This GMO-Free movement is what Jeffrey Smith calls the "tipping point" which will ultimately lead to the necessary restructuring of our food system, regulatory policies and eventually our entire healthcare paradigm, while mitigating the agricultural damages felt by our wildlife and our environment.

Inherently, the foundation of their business model and the blind trust of the public have allowed these entities to maintain unethical operations for decades, developing products that have failed to provide good results or value for the planet or mankind.

Now more than ever, it is time to speak up against the injustices plagued by Monsanto and company, since they have been given the genetic keys to our kingdom, rent-free. Walking in as if they owned the place, they have rearranged all the furniture (theoretically) and called it their own. Now they intend to sell it all back to us—fools, we are not.

As if they were gods, Monsanto acts as cavalier masters of the universe, dissecting and rearranging the biological components of our entire planet, furthering the original "Green Revolution" that brought us Monsanto's chemical pesticides, fertilizers and eventually GMOs. How *Green* is that?

Now we are waist deep in their new "genetic revolution." This has not been a revolution in the typical sense, but one of carnage nonetheless, as it contradicts our survival and the very foundation of our human and animal species. How will synthetic foods and toxic poisons feed the world or expand our ability to feed ourselves? Instead, it appears to be taking us on a crash course of fatal proportions. However, let me introduce you to some of the more powerful influences in your corner.

GMO-Free Unsung Heroes

Jeffrey Smith

Jeffrey Smith is the founder of Institute for Responsible Technology (IRT) and the author the book and documentary film *Genetic Roulette, The Gamble of Our Lives.*

In 1998, before most of us ever heard the term GMO, Jeffrey Smith was running for Congress in Iowa's First District on a platform opposing GMO farming. With hundreds of public appearances and presentations, Smith has received little attention from mainstream media in this colossal crusade to halt what appears to be a public health and environmental emergency. [5] Smith travels all over the world uniting the efforts of GMO-Free farmers, doctors, scientists, world and civic leaders as an ardent voice of reason, opposing genetically modified foods and the policies that allow them.

Jeffrey Smith continues to educate people and political figures all over the world, introducing them to the overwhelming evidence that he and other experts have gathered, assessed and imparted in this growing body of concern. Peer-reviewed published studies, compiled reports, legal proceedings and testimonials from every faction of science, medicine, farming and thousands of consumer complaints detail the growing threat from genetically modified organisms to our health and environment. [1]

Diana Reeves

During our 2015 interview, Diana Reeves talked to me about starting GMO FREE USA as a *Facebook* group:

We have grown to what is now a 501c3 non-profit with a social media presence. We reached 10.7 million people last week alone on Facebook and another two million plus on other social media platforms, including a new platform called TSU. We love it!

We started testing other products like we did with Kashi; and we will continue food testing. We are on a mission to change the food system by education and inspiring activism. We're all about food transparency and food justice. **We believe that you shouldn't have to be rich to afford safe and healthy food.**

The intent was to organize national boycotts of food companies that use GMO ingredients in their products and pressure them to remove those GMO ingredients. It started with a national call for the formation of at least 5,000 activists centralized into a *Facebook* group where actions would be directed. With the help of the nonprofit group, Organic Consumers Association, the GMO FREE USA grassroots initiative rapidly achieved its numbers, launching a campaign to Boycott Kellogg's GMOs.

GMO FREE USA and its dedicated volunteers, work tirelessly to achieve their mission which is to, "harness independent science and agro-ecological concepts to advocate for sustainable food and ecological systems." Member donations are pooled all together to provide third party lab testing on products suspected of being contaminated with GMOs.

GMO FREE USA presents: The Kashi Report

Diana explained the reasons why they chose Kellogg's for the boycott:

We've been targeting Kellogg's for a boycott for nearly three years. The reason they were chosen is because they market their products primarily to children. Children are vulnerable; children are growing and they should not be exposed to toxins. They are one of the worst offenders and they bought Kashi, which was a brand that had integrity and they destroyed it, basically. They took the wholesome ingredients they were using and replaced them with genetically engineered ingredients that are sprayed with herbicides, primarily with Roundup/glyphosate, which the World Health Organization recently concluded causes cancer in laboratory animals and probably causes cancer in people too.

These are not healthy ingredients and consumers have been calling the Kashi brand out for the past couple of years; and Kellogg's is making changes because they are forced to make changes, not because they care. Kellogg's spent 3.6 million dollars in the two years prior to 2014 on anti-labeling lobbying and they spent an additional two million dollars contributing to campaigns that pumped propaganda into the media in California, Washington, Oregon and Colorado.

This company, we believe, does not have integrity so we thought it would be prudent for us to test one of the Kashi cereals to see exactly what was in the box. The box we had tested was *not* in a box marked "Non-GMO Project Verified." We found out subsequently that the product Kashi Go Lean had been enrolled in the Non-GMO project.

We decided to release the results to the public regardless of the fact that it had (the product) been enrolled, because as recently as last week, when we were on the road, on tour with Neil Young, we found boxes of this particular cereal that were not verified, being mixed in with boxes on store shelves that had been Non-GMO Project verified. So we know the boxes are still out there; so consumers should be vigilant when making choices at the grocery store. We encourage everyone to boycott Kashi. We included it in the Kellogg's boycott.

What we found in that cereal was a level that was nearly six times higher than levels we previously detected on our test of a box of Kellogg's Fruit Loops. Their masquerading that this is their healthy brand and they say on their page, for consumers that are interested in Non-GMO products, we suggest that they buy Kashi. Well not only did we find this high level of Roundup/glyphosate in the package, we also found an even higher level of a chemical that is called AMPA, which is a breakdown, a metabolite of glyphosate. There has not been many studies done on it yet. It is prevalent in the environment in places as glyphosate breaks down where it is used. It has been identified as being toxic.

When AMPA and glyphosate are present together they are more toxic than either of them is alone. We found both it and glyphosate in the box and this is the first time any of our testing, which we send to an independent laboratory, detected AMPA; not only that, we found substantial levels of genetically engineered ingredients.

There are a lot of lessons to be learned here—a box created prior to Non-GMO Project verification, just because it is close to the date when the product was enrolled in the Non-GMO Project, doesn't mean that the product is safe. It does not mean that it is equivalent to a box that has gone through verification, and also the fact that we found GMOs and Roundup in that box is very worrying.

The corn that was detected was GMO, Bt corn, which is in its own right a pesticide that kills insects when they bite into it. It's registered with the EPA, regulated by the EPA. It produces up to six different versions within every cell of the plant and it does not wash off. The levels that are produced by these toxins are 1500-2000 times higher than what might be used in organic farming, because they'll tell you, the same thing is used in organic farming, but it isn't used the same way; in fact, it does break down and wash off in the way that it's used in organic farming. When it is genetically engineered into an ear of corn, it doesn't wash off and you're eating it whether you like it or not.

This is not about consumer choice. What they're trying to do, our wonderful government, is ramming GMOs and toxic pesticides down our throats and their also trying to push them on to the rest of the world. If anybody thinks our government is going to do the right thing and label genetically engineered foods in this country, voluntarily, and they're going to come through for us and protect us, they are sadly mistaken.

GMO FREE USA joins Neil Young for *The Monsanto Years*

I couldn't wait to hear about Diana's time on tour with Neil Young promoting his album, *The Monsanto Years.* It's thrilling when celebrity's raise dissent, voicing their opposition to injustice and Neil Young is a mighty defender of causes, and so I anticipated her return rather impatiently so I could share her experience with you:

We were contacted by Neil Young and invited to go on tour with him for his new studio album which is called *The Monsanto Years.* Neil is an activist at heart; he always has been. He's getting the message out there that these crops are not good for farmers and their not good for us, and mothers want to know what they're feeding their children.

The first unofficial stop was in Milwaukie, Wisconsin. There wasn't an activist village there, but we went because we wanted to take every opportunity to hand out information to the public about genetically engineered foods and educate as many people as possible. It was a really good platform for him promoting the new album. From there we went to Denver, Colorado and then we made our way to Lincoln, Nebraska, onto Cincinnati, Ohio and Detroit, Michigan. We had several stops along the East Coast with two stops in New York and one in New Jersey, Vermont, and Massachusetts.

During the tour, Neil had an activist village set up on the grounds that were primarily grassroots organizations educating the public about causes that are near and dear to Neil's heart. The focal area was genetically engineered food, which actually share much in common with many of the other issue areas which were represented there.

The heart of the matter is corporate personhood which considers corporations essentially like people. They aren't people and they shouldn't be treated like it, and that's the key to changing it.

We were in tents on-sight at the venues talking to people—handing out information. We made it a focus to talk to people about HR 1599, which outlaws GMO labeling on a state and federal level, which was sadly passed by Congress, known as the DARK ACT. It will overturn Vermont's GMO Labeling Law passed by the state and GMO crop bans that have been passed by counties at the local level. It is a bill written by industry, Monsanto, and the Grocer Manufacturer's Association to protect industry; people need to be made aware of what's going on.

We met so many people with heart-warming stories which really stayed with us. In Lincoln, Nebraska a man approached me saying, "my father has cancer, my cousin has cancer, my neighbors have cancer, nearly everyone in the heartland has cancer." We don't know statistically what's going on, but here he's telling us his experience, and it has to move you, because these are people that live in the middle of millions of acres of genetically engineered crops and their sick.

We actually approached a soy field, GMO obviously, that was bordering a rest stop; we took pictures of the crop. As I got closer I could smell the chemicals; I got a headache and I had to leave. That was within five minutes; I had to get out of there. This is a very real problem and to hear about it is really heart wrenching.

Another man came up to us in Cincinnati. He has a really close friend who is a farmer; he grows GMO crops, but he doesn't want to. He wants to make the switch, but he can't because they have a strangle-hold on him. He's surrounded by GMO fields and he knows that the pollen would drift on to his organic crop contaminating it and what then? What would happen is they would sneak onto his property in the middle of the night test his corn and find their gene, sue him and shut him down. That's what holds many farmers back from making the switch. It is very, very disturbing and sad. It puts our farmers on a chemical treadmill that they can't get off of. It's poison, poison in our food, poisoning these poor people buying it and putting it into our environment. It's all very disturbing.

We have 2029 studies on the *GMO FREE USA* website now. We are creating a database on the harmful effects of the GMOs themselves, the chemicals they are sprayed with, and Bt toxins. The whole thing is just one big batch of poison.

We believe everyone, irrespective of income level, should have access to clean food. By broadening this market and affecting supply and demand we help lower the costs of organic and non-GMO foods."

Please visit http://www.gmofreeusa.org/ to stay informed about GMO FREE USA and the GMO-Free movement. You can access recent food lab reports and a database of scientific evidence. Also, since they are a registered non-profit, you can add them as your chosen charity on your (free) *Amazon Smile* account. They will receive a small donation (it adds up) from qualified sellers, based on certain sales. I do a lot of shopping on *Amazon,* and because Diana uses those donations to test different food products in third party labs, I feel like I'm contributing to something very, very important. GMO FREE USA has become my favorite charity, along with the Institute for Responsible Technology (IRT) and the Center for Food Safety (CFS) which leads to our next unsung hero, Andrew Kimbrell.

Andrew Kimbrell

Andrew Kimbrell is the founder and executive director of the Center for Food Safety (CFS). As highly influential public interest attorney, Kimbrell has built the largest central legal and consumer advocacy group working in protection of our food rights. [2]

Kimbrell challenges companies like Monsanto, Dow, DuPont and Syngenta in court on behalf of farmers and consumer rights at the forefront of the GMO-Free movement. [2] CFS is running a strong campaign against the "DARK Act" and has championed GE food labeling bills for more than two decades, during which time over thirty states have introduced new laws requiring GMO labeling. They have helped 150 family farmers beat chemical companies in court, winning precedent-setting cases that protect family farmers from the detriments of genetically engineered crops. They have a variety of resources on their website, including GMO news updates, the latest scientific research and a database of information and tools to help you stay informed and ahead of the changes that are rapidly taking place in this country, without public knowledge. [2]

Ronnie Cummins

Ronnie Cummins is the co-founder and international director of the Organic Consumers Association (OCA), which is a non-profit consumer network dedicated to safeguarding our food supply and organic standards, along with their Mexican affiliate Via Organica. OCA's central strategy focuses on "national and global campaigns to promote health, justice and sustainability while integrating public education, marketplace pressure, litigation and lobbying against GMOs, factory farming and climate change." [3]

In October 2016, OCA and Cummins, with the help of various volunteers and activists, organized a tribunal against Monsanto to examine the evidence incriminating Monsanto for crimes against nature and humanity. [3]

Robyn Obrien

Robyn Obrien is the author of The *Unhealthy Truth* and founder of the AllergyKids Foundation, whose mission it is to "make clean and safe food affordable to all children." Robyn is a former financial and food industry analyst whose youngest child suffered a severe allergic reaction after she ate GMO food for breakfast one morning. Obrien has helped to perpetuate a national food awakening among consumers, food corporations and even political leaders. Companies like Kraft, Coca-Cola, Burger King, Chipotle and others continue to respond, as she educates consumers on the changing and challenging landscape of our food supply, policies and health outcomes. [4] One central goal of *AllergyKids* is to "restore the health of our children and the integrity of our food supply for families today and for future generations...we want to protect children from the additives—additives not used in children's foods in other developed countries." [4]

Zen Honeycutt

Zen Honeycutt is the founder of Moms Across America which prides itself as a "National Coalition of unstoppable moms." MAA is an organization of mother bears whose mission is to, "empower millions to educate themselves about GMOs and related pesticides, get GMOs labeled (as a first step to elimination) and offer GMO-Free and organic solutions." Their motto is "Empowered Moms, Healthy Kids." MAA commits to this, "by doing what we do best, CARING about our families and community and SHARING with them about food, GMOs, PESTICIDES and health." [5]

Honeycutt and MAA members reach thousands of families across the country by hosting in-person and virtual meetings, orchestrating marches, using petitions and educational endeavors. The MAA *Facebook* page is a great place to connect with and meet other GMO-Free moms, because they are passionate that families should know what is in their food and they should have the freedom to choose. [5]

Vandana Shiva

Vandana Shiva is an environmental activist from India and founder of Navdanya, a group of seed keepers and organic food producers. [6] She has published over 20 books, as one of the most powerful crusaders in the fight for food sovereignty. She was trained as a physicist at the University of Punjab, completing her Ph.D. in quantum theory from the University of Western Ontario, Canada.[6,7]

Shiva pushed her studies forward, transitioning over to inter-disciplinary research in science, technology and environmental policy. She attended the Indian Institute of Science and the Indian Institute of Management in Bangalore, India. She founded an independent institute in 1982, called the Research Foundation for Science, Technology and Ecology; "dedicated to high quality and independent research in order to address the most significant ecological and social issues of our times." [6, 7]

Shiva founded Navdanya to secure a national movement aimed at, "protecting the diversity and integrity of living resources—especially native seed—and to promote organic farming and fair trade." She combines her efforts with local communities and organizations, covering the past two decades, "serving more than 500,000 men and women farmers." Her diligence has "resulted in the conservation of more than 3000 rice varieties from across India, and the organisation has established 60 seed banks in 16 states across the country." [6, 7]

Time Magazine recognized Dr. Shiva as an "environmental hero" in 2003. *Asia Week* called her, "one of the five most powerful communicators in Asia," and in November 2010, *Forbes* acknowledged her, as one of the "Seven Most Powerful Women on the Globe."[7] Dr. Shiva is adament that,

> Monsanto has pushed GMOs in order to collect royalties from poor farmers, trapping them in unpayable debt and pushing them to suicide. Monsanto is largely responsible for the depletion of soil and water resources, species extinction and declining biodiversity, and the displacement of millions of small farmers worldwide...[8]

Goliath is Falling

2015 was a bad year for biotech's bottom line. Numerous lawsuits were launched against the corporation and the stock market was not finding favor in the poison products of Monsanto and company. [9] On the heels of public rejection, Monsanto announced massive job cuts in January 2016, as their markets fell in agricultural segments by a whopping 34 percent, hammering Monsanto's market shares substantially. [10]

GMO-Free Around the World

Most nations in the world do not trust that GMOs are safe to consume. More than 64 countries worldwide have placed serious restrictions and even outright bans on growing, importing producing and selling GMOs. [11] Hungary started burning GMO fields within their borders and even began cultivating a plan to criminalize GMO seeds as a felony possession, back in 2011. [12]

By the fall of 2015, headlines flooded over with crop bans spanning 19 countries across the EU including: Russia, France, Austria, Bulgaria, Croatia, Cyprus, Germany, Greece, Hungary, Italy, Latvia, Lithuania, the Netherlands, Poland, Slovenia, Wales and Scotland. [13]

January 2016 brought intelligent reports of a Taiwanese GMO ban in school lunches over substantial health concerns. To ensure food safety and protect student health, the lawmakers indicated that it was an imperative move to rid schools of GM foods served to school children. [14]

The spring thaw of 2016 generated even more international sanity with 38 countries affirming that they would not let their agricultural standards be degraded by GM contamination, they include:

Europe
Azerbaijan, Austria, Bosnia and Herzegovina, Bulgaria, Croatia, Cyprus, Denmark, France, Germany, Greece, Hungary, Italy, Latvia, Lithuania, Luxembourg, Malta, Moldova, the Netherlands, Northern Ireland, Norway, Poland, Russia, Scotland, Serbia, Slovenia, Switzerland, Ukraine, and Wales.

Asia
Bhutan, Kyrgyzstan, Saudi Arabia, and Turkey.

Americas
Belize, Ecuador, Peru, and Venezuela.

Africa
Algeria and Madagascar. [15]

The biotech plan is quickly losing ground and food security analysts are predicting that the international banning trend is likely to continue.

GMO-Free in the USA
The US is, by far, the biggest producer of genetically engineered

crops in the world, with around 73 million hectares (1 hectare is about 2.47 acres) of GE alfalfa, canola, cotton, maize, papaya, soybean, squash and sugarbeet, planted each year. [16]

Ahead of the "DARK Act", states were in position to place severe limitations on GM crops grown and sold within their borders.

Boulder, Colorado

In Colorado, Boulder County Commissioners began directing their county staff to draft out plans to phase out all planting of genetically engineered crops on farmlands owned by the county. [23] [17] Prior to this, the county's cropland policy allowed tenant farmers in Boulder County to grow certain varieties of genetically modified corn and sugar beets on the farmlands leased from the county. They said the previous policy would have remained in effect at least through the end of 2016. [17]

Their county lands total around 1,180 acres which are being leased to tenant farmers that would have had to phase out cultivation of GMO crops over a three-to-five year period if the "DARK Act" wouldn't have passed.

The Board of County Commissioners began the GMO-Free operation without a formal vote, although they were expecting support from at least two of the three other commissioners. [23] [17]

Jackson County, Oregon

EcoWatch said, "organic farmers are racking up new victories in the fight against "frankenfood," as a growing number of counties line up to bar genetically engineered (GE) crop cultivation throughout the country." [18] A federal judge in Oregon ruled to uphold a consent decree designating Jackson County a "GE-free zone." The decision was designed to protect the decree from being appealed and granted new protections to area farmers, consumers and the environment. Voters approved the ban by ballot measure in 2014, and Monsanto has been fighting it ever since, thus, we now see the passage of the new "DARK Act," quashing the voice and rights of every American. [19] The battle lines have been drawn and United States citizens, and those around the world, have made it crystal clear that they have serious doubts as to the safety of re-engineered food-crops and animals. Increasingly, the "genetic revolution" has evolved into a sonic boom of dissatisfied customers, marching against the soiled tempo of Monsanto's poison drum.

Decades of Failure

Greenpeace revealed a 40-page report called, "Twenty Years of Failure—Why GM Crops Have Failed to Deliver On Their Promises." [20] EU's Greenpeace Food Policy Director Franziska Achterberg said,

> Over the past 20 years, GM technology has only been taken up by a handful of countries for a handful of crops, so no wonder two thirds of Europe have decided to ban it. Where GM crops are grown, they lead to increased pesticide use and the entrenchment of industrial farming systems that in turn exacerbate hunger, malnutrition and climate change. [20, 21]

Greenpeace continues to highlight the many, many complications we've seen associated with GM crops, which are mainly cultivated in just four major countries including the US, Brazil, Argentina and Canada, the Greenpeace report says. [20 21]

One by one the authors unravel the conventional myths associated with GM crops that have been perpetuated by biotech producers in order to increase market shares. Although they claim that planting GMO crops decreases long-term production costs, the report finds just the opposite:

> In principle, Roundup Ready and other herbicide- resistant crops reduce labor costs by allowing singular pesticide treatments across large areas, while pesticide-producing crops can reduce the need to spray insecticides. This should bring down expenses on pesticides as well as labor costs. [However,] the emergence of super-weeds can rapidly erode these benefits, requiring farmers to ramp

up pesticide applications and upgrade to more expensive 'stacked trait' GM crops. [20 21]

Driving it home, they further illustrate that,

In 2004, after several years of commercialization, GM cotton farmers in China were spending $101/ hectare on pesticides, almost as much as conventional farmers, and were spraying pesticide nearly three times more often than in 1999—suggesting that labor savings can also be swiftly eroded. [20 21]

Another investigation, this one by GE-Free New Zealand, reports on, "Genetically Engineered Animals—The First Fifteen Years," unveiling a deceptive history of selective reporting and omissions of vital research data. The researchers have been allowed to continue experimenting with transgenic cows, while avoiding any public examination or media scrutiny of tragic outcomes being caused in these animals. "There are serious gaps in the management of the experiments and a collective silence on the treatment of animals," says Jon Carapiet, a spokesperson for GE Free NZ. [22]

The authors reveal that the cows are being bred to express one specific trait out of six potential protein traits in their milk for use as bio-pharmaceutical products, termed biologics. The company, AgResearch, has carried out these 'bio-pharming' trials for the past fifteen years, 2000-2015, at their Ruakura facility in Hamilton, New Zealand." [22]

The information they got was obtained from Official Information Act (OIA) requests and AgResearch reports, submitted every year to the Environmental Protection Authority (EPA):

These annual reports catalogue a sad and profoundly disturbing story of illness, reproductive failure and birth deformities that have consistently afflicted the genetic engineering (GE) trials. Both the surrogate and transgenic cows suffer from chronic illness, reproductive losses, sudden unexplained deaths and severe deformities, relating to the foreign DNA inserted in the embryos used in the artificial insemination programme...most of the transgenic cows are not able to reproduce past the first generation. The transgenic cows that have produced a second generation have borne sterile offspring. After fifteen years of experimentation, from the many thousands of transgenic embryos the cows have carried, the average live birth rate has ranged from 0—7%. These embryos have been predominately developed offshore in the private partnership laboratories. By December 2014, there were just 19 transgenic cows surviving at the Ruakura facility."[22]

The fact is, we do not need GMOs to feed the world and Monsanto is getting a clear indication of that from people across the globe. The whole agenda is simply a matter of designed control over the reproduction and manifestation of nature's bounty.

National Academy of Sciences—Missed Conduct

As I prepare the final manuscript for my publisher, mainstream media is again spewing biased misinformation on behalf of the biotech agenda regarding a "new research" paper from the National Research Council (NRC), part of the National Academy of Sciences. The paper titled "Genetically Engineered Crops—Experiences and Prospects," has been heavily criticized by independent scientists for its obvious lack of objectivity and balanced reporting. [23]

Food & Water Watch is an influential Washington D.C. based advocacy group. They say the NRC has a long-standing reputation as an, "elite scientific body" in the US, acting as an independent institution, often commissioned by Congress for "impartial" scientific judgment on topics like GMOs to establish government policies. The group says, NRC is mandated under the Federal

Advisory Committee Act to minimize and report any potential conflicts of interest that might interfere with providing a sound and reasonable assessment of the scientific evidence. However, the panel's membership does not uphold that standard, says Food & Water Watch, and it appears to have a direct aversion to sound evidence from opposing authorities. Additionally, they disclose that, "A wide body of literature shows that when industry plays a role as an author or funder of scientific research, it tends to produce results favorable to industry." In turn, they caution that the NRC is an organization that has accepted millions of dollars from corporations like Monsanto and DuPont, allowing corporate representatives to sit on high-level boards, directing NRC's projects.

Scientific communities throughout the world have slammed the NRC, over the years, for maintaining unspoken revolving door policies for industry (mis)-aligned researchers. The panel's key staffers promote a biotech agenda, marginalizing and discounting research that opposes corporate intentions. [23]

Science Magazine even mentions that the NRC authors simply, "picked through hundreds of research papers to make generalizations about GE varieties already in commercial production." The NRC paper concludes that there is "reasonable evidence that animals were not harmed by eating food derived from GE crops," and that there is no proof of an increase in cancer or any other health problems, because they entered the market. [24]

Okay, time out! I would like take this moment to reiterate the major glitch in their assumption and that is their conclusion is simply just that, pure assumption; because we know - *If you can't track it, you can't control it.* The infrastructure was deliberately put in place absent of a tracking system with two motives in mind. First, if you don't know what you're eating and when you're eating it, then you don't know if it's making you sick. Without labels we are unable to trace it back to them. They know it and they think we're too dumb to figure it out. The NRC pawns know perfectly well that lack of evidence, in-and-of itself, does not constitute proof of non-existence in any scientific arena.

Food & Water Watch preempted the NRC report with a brief of their own, declaring that

> More than half of the invited authors of the new NRC study are involved in GMO development or promotion or have ties to the biotechnology industry—some have consulted for, or have received research funding from, biotech companies. NRC has not publicly disclosed these conflicts. [23]

Furthermore, the brief clearly demonstrates how, "NRC routinely arrives at watered-down scientific conclusions on agricultural issues based on industry science." In addition, they note that NRC's 2000 report on GMOs was peppered with heavy influences by eight panel members (out of 12), with certain financial interests in the final outcome. The 2010 report, released by the same panel, is said to indicate similar conflicts of interest, undoubtedly, affecting the reliability of its own conclusions. Another aspect of the brief covers a controversial *Frontline* investigation, revealing how much political influence chemical companies have had on the National Academy of Sciences. The story details the dismissal of former NRC Director Charles Benbrook, after his criticisms of the pesticide industry. [23]

As if to maintain a picture of integrity, NRC researchers do acknowledge the only points that evidence could not dispute, that is GMOs, do indeed, promote a "heavy reliance on the chemical" [glyphosate] and new resistant weeds, they admit, are presenting major problems for growers. They indicate that genetically engineered crops might be generally saving farmers money, but they don't appear to increase product yields. [25, 26] Finally, the report determines that no monarch butterfly populations have been harmed in the making of this alternate reality. [25, 26]

The sticky point of contention seems to be that these transgenic crops are still somehow worthwhile in spite of these meaningful cons. They continue to deny any notion of biological senses, rejecting the GMO elephant in the trees, as they invalidate every notion that their experimental trials have gone horribly awry.

To recap, their own NRC report says GMOs do not appear to increase crop yields, tend to expand use of glyphosate-based chemicals, and encourage proliferation of super weed invasions which inhibit major growth factors that were marketed as being main benefits of GMO crops, in the first place. [25, 26] Tell me again how they intend to feed the world.

Bait and Switch

Now as our markets prepare for yet another eruption of newly developed GMO crops produced with a new "precise" gene-editing technology called "CRISPR," regulators are setting the stage to redefine what constitutes a genetically modified organism. The more immediate concern, says *Science Magazine* involves, *"what to do with gene-edited plants that won't always fit the technical definition of a regulated GE crop."* [24] BINGO!

If you recall, with my *Salem-News* article "Contamination without Representation," *I* exposed the political intention to federally redefine the term genetically modified organism back in 2011. (See the ag hearing video in "GMO-Free Data Sources"—Chapter 1)

This may be why state regulators *appear* to have reluctantly caved on the matter of GMO labeling. It may simply be another tactic designed to manipulate and pacify the people back into the lull of quiet discontent. They have no intention of reversing current GMO trends in favor of more sustainable alternatives, because they have dug themselves so deep into biotech pockets that there is no logistical sense of direction, regardless of the dead end cliffs present at the end of their GMO revolutionary road.

They do not want us to know what we are feeding our children and they will do anything to facilitate and maintain that secrecy, even to the point of full contamination and redefinition of nature itself within the entire food scheme. Case in point:

The Safe and Accurate Food Labeling Act - "DARK Act"

At first glance, Congress moved to reject the illusionary factors of the Safe and Accurate Food Labeling Act, in March 2016. Senator Bernie Sanders commended Congress for the bill's defeat:

> Congress stood up to the demands of Monsanto and other multi-national food industry corporations and rejected this outrageous bill. Today's vote was a victory for the American people over corporate interests. Senator Roberts' legislation violates the will of the people of Vermont and the United State who overwhelmingly believe that genetically modified food should be labeled ... all over this country, people are becoming more conscious about the food they eat and the food they serve their kids. When parents go to the store and purchase food for their children, they have a right to know what they are feeding them. GMO labeling exists in 64 other countries. There is no reason it can't exist here. [27]

Food advocates shared a breath of relief over the close call, as Monsanto narrowly missed the 60 legislative votes needed to move the plan forward. [27] Within days of the decision, cereal giant General Mills surrendered with new plans to label products containing genetically modified ingredients, to comply with Vermont's new state law. The Executive Vice President and Chief Operating Officer Jeff Harmening conceded: "As the discussions continue in Washington, one thing is very clear: Vermont state law requires us to start labeling certain grocery store food packages that contain GMO ingredients or face significant fines." [28] That appeared on the heels of Campbell's announcement, coming clean about GMO ingredients in their products with promises to label. [29]

What caused them to flip-flop midstream? Why the sudden commitment to GMO labeling and even federal legislation that would require all foods and beverages to be labeled? Why the sudden change of heart; did the ghost of fortitude come to call?

As it turns out, we weren't quite free of the "DARK" woods yet. It was simply a reflective measure, stalling to allow ample opportunity to repackage and remodify, because just a few short months later, it reappeared and cleared, breezing through the coddling doors of Congress right into the trembling hands of Obama dedicating it to our dismay in July 2016. Obama didn't waste a breath before he signed, even after the civil rights leader Reverend Jesse Jackson sent him a letter urging him to veto the measure:

> [The] law's principal thrust is to rely on QR codes which shoppers will scan to gain product information relative to GMOs. However, 100,000,000 Americans, most of them poor, people of color and elderly either do not own a smart phone or an iPhone to scan the QR code or live in an area of poor internet connectivity…as someone who like yourself, has traversed the rocky upward path to social and economic justice on behalf of those at the other side of society's great divides, racial, social and economic—I want to call to your attention serious inequities on GMO labeling legislation coming soon to your desk. [30]

Bloomberg Politics also took issue with the hasty decision stating that,

> Under the legislation, which has been pushed for by companies including Monsanto, Wal-Mart Stores Inc. and groups including the National Corn Growers Association, consumers may still find it hard to figure out if the food they are buying is genetically modified, leading opponents to dub the bill the DARK Act. [31]

This rogue congressional decision clears the legislative path to undercut state's rights, while invalidating local efforts to regulate GMOs via product labeling. Whereas the fact remains that 91% of polled American consumers said they wanted GMOs labeled (2012

Mellman Group). [32] Why then, does Congress insist on ignoring the rights of the people in favor of corporate interests?

A United Front - Rise of the "Food Reich"

In the hail of the storm, Monsanto seeks German asylum with emerging prospects of a new "Food Reich." This modern empire may just be born from the salivating glands of anti-trust lawyers in a 66-billion dollar Bayer-Monsanto mega-merger, promising to revive the murky shadows of Germany's holocaustic past. [33]

Let's take a quick jaunt down death row: At the end of World War II, dozens of Nazi war criminals were brought to trial for crimes against humanity in connection to the Nazi death camps directed by Adolf Hitler. Two dozen company officials from IG Farben (now Bayer) were charged with war crimes that included torture, slavery and genocide, among many others. The IG Farben cartel was the biggest chemical and pharmaceutical giant in the world. The founder's son and board director, chemist Dr. Fritz ter Meer served only four years, of a seven year prison term, for his part in the human experiments and for development of the nerve gas Zyklon-B that was used to kill millions of Jews. [34]

US Chief Prosecutor Colonel Telford Taylor prosecuted the war criminals during the Nuremberg Trials, concluding that the Nazi war efforts would have failed without the company's chemical hand. This group, later deemed the "Devil's Chemists," used live death camp inmates to test their toxic formulas, pharmaceuticals, and vaccines as unwilling victims, tens of thousands died. After prison, the infamous doctor returned for work at Bayer as a company chairman, where he stayed for next 10 years, until he retired in 1961. [34] The original source remains unclear, but several online articles mention that the doctor was asked whether he considered the human medical experiments at Auschwitz to be justified. Apparently, he responded that it was irrelevant since, "They were prisoners thus no particular harm was inflicted, as they would have been killed anyway." [35]

Two decades later, Bayer still lacked any moral compass as they sold, what they knew to be, tainted blood supplies banned in the US. Their blood-clotting product was contaminated with the AIDS virus and instead of destroying its reserves the company sent multiple shipments of the drug to hemophiliacs in Japan, Italy and France. [36]

In 2011, *CBS News* reiterated a French report by the *Agence France Press* (using Google translation): "The German group Bayer and three other labs will pay tens of millions of euros to hemophiliacs who accused them of having sold in the 1980s blood products contaminated with HIV, a source close to the deal told AFP." Around 20,000 people contracted the virus and many of them were children. [36] Does this sound like a company we can trust with our future?

2016 may bind the unholy marriage of two of the biggest industrial villains in all of our history. Will we forever be wiping away the after-birth of a new genetic holocaust from the biotech babes the new "Food Reich"?

Food Democracy Now!

Food Democracy Now! is a grassroots community advocating for a sustainable food system. They call on all governments of the world to sit up and take notice of this situation. [37]

Reports say that Monsanto admits to filing 150 lawsuits against America's family farmers whose Non-GMO crops have been contaminated by their GMO varieties. They've also settled another 700 lawsuits out of court, while investigating an average of 500 family farmers every year. [37]

The controversy and subsequent protest have spread around the world, raising the voices of the oppressed and shining the light of accountability on the intimidating tactics of Monsanto against the cultures and people of the world.

Farmer suicides in India have resulted from widespread crop failures from super weed infestation and bugs that were guaranteed not to of concern. Farmers have no recourse if GMO crops fail. They have to repurchase new seeds every year, or they are infringing on Monsanto's patent rights. They are unable to save seeds for reuse and so failed crops in just one season will drive a small, poor farmer into bankruptcy, especially in countries where people have very little resources. [38]

In his *Mother Jones* article, "No, GMOs Didn't Create India's Farmer Suicide Problem, But...," the author Tom Philpot seems to be unclear about which side he's on; while he denies GMOs involvement in the farmer suicides, he seems to make the case for the opposition. Case in point, he illustrates a study that shows, "65 percent of India's cotton crop comes from farmers who rely on rain, not irrigation pumps," and "reliance on pesticides and the higher cost of the seeds increase the risk of bankruptcy and thus suicide." In addition, Philpot says, "the smaller and more Bt-reliant the farm in these rain-fed cotton areas, the higher the suicide rate." I fail to see where this justifies his original premise that GMOs were not the culprit here. He simply solidifies this point. [38]

In Guatemala and countries like it, the GMO push endangers the cost of food production, contributing to the detriments of an already impoverished nation and worsening a food crisis already in full swing. [25]

By the fall of 2015, gathering voices of indigenous people were joined by farmers, social movements, trade unions and women's organizations, all protesting to overturn the "Monsanto Law." The law was designed to allow exclusive rights on patented seeds for a few corporations, undermining the agricultural heritage of those farmers dedicating their lives to small family farms. [39]

The food war is about justice, sovereignty and the ability to feed ourselves and allow future generations to have access to conventional seeds that they can grow and harvest year after year, season after season, because as human beings we should have that inherent right.

The fact remains, many GMO seeds require significantly more water to grow and the seeds cost more than conventional ones, plus you have to repurchase the seeds and chemicals that go along with them every season. They cost more and when they fail they can take the whole farm, family and often the community down with them. This agricultural system of GMOs and glyphosate quickly becomes a dangerous and unsustainable cycle, in which farmers can't escape. [40]

Farmers become trapped in a revolving door of chemicals and toxic farming practices, depleting the life force from the soil, until it can't grow anymore. And even when they decide they want to go organic, often they can't because their neighbors are growing GMO varieties that threaten to contaminate and destroy their marketing prospects every time the wind blows.

Generations upon generations of family farmers and their communities have relied upon the land to bear fruit and feed for thousands of years. Now in recent decades, with the drastic agricultural overhaul and remanufacturing of nutrition, we find incredible surges in disease epidemics, along with a political scheme that threatens to destroy the very fabric of American culture and any perception of freedom and independence from a nation of dictators and oppressors.

GMOs have devastated our ability to feed ourselves and our children healthy, wholesome foods that will nourish their bodies and perpetuate a life worth living.

No Force of Hand Controls Our Lands

We have to ask, what is the real agenda behind the "GMO Rubik's Cube" and why such hesitation to track the consumption of their genetically modified organisms? Obviously, they don't want controls in place that would limit their infiltration of the world's food systems. Isn't it likely that they are very well aware of the results of published independent animal feeding studies and the ensuing public health crisis they knew would follow? Why would I say something so outrageous? Am I actually insinuating that they are making people sick on purpose? Does the GMO shoe fit?

Why then, would they refuse to track the long-term health effects of GMO consumption on humans and why are they refusing to grant permission to scientists who want to find out? Wouldn't you think that valuable marketing data could be collected from suitable tracking methods, perhaps even a strategic and competitive edge, if they were to validate their underlying safety claims?

With our children's health in rapid decline, the GMO relationship must be critically examined and considered as a plausible cause for concern in relation to these widespread conditions plaguing our young (and old) populations. No stone should be left unturned in the ruthless hunt for the root source of this suffering. Our children deserve the very best chance at a healthy life, anything obstructing that potential should be pursued and destroyed, with all fervor.

Time and again, we have been coerced as a "free nation" to go along with agendas that are not the will of the people. They have taken our freedom, our liberties and our constitutional inheritance, flushing it away in a corporate façade of "democratic choice." A choice it is not. Justice does not represent the voices of the afflicted, gagged and bound to a system that doesn't hear them. So I ask you, is it not reasonable to pursue the path of least destruction, rather than that of least resistance?

With that, my friend, please go forth and do well. Be wary of the snake oil salesman of today. Thank you for your commitment and dedication to end this monstrosity. I believe that you will find this the most worthy of causes, because it's really just:

~ The beginning ~

One Final Thought

No mother should ever feel concerned, each and every time they feed their child. The very thing they need to sustain their lives should not be questionable and no parent should ever have to choose between paying the rent and poisoning their children with the food they eat.

The body does not recognize synthetic forms of food as

nutrition, no matter how much the eye is convinced of its authenticity.

As a nation, we have been fooled into believing that they could falsify nature and remain adherent to the genetic structure and all of the intricate and inherent complexities of life itself.

The very core of the biotech belief system is scientifically and foundationally flawed and irrational. Their misdirected assumptions have collapsed under the scientific test of time and trial. The recurrent rate of failure surrounding these toxic products and the obliviousness in which they render their reckless determinations continues the assault on our children, our environment and our planet. They choose to trespass over the rights of humanity, as if the world belongs exclusively to them, because they have more shreds of green paper!!

It has become my life's errand, and that of those whom are educated in the nuances of these matters, to prevent further harm and impending certainty of doom and devastation from what is entirely preventable outcomes.

This GMO experiment is based upon a categorically false and foolish endeavor that has been designed simply as a tool to manipulate you out of your money, while they redesign nature and OUR WORLD and sell it back to us, as the oblivious sheep they think we are.

AS A LOYAL CITIZEN OF THE UNITED STATES OF AMERICA, BEING A TRUE AND FREE CITIZEN, I DO DEMAND THAT THIS GMO EXPERIMENT BE HALTED AND HELD SUSPECT, AS IT MAY BE IMPICATED IN THE CHRONIC CONDITION AND DETERIORATIN OF OUR PUBLIC HEALTH SITUATION AND MAY BE CONSIDERED A SERIOUS HEALTH HAZARD TO THE PEOPLE OF THIS NATION AND OTHERS.

FURTHERMORE, I DEMAND THAT THIS UNITED STATES GOVERNMENT AND ALL ITS JUDICIARIES

REVIEW AND REVOKE ANY AND ALL PATENTS ON LIFE, LIVING SUBJECTS OR MATTERS OF NATURE AND THEIR DESCENTDANTS.

UNDER THE DIRECTION OF THE FDA, USDA AND EPA, I DEMAND DESIGNATION AND FULL IMPLE-MENTATION OF THE SENSIBLE FEATURES OF THE PRECAUTIONARY PRINCIPLE, IN LIGHT OF THESE MATTERS OUTLINED IN THIS TEXT AND BY THOSE THAT HAVE STUDIED AND WITNESSED THE DAMAGING HEALTH EFFECTS, NOT CONSIS-TENT WITH THE CLAIMS OF THE BIOTECH RUSE.

With all sincerity,

April Scott
The *Cleanfood* Advocate

GMO-Free Child Data Sources

Introduction

1. "The Future of Food." Dir. Deborah Koons Garcia. *Lily Films*, 2004. Film <http://www.thefutureoffood.com/onlinevideo.html>

2. Obrien, Robyn. "Defining Food Allergies." AllergyKids. *Allergykids.com*, n.d. Web. Mar. 2016. <http://www.allergykids.com/>

Rubik's Cube

1. Olshansky, Jay S., Douglas J. Passaro, and M.D., Ronald C. Hershow and et al. "A Potential Decline in Life Expectancy in the United States in the 21st Century." New England Journal of Medicine. *NEMJ.org*, Mar. 2005. Web. July. 2015. **<http://www.nejm.org/doi/full/10.1056/ NEJMsr043743 >**

Chapter 1 Why GMO?

1. "The Future of Food." Dir. Deborah Koons Garcia. *Lily Films*, 2004. Film <http://www.thefutureoffood.com/onlinevideo.html>

2. GMO Awareness. "GMO Defined." *GMO-Awareness.com*, n.d. Web. Mar. 2016. <http://gmo-awareness.com/all-about-gmos/gmo-defined/>

3. Freedman, David H. "The Truth About Genetically Engineered Food." Scientific American. *Scientificamerican.com*, Sept. 2013. Web. Mar. 2016. <http://www.scientificamerican.com/article/genetically-modified-crop/>

4. Wilson, Allison K., Jonathan R. Latham and et al. "Transformation-induced mutations in transgenic plants: Analysis and biosafety implications." Bioscience Resource Project, Biotechnology and Genetic Engineering Reviews—Vol. 23, Dec. 2006 <http://bsr.wpengine.com/wp-content/uploads/2012/02/BSR-2-BGERvol23.pdf>

5. Prakash, Dhan, Sonika Verma, Ranjana Bhatia, and B. N. Tiwary. "Risks and Precautions of Genetically Modified Organisms." ISRN Ecology 2011 (2011): 1-13. Web. <http://www.hindawi.com/journals/isrn/2011/369573/>

6. "Bought, The Truth Behind Big Pharma, Vaccines and your Food." Dir. Bobby Shehan. Capstone Entertainment, *Boughtmovie.com*, 2014. Film. July. 2015. <http://www.boughtmovie.com/ >

7. "Everything You Never Wanted to Know About Monsanto's Modus Operandi (M.O.)." *Mindfully.org*, n.d. Web. Aug. 2015. <http://www.mindfully.org/Pesticide/Monsanto-Roundup-Glyphosate.htm>

8. "Human Rights." Monsanto. *Monsanto.com*, April. 2006. Web. July 2015. <*http://www.monsanto.com/whoweare/pages/human-rights.aspx*>

9. Edwards Terral, John Faerber, et al. "Benefits of GM Foods." University of California, Santa Cruz. Basken School of Engineering. *classes.soe.ucsc.edu*, 2005. Web. July. 2015. <https://classes.soe.ucsc.edu/cmpe080e/Spring05/projects/gmo/benefits.htm >

10. "The Future of Food." Dir. Deborah Koons Garcia. *Lily Films*, 2004. Film. <http://www.thefutureoffood.com/onlinevideo.html>

11. Michaelis, Kristen. "Hybrid Seeds VS. GMOs." Food Renegade. *foodrenegade.com*, n.d. Web. July. 2015. <http://www.foodrenegade.com/hybrid-seeds-vs-gmos/>

12. "The Difference Between Open Pollinated Seeds, Hybrids and GMOs." Small Footprint Family. *Smallfootprintfamily.com*, n.d. Web. July. 2015. <http://www.smallfootprintfamily.com/hybrid-seeds-vs-gmos#ixzz3s3t0plef>

13. Fairholm, Rebsie. Adventures in experimental Horticulture "F1 hybrids: what every gardener should know." Daughter of the Soil. *Daughterofthesoil.blogspot.com*, 7 July. 2006. Web. July. 2015. <http://daughterofthesoil.blogspot.com/2006/07/f1-hybrids-what-every-gardener-should.html>

14. "One Man, One Cow, One Planet." Dir. Thomas Burstyn. *Cloud South Films*, 2007. Film <http://www.cloudsouth.co.nz/project/one-man- one-cow/>

15. Malone, Andrew. "The GM genocide: Thousands of Indian farmers are committing suicide after using genetically modified crops." Daily Mail. *dailymail.co.uk*, 2 Nov. 2008. Web. July 2015. <http://www.dailymail.

co.uk/news/article-1082559/The-GM-genocide-Thousands-Indian-farm-ers-committing-suicide-using-genetically-modified-crops.html>

16. Link removed <http://www.tendmagazine.co.uk/home/we-need-to-know-about-seeds>

17. "What Is Happening To Biodiversity?" Food and Agriculture Organization of the United Nations. *Fao.org*, n.d. Web. Oct. 2015. <http://www.fao.org/docrep/007/y5609e/ y5609e02.htm>

18. Mattern, Vicki. "Hybid Seeds vs. GMOs." Mother Earth News. 16 Jan. 2013. *Motherearthnews.com*, Web. Oct. 2015. <http://www.motherearth-news.com/real-food/hybrid-seeds-vs-gmos-zb0z1301zsor.aspx>

19. Scott, April. "Genetically Engineered Salmon... Speak Now or Forever You're your Fish." Salem-News. *Salem-news.com*, 06 Sept. 2010. Web. Oct. 2015. <http://www.salem-news.com/articles/september062010/ge-salm-on-as.php>

20. "Genetic Roulette: The Gamble of Our Lives." Dir. Jeffrey M. Smith. The Institute for Responsible Technology. *geneticroulettemovie.com*, 1 Jan. 2012. Web. July 2015. <http://geneticroulettemovie.com/>

21. Halstead, Bruce W. "Poison." Encyclopedia Britannica. *britannica.com*, n.d. Web. Oct. 2015. <http://www.britannica.com/science/poison-biochemistry/Types-of-poison#ref396534>

22. "History Of Pesticide Use." Oregon State University. *people.oregonstate.edu*, n.d. Web. Oct. 2015. <http://people.oregonstate.edu/~muirp/pesthist.htm>

23. "Paul Hermann Muller." Encyclopedia Britannica. *britannica.com*, n.d. Web. Oct. 2015. <http://www.britannica.com/biography/Paul-Hermann-Muller>

24. "The Story of Silent Spring." Natural Resources Defense Council. *nrdc.org*, 5 Dec. 2013. Web. Oct 2015. <http://www.nrdc.org/health/pesti-cides/hcarson.asp>

25. Griswold, Eliza. "How 'Silent Spring' Ignited the Environmental Move-ment." The New York Times Magazine. *Nytimes.com*, 21 Sep. 2012. Web. Oct. 2015 <http://www.nytimes.com/2012/09/23/magazine/how-si-lent-spring-ignited-the-environmental-movement.html?_r=0>

26. "DDT—A Brief History and Status." United States Environmental Protection Agency. *Epa.gov*. n.d. Web. Oct. 2015. <http://www2.epa.gov/ingredients-used-pesticide-products/ddt-brief-history-and-status>

27. "Glyphosate Facts. Industry Task Force on Glyphosate." *glypho-sate.eu*, Oct. 2012. Web. Oct. 2015. <http://www.glyphosate.eu/history-glyphosate>

28. Irani, Riyad Rida. "Aminophosphonate Herbicides." Monsanto Co. assignee. Patent US3455675. 25 June 1965. Web. Dec. 2015. http://www.google.com/patents/US3455675

29. Pollack, Andrew. "E.P.A. Revokes Approval of New Dow Herbicide for G.M.O. Crops." New York Times. *nytimes.com*, 25 Nov. 2015. Web. Dec. 2015. <http://www.nytimes.com/2015/11/26/business/epa-revokes-approval-of-new-dow-herbicide.html?_r=0>

30. *The World According to Monsanto*. Dir. Marie-Monique Robin. National Film Board of Canada, 2008. <https://www.youtube.com/watch?v=2g4L-N9xGdng >

31. Meyer, Nick. "These Politicians Bend Over Backwards to Help Monsanto, But Insist on Organic at Home. "Althealth Works. *Althealthworks. com*, 28 Feb. 2016. Web. Feb. 2016. <http://althealthworks.com/3921/doeshillaryeatorganic-obamagmo-clintongmo-bushorganic-eatorganicorgmo/#sthash.BID9uhwt.dpuf>

32. Lendman, Stephen. "Hillary Clinton Endorses GMOs. White House Meals Are Organic. Organic." Consumers Association. *Organicconsumers. org*, June. 1. 2015. Web. Oct. 2015. <https://www.organicconsumers.org/news/hillary-clinton-endorses-gmos-white-house-meals-are-organic>

33. Miller, S.A. "Hillary's agribusiness ties give rise to nickname in Iowa: 'Bride of Frankenfood'." The Washington Times. *washingtontimes.com*, 17 May. 2015. Web. Oct. 2015. <http://www.washingtontimes.com/news/2015/may/17/hillary-clinton-gmo-support-monsanto-ties-spark-ba/?page=all>

34. NAFTA signed into law. A&E Television Networks, LLC. *history.com*, n.d. Web. Oct. 2015. <http://www.history.com/this-day-in-history/nafta-signed-into-law>

35. Sealing, Keith. "Indigenous Peoples, Indigenous Farmers: NAFTA's Threat to Mexican Teosinte Farmers and What Can be Done About It." American University International Law Review 18, no. 6 (2003) 1383-1398. Web. Oct. 2015. <http://digitalcommons.wcl.american.edu/cgi/viewcontent.cgi?article=1204&context=auilr>

36. Hansen-Kuhn, Karen. "NAFTA at 20: State of the North American Famer." Foreign Policy In Focus. *Fpif.org*, 20 Dec. 2013. Web. Oct. 2015. <http://fpif.org/nafta-20-state-north-american-farmer/>

37. "GM Crops Now Banned in 38 Countries Worldwide—Sustainable Pulse Research." Sustainable Pulse. *Sustainablepulse.com*, 22 Oct. 15. Web. Oct 2015. <http://sustainablepulse.com/2015/10/22/gm-crops-now-banned-in-36-countries- worldwide-sustainable-pulse-research/#.VoSQd_krLIU>

38. Swanson, Nancy. "The Poisoning of our food supply." AXS Network. *examiner.com*, 5 Mar. 2014. Web. Oct. 2015. <http://www.examiner.com/article/the-poisoning-of-our-food-supply>

39. Abate, Tom. "Going Backwards: Clinton Administration Appoints A Former Monsanto Corp. Lobbyist To Represent US Consumers On Genetically Engineered Food Issues." San Francisco Chronicle. *sfgate.com*, 24 July. 2000. Web. Oct. 2015. <http://www.commondreams.org/headlines/072600-03.htm>

40. Philpott, Tom. "Does Monsanto Man Mitt Romney Secretly Eat Organic?" Mother Jones and the Foundation for National Progress. *Motherjones.com*, 26 Sep. 2012. Web. Oct. 2015. <http://www.motherjones.com/tom-philpott/2012/09/report-monsanto-man-mitt-romney-eats-organic>

41. Vidal, John. "GM lobby takes root in Bush's cabinet." Guardian News and Media. *theguardian.com*, 31 Jan. 2001. Web. Oct. 2015. <http://www.theguardian.com/science/2001/feb/01/gm.food>

42. "Racketeering Charges Filed Against Donald Rumsfeld & Monsanto." Organic Consumers Association. *organicconsumers.org*, 7 Nov. 2006. Web. Oct. 2015. <https://www.organicconsumers.org/news/racketeering-charges-filed-against-donald-rumsfeld-monsanto>

43. "Organics program weakened under Bush administration changes, activists say." Grist. *Grist.org*, 19 May. 2004. Web. Oct. 2015. <http://grist.org/article/griscom-organic/>

44. Chua, Jasmin Malik. "USDA Waters Down Organic Standard. Narrative Content Group." *Treehugger.com*, 27 June. 2007. Web. Oct. 2015. <http://www.treehugger.com/green-food/usda-waters-down-organic-standards.html>

45. Corley, Matt. "Bushes Feast On Organic Food But Undermines Same Opportunity For American Families." Center For American Progress Action. *Thinkprogress.org*, 15 Jan. 2009. Web. Oct. 2015. <http://thinkprogress.org/politics/2009/01/15/34854/laura-bush-organic/>

46. "These Politicians support GMOs, but eat Organic at Home." VAN. *Viralalternativenews.com*, 12 Nov. 2015. Web. November. 2015. <http://www.viralalternativenews.com/2015/11/these-politicians-support-gmos-but-eat.html>

47. CENTER FOR FOOD SAFETY, ORGANIC SEED ALLIANCE, SIERRA CLUB AND HIGH MOWING ORGANIC SEEDS Vs. Thomas J. Vilsack, UNITED STATES DISTRICT COURT FOR THE NORTHERN DISTRICT OF CALIFORNIA SAN FRANCISCO DIVISION § Civil Action No 08-0484-JSW (2009). PDF. <https://www.sustainablefoodnews.com/userfiles/file/gm%20sugar%20beet%20no%20change%20at%20USDA.pdf >

48. "Obama signs Monsanto Protection Act! Betrays America—It's Time to Label GMOs!" Food Democracy Now. *Fooddemocracynow.org*, 27 Mar. 2013. Web. Oct. 2015. <http://www.fooddemocracynow.org/blog/2013/mar/27/obama_signs_monsanto_protection_act>

49. Shen, Aviva. "The Real Monsanto Protection Act: How The GMO Giant Corrupts Regulators And Consolidates Its Power." Center For American Action Fund. *Thinkprogress.org*, 10 Apr. 2013. Web. Oct. 2015. <http://thinkprogress.org/health/2013/04/10/1832621/monsanto-protection-act-power/>

50. Alman, Ashley. Monsanto Protection Act' To Expire, Won't Be Part Of

Continuing Resolution. HuffPost Politics. Huffingtonpost.com, 24 Sept. 2013. Web. Oct. 2015. <http://www.huffingtonpost.com/2013/09/24/monsanto-protection-act-expire_n_3985673.html>

51. Shen, Aviva. "The Real Monsanto Protection Act: How The GMO Giant Corrupts Regulators And Consolidates Its Power." Center For American Action Fund. *Thinkprogress.org*, 10 Apr. 2013. Web. Oct. 2015. <http://thinkprogress.org/health/2013/04/10/1832621/monsanto-protection-act-power/>

52. "Obama signs Monsanto Protection Act! Betrays America—It's Time to Label GMOs!" Food Democracy Now. *Fooddemocracynow.org*, Mar. 27. 2013. Web. Oct. 2015. <http://www.fooddemocracynow.org/blog/2013/mar/27/obama_signs_monsanto_protection_act>

53. United States Congress. House—Energy and Commerce; Agriculture | Senate—Agriculture, Nutrition, and Forestry. Congress.gov. Rep. Pompeo, Mike [R-KS-4], 23 July 2015. Web. Oct. 2015. <https://www.congress.gov/bill/114th-congress/house-bill/1599>

54. Walia, Arjun. "Monsanto Protection Act Part 2? New Bill Introduced Spells Bad News For GMO Activists." Collective Evolution. *Collective-evolution.com*, 21 June. 2015. Web. Oct. 2015. <http://www.collective-evolution.com/2015/06/21/monsanto-protection-act-part-2-new-bill-introduced-spells-bad-news-for-gmo-activists/>

55. "State Labeling Initiatives." Center For Food Safety *Centerforfoodsafety.org*, n.d. Web. Oct. 2015. <http://www.centerforfoodsafety.org/issues/976/ge-food-labeling/state-labeling-initiatives>

56. "Public Pressure and Allies in Congress Keep "Rider" Blocking State Labeling of GMOs Out of Spending Bill." Center For Food Safety. *Centerforfoodsafety.org*, 16 Dec. 2015. Web. Dec. 2015. <http://www.centerforfoodsafety.org/press-releases/4171/public-pressure-and-allies-in-congress- keep-rider-blocking-state-labeling-of-gmos-out-of-spending-bill>

57. Gucciardi, Anthony. "Senate Passes TPP 'Fast-Tracking' That Could Make GMO Labeling Illegal." Natural Society. *naturalsociety.com*, 24 June. 2015. Web. Oct. 2015. <http://naturalsociety.com/senate-passes-tpp-fast-tracking-gmo-labeling-illegal/#ixzz3uoFO6jEV>

58. Kaminski, Margot E. "Don't Keep the Trans-Pacific Partnership Talks Secret." The New York Times. *nytimes.com*, April. 14. 2015. Web. Oct. 2015. <http://www.nytimes.com/2015/04/14/opinion/dont-keep-trade-talks-secret.html?_r=0>

59. Stone, Jeff. "TPP Trade Deal Would Curb Freedom of Speech Online, Internet Activists Warn." International Business Times. *ibtimes.com*, 17 April. 2015. Web. Oct. 2015. <http://www.ibtimes.com/tpp-trade-deal-would-curb-freedom-speech-online-internet-activists-warn-1883780>

60. Lendman, Stephen. "Hillary Clinton Endorses GMOs. White House Meals are Organic." Global Research. *Globalresearch.ca*,

25 May. 2015. Web. Oct. 2015. <http://www.globalresearch.ca/hillary-clinton-endorses-gmos-white-house-meals-are-organic/5451481>

61. "PA: Hillary Clinton Fights Obama, Unions, Labor & US Jobs." YouTube. *YouTube.com*, 13 Feb. 2008. Web. Oct. 2015. <https://www.youtube.com/watch?v=sigkAd3SxxI>

62. "Children Found Sewing Clothing For Wal-Mart, Hanes & Other U.S. & European Companies. " The Labor and Worklife Program at Harvard Law School. *Law.harvard.edu*. n.d. Web. Oct. 2015 <http://www.law.harvard.edu/programs/lwp/NLC_childlabor.html>

63. Clinton, William J. "Hillary Rodham Clinton." National Archives. *Nara.gov*, n.d. Web. Oct 2015 <*http://clinton2.nara.gov/WH/glimpse/firstladies/html/hc42.html*>

64. Miller, S.A. "Hillary's agribusiness ties give rise to nickname in Iowa: 'Bride of Frankenfood'." The Washington Times. *washingtontimes.com*, 17 May. 2015. Web. Oct. 2015. <http://www.washingtontimes.com/news/2015/may/17/hillary-clinton-gmo-support-monsanto-ties-spark-ba/?page=all>

65. McMorris-Santoro, Evan. "Sanders Claims CBS Canceled Agriculture Interview Because Monsanto Was 'Threatening' To Sue." Buzzfeed Inc. *buzzfeed.com*, Nov. 21. 2015. Web. Nov. 2015. <http://www.buzzfeed.com/evanmcsan/sanders-claims-cbs-canceled-agriculture-interview-because-mo#.sfjjkzdLR>

66. "CNN: Millions protest genetically modified food, Monsanto, organizers say." Occupymonsanto.com, 28 May. 2013. <**http://occupy-monsanto.com/tag/bernie-sanders/**> VIDEO

67. Frankel, Judy. "Hillary vs. Bernie on Frankenfood." HUFFPOST POLITICS *Huffingtonpost.com,23* June. 2015. Web. Oct. 2015. <http://www.huffingtonpost.com/judy-frankel/hillary-vs-bernie-on-fran_b_7638846.html>

68. Easley, Jason. "Bernie Sanders Calls Out Monsanto for Killing His GMO Labeling Amendment." PoliticusUSA. *Politicususa.com*, 15 June. 2013. Web. Oct. 2015. <http://www.politicususa.com/2013/06/15/bernie-sanders-calls-monsanto-killing-gmo-labeling-amendment.html>

69. Frankel, Judy. "Hillary vs. Bernie on Frankenfood." HUFFPOST POLITICS. *Huffingtonpost.com*, 23 June. 2015. Web. Oct. 2015. <http://www.huffingtonpost.com/judy-frankel/hillary-vs-bernie-on-fran_b_7638846.html>

70. "Michael R. Taylor, JD., Deputy Commissioner for Foods and Veterinary Medicine." US Food and Drug Administration. *Fda.gov*, n.d. Web. Oct. 2015. <http://www.fda.gov/AboutFDA/CentersOffices/OfficeofFoods/ucm196721.htm>

71. "Taylor, Michael R. The Center For Responsive Politics." *Opensecrets.org*,

n.d. Web. Oct. 2015. <https://www.opensecrets.org/revolving/rev_summary.php?id=20919>

72. Swanson, Nancy "The Poisoning of our food supply." AXS Digital Group, LLC. *examiner.com*, March. 5. 2014. Web. Oct. 2015. <http://www.examiner.com/article/the-poisoning-of-our-food-supply>

73. "The Delaney Clause." The Center on Congress, *Centeroncongress.org,* n.d. Web. Oct. 2015. <http://centeroncongress.org/delaney-clause>

74. <http://www.chemheritage.org/discover/collections/oral- histories/details/tsca-fisher.aspx> BROKEN LINK

75. Upholding Values, Managing the Network, and Driving Excellence. DuPont. *Dupont.com,* n.d. Web. Oct. 2015. <http://www.dupont.com/corporate-functions/our-company/leadership/senior-leadership/articles/fisher.html>

76. North, Rick. "Recombinant Bovine Growth Hormone (rBGH or RBST)." Physicians for Social Responsibility, *Noharm.org.* n.d. Web. Oct. 2015. <http://noharm.org/lib/downloads/nurses/presentations/rBGHin_Dairy.pdf>

77. "Mickey Kantor." Washington Speakers Bureau. *Washingtonspeakers.com,* n.d. Web. Oct. 2015. <http://www.washingtonspeakers.com/speakers/biography.cfm?SpeakerID=2077>

78. South Carolina Bureau. "Hale leaving White House post." The Augusta Chronicle. *Chronicleagusta.com,* 20 May. 1997. Web. Oct. 2015 <http://chronicle.augusta.com/stories/1997/05/20/met_208646.shtml#.Vm3lSEorLIU>

79. "Michael A. Friedman, M.D. President and Chief Executive Officer City of Hope Medical Center." Tulane University. *Tulane.edu,* n.d. Web. Oct. 2015. <https://tulane.edu/presidentialsearch/michael-friedman.cfm>

80. Pantsios, Anastasia. "GMO Labeling Nation's 'Biggest Food Fight' Hits DC." EcoWatch. *Ecowatch.com,* 25 Mar. 2015. Web. Oct. 2015. <http://ecowatch.com/2015/03/25/gmo-labeling-hits-dc/>

81. "Biography of William D. Ruckelshaus: First Term." United States Environmental Protection Agency. *Epa.gov,* n.d. Web. Oct. 2015. <http://www.epa.gov/aboutepa/biography-william-d-ruckelshaus-first-term>

82. Mulkern, Anne C. "Revolving Door." Denver Post. *Mindfully.org, 23* May. 2004. Web. Oct. 2015 <http://www.mindfully.org/GE/Revolving-Door.htm>

83. Sager, Josh. "Justice Clarence Thomas and Monsanto." *Theprogressivecynic.com,* July. 2013. Web. Oct. 2015. <https://theprogressivecynic.com/2013/07/15/justice-clarence-thomas-and-monsanto/>

84. "Donald Rumsfeld." Wikimedia Foundation, Inc. *Wikipedia.org,* n.d. Web. Oct. 2015. <https://en.wikipedia.org/wiki/Donald_Rumsfeld>

85. "108 Corporations depart ALEC" ALEC Exposed. Center for Media and

Democracy. *Alecexpsed.org*. n.d. Web. Oct. 2015. <http://www.alecex-posed.org/wiki/ALEC_Exposed>

86. What Is The Basis For Corporate Personhood? Oregon Public Broadcasting NPR. *Npr.org*, 24 Oct. 2011. Web. Oct. 2015. <http://www.npr.org/2011/10/24/141663195/what-is-the-basis-for-corporate-personhood>

87. Scott, April. "Genetically Modified Crops—Contamination without Representation." Salem-News.com. *salem-news.com*, 17 Nov. 2011. Web. Oct. 2015. <http://www.salem-news.com/articles/november172011/gm-beets-as.php>

88. "U.S House of Representatives, Committee on Agriculture Forum on GM Alfalfa." *Agriculture.house.gov*, 20 Jan. 2011. Video hearing transcript. Oct. 2015. https://agriculture.house.gov/sites/republicans.agriculture.house.gov/files/pdf/publicforum/forumcommitteeprint110120.pdf>

   88a. Original video hearing: http://agriculture.house.gov/hearings/hearingdetails.aspx?NewsID=1269> BROKEN LINK—**removed from public access**.

89. "U.S House of Representatives, Committee on Agriculture Forum on GM Alfalfa." Adapted by: GMO-FREE Portland and retitled; "Inappropriate Manipulation by House Ag Committee." GMOreform. *YouTube*, 20 Oct. 2011. Web. Oct. 2015. <https://www.youtube.com/watch?v=83gIyaEpWJY>

90. "World Food Prize goes to Monsanto." GM Watch. *gmwatch.org*, 26 June. 2013. Web. Oct. 2015. <http://www.gmwatch.org/news/archive/2013/14786-world-food-prize-goes-to-monsanto>

91. Heinemann, Jack A., Melanie Massaro, Dorien S. Coray, Sarah Zanon Agapito-Tenfen, and Jiajun Dale Wen. "Sustainability and Innovation in Staple Crop Production in the US Midwest." *International Journal of Agricultural Sustainability* 12.1 (2013): 71-88. <http://www.tandfonline.com/doi/full/10.1080/14735903.2013.806408>

92. Richardson, Jill. "Research Shows That Monsanto's Big Claims for GMO Food Are Probably Wrong." The Cornucopia Institute. Cornucopia.org, 28 June 2013. Web. Oct. 2015. <http://www.cornucopia.org/2013/06/research-shows-that-monsantos-big-claims-for-gmo-food-are-probably-wrong/>

93. Genetically Engineered Foods Q & A. USA Today. *usatoday.com*. Oct 28. 2012. Web. Oct. 2015. <www.usatoday.com/story/news/nation/2012/.../gmo.../1658225/>

94. Philpott, Tom. "Could Prop. 37 Kill Monsanto's GM Seeds?" Foundation for National Progress. *Motherjones.com*, Oct. 10. 2012. Web. Oct. 2015. <http://www.motherjones.com/environment/2012/10/california-prop-37-monsanto-gmo-labeling>

95. Kelly, Margie. "Top 7 Genetically Modified Crops." HUFFPOST GREEN. *Huffingtonpost.com*, 30 Oct. 2012. Web. Oct. 2015. <http://www.

huffingtonpost.com/margie-kelly/genetically-modified-food_b_2039455.
html>

96. Ho, Mae-Wan and Sirinathsinghji. Eva. "Ban GMOs Now Health &
    Environmental Hazards." The Institute of Science in Society, *i-sis.org.
    uk,* 05 May 2013. Web. Oct. 2015. <http://www.i-sis.org.uk/Ban_GMOs_
    Now.php>

97. Mertens, Martha. *Assessment of Environmental Impacts of Genetically Modified
    Plants: Implementation of the Biosafety Protocol Development of Assessment Bases*
    FKZ 201 67 430/07. Bonn: BN—*Institute for Biodiversity,* 2008. Bundes-
    samt Für Naturschutz. 2008. PDF. Oct. 2015. <https://www.bfn.de/
    fileadmin/MDB/documents/service/skript217.pdf>

98. Johnson, David and O'Connor, Siobhan. "These Charts Show Every
    Genetically Modified Food People Already Eat in the U.S." Time, inc.
    Time.com, 30 April. 32015. Web. Oct. 2015. <http://time.com/3840073/
    gmo-food-charts/>

99. "WHAT IS GMO?" NON-GMO PROJECT, *Nongmoproject.org,* n.d. Web.
    Oct. 2015. <http://www.nongmoproject.org/learn-more/what-is-gmo/>

100. Satran, Joe. "Greening-Resistant GMO Oranges Come One Step Closer
     To Market. Here's Why You Should Care." HUFFPOST GREEN.
     *Huffingtonpost.com,*14 May 2015. Web. Oct. 2015. <http://www.
     huffingtonpost.com/2015/05/14/gmo- oranges-citrus-greening-south-
     ern-gardens_n_7244858.html>

101. "Invisible GM Ingredients." Institute for Responsible Technology. *Nong-
     moshoppingguide.com.* n.d. Web. Oct. 2015. <http://nongmoshoppingguide.
     com/brands/invisible-gm-ingredients.html>

Chapter 2 Independent Science

1. Ho, Mae-Wan. "Open Letter from World Scientists to All Governments."
   Institute for Science in Society. *I-sis.org,* Feb. 1999. Web. Aug. 2015.
   <http://www.i-sis.org.uk/list.php>

   1a. Ho, Mae-Wan. "The Independent Science Panel on GM Final
       Report." Institute for Science in Society. *I-sis.org,* May. 2003. Web.
       Aug. 2015 <http://www.i-sis.org.uk/ispr-summary.php>

   1b. Ho, Mae-Wan and Lim Li Ching. "The Case for a GM-Free Sustain-
       able World." Institute for Science in Society. *I-sis.org,* 15 June 2003.
       Web. Aug. 2015 <http://www.i-sis.org.uk/TheCaseforAGM- FreeSus-
       tainableWorld.php> or <*http://www.psrast.org/caseforGMfreeW.pdf* >

   1c. Ho, Mae-Wan, Eva Sirinathsinghji. "Ban GMOs Now." The Insti-
       tute of Science in Society. *i-sis.org.uk,* 24 May 2013. Web. Aug. 2015.
       <http://www.isis.org.uk/Ban_GMOs_Now.php>

   1d. Independent Scientists Manifesto on Glyphosate." The Institute of

Science in Society. *i-sis.org.uk,* 6 Aug. 2015. Web. Aug. 2015. <http://www.isis.org.uk/Independent_ Scientists_Manifesto_on_Glyphosate.php>

2.   "About Us." Union of Concerned Scientists. *ucsusa.org,* n.d. Web. Aug. 2015 < http://www.ucsusa.org/about-us#.V9snMSgrLIU>

    2a. "Genetic Engineering Risks and Impacts." Union of Concerned Scientists. *ucsusa.org,* n.d. Web. Aug. 2015. < http://www.ucsusa.org/food_and_agriculture/ our-failing-food-system/genetic-engineering/risks- of- genetic-engineering.html#.V66LF4-cFMs>

    2b. "The Healthy Farm-A Vison for U.S. Agriculture. "Union of Concerned Scientists Policy Brief. *Ucsusa.org,* 2013. PDF. Aug. 2016 <http://www.ucsusa.org/food_and_agriculture/ solutions/advance-sustainable- agriculture/healthy-farm-vision.html#.V7JqU4- cHIU>

3.   Leary. Warren E. "Genetic Engineering of Crops Can Spread Allergies, Study Shows." The New York Times. Nytimes.com, 14 Mar. 1996. Web. Aug. 2015 <http://www.nytimes.com/1996/03/14/us/genetic-engineering-of-crops-can-spread-allergies-study-shows.html>

4.   "More Americans getting multiple chronic illnesses." Reuters, *Reuters. com,* 6 Jan. 2009. Web. Aug. 2015._<http://www.reuters.com/article/us-usa-chronic-idUSTRE5050S920090106>

5.   Smith, Jeffrey. "10 Reasons to Avoid GMOs." Institute for Responsible Technology. *Responsibletechnology.org,* 25 Aug. 2011. Web. Aug. 2015. <http://responsibletechnology.org/10-reasons-to-avoid-gmos/>

6.   Scott, April. "While We Were Sleeping...GM Food and the Brink of No Return." Salem-News. Salem-news.com, 1 Mar. *2010. Web. Aug. 2015.* <http://www.salem-news.com/articles/march012010/monsanto_as.php >

7.   Rowell, Andy. "Don't Worry (It's Safe to Eat): The True Story of GM Food, BSE and Foot and Mouth." Earthscan Publications, New York, 2003. *78-97.* Print. Aug. 2015. <http://www.powerbase.info/index.php/Arpad_Pusztai >

8.   Engdahl, F. William. "Seeds of Destruction. The Hidden Agenda of Genetic Manipulation" Global Research, Centre for Research on Globalization. Montreal, Canada. 2007. PDF. Aug. 2015. <https://media.8ch.net/tdt/src/1445315187664.pdf >

9.   Rowell, Andy. "Don't Worry (It's Safe to Eat): The True Story of GM Food, BSE and Foot and Mouth." Earthscan Publications, New York. 2003. *78-97.* Print. Aug. 2015. <http://www.powerbase.info/index.php/Arpad_Pusztai >

10. "Arpad Pusztai to receive Stuttgart Peace Prize." GMWatch, *GMWatch. org,* 11 Dec. 2009. Web. Aug. 2015. <http://www.gmwatch.org/news/archive/2009/11801-pusztai-to-receive-stuttgart-peace-prize>

11. "Fifteen years too late—when will Pusztai get an apology from those

who destroyed his career?" GM-FREE Cymru. gmfreecymru.org, 23 April 2014.Web. Aug. 2015. <http://www.gmfreecymru.org/documents/pusztai-fifteen-years-too-late.html>

12. "Republication of Seralini Study: Science Speaks for Itself." Sustainable Pulse. *GMO Seralini.org*, 24 June 2014. Web. Sept. 2015. <http://www.gmoseralini.org/republication-seralini-study-science-speaks/>

13. Sarich, Christina. "Huge: Seralini Wins Defamation Forgery Court Cases Over GMO Research." Natural Society, *Naturalsociety.com*, 1 Dec. 2015. Web. Sept. 2015. <http://naturalsociety.com/huge-seralini-wins-defamation-forgery-court-cases-gmo-research/>

14. Miller, Henry I. "Scientists Smell a Rat in Fraudulent Genetic Engineering Study." Forbes Opinion. *Forbes.com*, 25 Sept. 2012. Web. Aug. 2015. <http://www.forbes.com/sites/henrymiller/2012/09/25/scientists-smell-a-rat-in-fraudulent-genetic-engineering-study/#3e170c9f1ff1>

15. Séralini, Gilles-Eric, et al. Republished study: Long-term Toxicity of a Roundup Herbicide and a Roundup Tolerant Genetically Modified Maize. Environmental Sciences Europe, *enveurope.com*, (2014): 26:14. Web. Aug. 2015. <http://www.enveurope.com/content/26/1/14>

16. Shilhavy, Brian. "Glyphosate Causes Cancer: EPA "Trade Secret" Sealed Files Reveal Cancer Link Known Back in the 1970s." Health Impact News. *healthimpactnews.com*, 29 May 2015. Web. Aug. 2015. <http://healthimpactnews.com/2015/glyphosate-causes-cancer-epa-trade-secret-sealed-files-reveal-cancer-link-known-back-in-the-1970s/#sthash.7JsSxNsy.dpuf>

17. Polansek, Tom. "Monsanto weed killer can 'probably' cause cancer: World Health Organization." Reuters. *Reuters.com*, 20 Mar. 2015. Web. Aug. 2015. <http://www.reuters.com/article/us-monsanto-roundup-cancer-idUSKBN0MG2NY20150320>

18. Samsel, A. and S. Seneff. "Glyphosate's Suppression of Cytochrome P450 Enzymes and Amino Acid Biosynthesis by the Gut Microbiome: Pathways to Modern Diseases." Entropy. *Mdpi.com*, 2013, 15, 1416-1463; doi:10.3390/e15041416. Web. Aug. 2015. <http://www.mdpi.com/1099-4300/15/4/1416>

18a. Samsel, A. and S. Seneff. "Glyphosate, pathways to modern diseases II: Celiac sprue and gluten intolerance." Interdiscip Toxicol. (4):159-84. doi: 10.2478/intox-2013-0026. 6 Dec. 2013 <http://www.ncbi.nlm.nih.gov/pubmed/24678255>

18b. Samsel, A. and S. Seneff. "Glyphosate, pathways to modern diseases III: Manganese, neurological diseases, and associated pathologies." Surgical Neurology International. 6(1):45 ·DOI: 10.4103/2152-7806.153876. March 2015 <https://www.researchgate.net/publication/274005953_Glyphosate_pathways_to_modern_diseases_III_Manganese_neurological_diseases_and_associated_pathologies>

18c. Samsel A and S. Seneff. "Glyphosate, pathways to modern diseases

IV: cancer and related pathologies." Journal of Biological Physics and Chemistry. 15(3):121-159 · January 2015 DOI: 10.4024/11SA15R. jbpc.15.03 <https://www.researchgate.net/publication/283490944_ Glyphosate_pathways_to_modern_diseases_IV_cancer_and_ related_pathologies>

18d. Samsel A and S. Seneff. "Glyphosate, pathways to modern diseases V: Amino acid analogue of glycine in diverse proteins." Journal of Biological Physics and Chemistry 2016;16:9-46. < https://www.researchgate.net/publication/305318376_Gly-phosate_pathways_to_modern_diseases_V_Amino_acid_ analogue_of_glycine_in_diverse_proteins>

19. Francis, Raymond. "Inflammation a Common Denominator of Disease. Wellbeing Journal." Nov/Dec. 2008. Reprinted by Arizona Center for Advanced Medicine. *Arizonaadvancedmedicine.com*, 26 June 2013. Web. Aug. 2015. <http://www.arizonaadvancedmedicine.com/Articles/2013/ June/Inflammation-A-Common-Denominator-of-Disease.aspx>

20. Suzuki, David. "Biography." David Suzuki Foundation. *davidsuzuki.org*, n.d. Web. Sept. 2015. <http://www.davidsuzuki.org/david/>

21. Fenlon, Brodie. "Professor David Suzuki Speaks Out Against GMOs." Canadian Broadcast Company (CBC). *cbc.ca*, Oct.17.2001. TV. Sept. 2015. <http://www.cbc.ca/archives/entry/ david-suzuki-speaks-out-against-genetically-modified-food>

22. "What are Roundup Ready & Bt Pesticide GMO crops? You need to know!" Michael Trout. YouTube. *Youtube.com, Nov. 3. 2012. Video. Sept. 2015.* <https://www.youtube.com/watch?v=9hjy-CJlzbM>

23. Walia, Arjun. "Confirmed: DNA from Genetically Modified Crops Can Be Transferred To Humans Who Eat Them." Collective Evolution. *collective-evolution.com*, 9 Jan. 2014. Web. Sept. 2015. <http:// www.collective-evolution.com/2014/01/09/confirmed-dna-from-genet-ically-modified-crops-can-be-transfered-to-humans-who-eat-them-2/ comment-page-3/>

24. Fenlon, Brodie. "Professor David Suzuki Speaks Out Against GMOs." Canadian Broadcast Company (CBC). cbc.ca, 17 Oct. 2001. TV. Sept. 2015. <http://www.cbc.ca/archives/entry/ david-suzuki-speaks-out-against-genetically-modified-food>

25. N/A

26. Scott, April. "GM Food...Feeding the Hungry or Population Control?" Salem-News. *Salem-news.com*, 26 April 2010. Web. Sept. 2015. <http:// www.salem-news.com/articles/april262010/gm-food-as.php>

27. Baranov AS, Chernova OF, Feoktistova NY and Surov AV. "A new example of ectopia:oral hair in some rodent species." *ncbi.nlm.nih.gov*, Dokl Biol Sci, 2010 Mar-Apr; 431:117-20. PubMed PMID: 20506849. Web. Sept. 2015. <http://www.ncbi.nlm.nih.gov/pubmed/20506849>

28. Smith, Jeffrey. "Genetically Modified Soy Linked to Sterility, Infant Mortality in Hamsters." Huffington Post. *Huffingtonpost.com*, 9 Aug. 2010/25 May 2011.Web. Sept. 2015 .<http://www.huffingtonpost.com/jeffrey-smith/genetically-modified-soy_b_544575.html>

29. Swanson, Nancy. "Nancy Swanson." GMO Experts. GMO-FREE Washington. *gmofreewashington.com*, n.d. Web. Sept. 2015. <http://gmof-reewashington.com/our-experts/nancy- swanson/ >

30. Swanson, Nancy, et al. "Genetically engineered crops, glyphosate and the deterioration of health in the United States of America." Journal of Organic Systems, 9(2), *Organic-systems.org*, 2014. PDF. Sept. 2015. <http://www.organic-systems.org/journal/92/JOS_Volume-9_Number-2_Nov_2014-Swanson-et-al.pdf>

31. Huber, Don. "Dr. Don Huber's Cover Letter to EU and UK Commissions. "Food Democracy Now. *fooddemocracynow.com*, 6 April 2011. Web. Sept. 2015. <http://www.fooddemocracynow.org/blog/2011/apr/6/don-hubers-cover-letter-euuk-commissions>

32. Huber, Don. "Why We Need to KO GMOs." Bulletproof Radio. *Bulletproofexec.com*, 2013. PDF. Oct. 2015. <https://www.bulletproofexec.com/wpcontent/uploads/2016/06/Transcript-DonHuber.pdf >

33. Obrien, Robyn. "A Former GMO Scientist Sends an Open Letter to Canada's Minister of Health." Robyn Obrien. *robynobrien.com*, 2 Nov. 2014. Web. Oct. 2015. <http://robynobrien.com/a-former-gmo-scientist-sends-an-open-letter-to-canadas-minister-of-health/ >

34. Vrain, Thierry. "GMOs and the Roundup Chemical Glyphosate." Watershed Sentinel. *Watershedsentinel.ca*, Mar-April. 2015. Vol. 25-2. Web. Oct. 2015. <http://www.watershedsentinel.ca/content/gmos-and-round-up-chemical-glyphosate >

35. Gasnier, Celine, Coralie Dumont, Nora Benachour, Emilie Clair, Marie-Christine Chagnon and Gilles-Eric Seralini. "Glyphosate based herbicides are toxic and endocrine disrupters in human cell lines." *ncbi.nlm.nih.gov*. Toxicology Vol 262, Issue 3, 21 Aug. 2009, Pages 184-191. Oct. 2015. <http://www.ncbi.nlm.nih.gov/pubmed/19539684>

36. Zimmermann, Kim Ann. "Endocrine System: Facts, Functions and Diseases." LiveScience. *Livescience.com*, March.11.2016. Web. *Oct. 2015.* <http://www.livescience.com/26496-endocrine-system.html>

37. Vrain, Thierry. "Dr. Thierry Vrain." GE FREE Comax Valley, GE Free Comax Valley. *gefreecomoxvalley.wordpress*. n.d. Web. Oct. 2015. <https://gefreecomoxvalley.wordpress.com/dr-thierry-vrain/>

38. Vrain, Thierry. "Former Pro-GMO Scientist Speaks Out On The Real Dangers Of Genetically Modified Food." GMO Empowerment. *gmosummit.org*, n.d. Web. Oct. 2015. <http://gmosummit.org/former-pro-gmo-scientist/>

39. Edwards, Rob. "Eating GM Food Could Give You Cancer Says Scientist."

Rense.com. via the Sunday Herald, 9 Dec. 2000. Web. Oct. 2015. <http://www.rense.com/general32/Eating.htm>

40. Smith, Jeffrey. "Most Offspring Died When Mother Rats Ate Genetically Engineered Soy." Institute for Responsible Technology. *responsibletechnology.org*, n.d. Web. Oct. 2015. <http://responsibletechnology.org/allfraud/most-offspring-died-when-mother-rats-ate-genetically-engineered-soy/>

41. Smith, Jeffrey M. "Doctors Warn Avoid Genetically Modified Food." *Rense.com*, 22 July 2009. Web. Oct. 2015. <http://www.rense.com/general86/doct.htm>

42. *Scientists for a GMO Free Europe*. Institute for Science in Society, *i-sis.or.uk*. Nov. 6. 2011. Web. Oct. 2015. <http://www.i-sis.org.uk/GM_Free_Europe.php>

43. Sarich, Christina. "Lobbyists At It Again: GMO Labeling Fight Likely To Resume In New Year. "*naturalsociety.com*. Natural Society, 27 Dec. 2015. Web. Jan.2016. <http://naturalsociety.com/lobbyists-at-it-again-gmo-labeling-fight-likely-to-resume-in-new-year/>

44. Smith, Jeffrey. "Spilling the Beans: Unintended GMO Health Risks." *organicconsumers.org*. Organic Consumers Association, 1 Mar. 2008. Web. Oct. 2015. <https://www.organicconsumers.org/news/spilling-beans-unintended-gmo-health-risks>

45. Ermakova, Irina V. "Influence of Genetically Modified-SOYA on the Birthrate and Survival of Rat Pups: Preliminary Study. " *Mindfully.org*, 10 Oct. 2005. Web. Oct. 2015. <http://www.mindfully.org/GE/2005/Modified-Soya-Rats10oct05.htm>

46. Smith, Jeffrey. "Suppression of the truth about GMO hazards." Physicians and Scientists for Responsible Application of Science and Technology, *psrast.org*. n.d. Web. Oct. 2015. <http://www.psrast.org/criticssuppr.htm>

47. Ayyadurai, V.A. Shiva and Prabhakar Dionikar. "Do GMOs Accumulate Formaldehyde and Disrupt Moleculars Equilibria? Systems Biology May Provide Answers." Systems Biology Group, International Center for Integrative Systems, Agricultural Sciences. 2015, 6, 630-662. *Prnewwire.com*, July 2015 Print. Oct. 2015. <http://www.prnewswire.com/news-releases/systems-biology-group-international-center-for-integrative-systems-gmo-soy-accumulates-formaldehyde—disrupts-plant-metabolism-suggests-peer-reviewed-study-calling-for-21st-century-safety-standards-300112959.html>

47a. Ayyadurai, V.A. Shiva and Prabhakar Dionikar. "Do GMOs Accumulate Formaldehyde and Disrupt Moleculars Equilibria? Systems Biology May Provide Answers." Systems Biology Group, International Center for Integrative Systems, Agricultural Sciences. 2015, 6, 630-662. *integrativesystems.org*. July 2015 in SciRes. Print. Oct. 2015. <http://www.integrativesystems.org/systems- biology-of-gmos/ >

48. Engdahl, F. William. "A Killer-Diller: GMO Soy Makes Form-aldehyde in Our Gut." New Eastern Outlook. *journal-neo. org,* 27 July 2007. Web. Oct. 2015. <http://journal-neo. org/2015/07/27/a-killer-diller-gmo-soy-makes-formaldehyde-in-our-gut/>

49. Mesnage, Robin, Matthew Arno, Manuela Costanzo, Gilles-Eric Ser-alini and Michael N. Antoniou. 'Transcriptome profile analysis reflects rat liver and kidney damage following chronic ultra-low dose Roundup exposure'. Environmental Health Journal, 14:70. DOI: 10.1186/s12940-015-0056. 25 Aug. 2015. Print. Oct. 2015. <http://www.ehjournal.net/ content/pdf/s12940-015-0056-1.pdf%20(open%20access) >

50. Antoniou, Michael N, Claire Robinson and John Fagan. "GMO Myths and Truths, an evidence based examination of the claims made for the safety and efficacy of genetically modified crops." Earth Open Source. *earthopensource.org,* June 2012. Web. Oct. 2015. <http://responsibletech-nology.org/media/docs/GMO_Myths_and_Truths_1.3b.pdf>

51. "New Report Challenge GM Industry Myths." Farming Online. *farming. co.uk,* 19 June. 2012. Web. Oct. 2015. <http://www.farming.co.uk/news/ article/6711>

52. "Seeds of Information, Twelve Years of GM Soya in Argentina—a Disaster for People and the Environment, Seedling." GRAIN, *grain. org,* 4 July 2009. Web. Oct. 2015. <https://www.grain.org/article/ entries/750-seeds-of-information?print=true>

53. Smith, Jeffrey. "GMO Researchers Attacked, Evidence Denied, and a Population at Risk." Global Research. *globalresearch.ca,* 19 Sept. 2012. Web. Oct. 2016. <http://www.globalresearch.ca/gmo-researchers-at-tacked-evidence-denied-and-a-population-at-risk/5305324?print=1>

54. Carman, Judy. Interview with Simon Lauder. "Study casts doubt on safety of GM Foods." ABC. PM. *Abc.net.au,* Australia: 12 June 2013. Radio. Oct. 2016. <http://www.abc.net.au/pm/content/2013/s3780391. htm>

55. Carman, Judy. "A long-term toxicology study on pigs fed a mixed GM diet. Adverse effects of GM crops found." Sustainable Pulse. *gmojudy-carman.org,* 11 June. 2013. *Web. Oct. 2016.* <http://gmojudycarman.org/ wpcontent/uploads/2013/06/Clear-English-explanation-of-the-study-for-website-11Jun13.pdf>

56. Carman, Judy A, et al. "A long-term toxicology study on pigs fed a com-bined genetically modified (GM) soy and GM maize diet." Journal of Organic Systems, *Organic-systems.org.* (2013): 8 (1): 38-54. Open access full text. PDF. Oct. 2015. <http://www.organic-systems.org/journal/81/ 8106. pdf>

57. Smith, Jeffrey. "Please Stop All Dangerous Attacks on Independent GMO Researchers." Food Consumer (As submitted to the French Courts). *foodconumer.org,* Nov. 2010. Web. Oct. 2015. <http://www.

foodconsumer.org/newsite/Politics/Politics/gmo_researchers_0409110105.
html>

58. "Do Seed Companies Control Crop Research?" Scientific American. *scientificamerican.com*, 1 Aug. 2009. Print. <**http://www.scientificamerican.com/article/do-seed-companies-control-gm-crop-research/**>

59. Wirz, Johannes. "The Case of Mexican Maize." The Nature Institute, In Context #9. (Spring, 2003, pp. 3-5). *Natureinstitute.org*, Web. Oct. 2015. <http://natureinstitute.org/pub/ic/ic9/maize.htm>

60. Smith, Jeffrey. "Suppression of the truth about GMO hazards." Physicians and Scientists for Responsible Application of Science and Technology. *psrast.org*, n.d. Web. Oct. 2015. <http://www.psrast.org/criticssuppr.htmhttp://www.psrast.org/criticssuppr.htm>

61. N/A

62. Steinman, Jon "The GMO Trilogy—Hidden Dangers in Kids Meals." Podcast with Sue Kedgley. Kootenay Co-op Radio CJLY. *deconstructingdinner.com*, 26 Sept. 2006. Online. Oct. 2015. < <http://www.deconstructingdinner.com/podcast-speaker/sue-kedgley/> >

63. Smith, Jeffrey M. "Whistle Blowers Threats and Bribes." Council for Responsible Genetics, *Councilforresponsbilegenetics.org*, n.d. Web. Oct. 2015. <http://www.councilforresponsiblegenetics.org/ViewPage.aspx?pageId=125>

64. Smith, Jeffrey M. "Got Hormones?" Say No to GMOs! *saynotogmos.org*, 1 Dec. 2004. Web. Oct. 2015. <http://www.saynotogmos.org/ud2004/udec04.html>

65. Smith, Jeffrey M. Seeds of Deception: Exposing Industry and Government Lies about the Safety of the Genetically Engineered Foods You're Eating. Fairfield, IA: Yes, 2003. Print. <https://archive.org/stream/pdfy-JME_cHRxUJWJdqmi/Seeds%20of%20Deception%20(GMO%20FOOD)_djvu.txt>

66. Smith, Jeffrey M. "FDA Promotes Unsafe Milk Due to Industry Pressure." The Huffington Post. *huffingtonpost.com*, 25 May 2011. Web. 22 Apr. 2016. <http://www.huffingtonpost.com/jeffrey-smith/fda-promotes-unsafe-milk_b_184886.html>

67. Moody, Robin J. "Is Monsanto milking it?" Portland Business Journal. *Bizjournals.com*, 27 Feb. 2005. Print. Oct. 2015 <http://www.bizjournals.com/portland/stories/2005/02/28/tidbits1.html>

68. Hilbeck, Angelika, et al. "No consensus on GMO safety." Environmental Sciences Europe. *Enveurope.springeropen.com*, 27:4 24 Jan. 2015. Web. Oct. 2015. <http://www.ensser.org/media/> <http://www.gmwatch.org/news/archive/2013/15139-developer-of-first-commercialised-gm-food-says-debate-isn-t-over>

69. Hansen, Lauren. "7 genetically modified animals that glow in the dark." The Week.

theweek.com, 30 April. 2013. Online. Oct. 2016. <http://theweek.com/articles/464980/7-genetically-modified-animals-that-glow-dark>

70. "GM Foods Are Not Safe." Institute for Responsible Technology, n.d. Online. *Responsiblitytechnology.org*, 24 Mar. 2016. <http://responsibletechnology.org/docs/gmos-are-not-safe.pdf>

71. Ho, Mae-Wan. "Horizontal Gene Transfer—The Hidden Hazards of Genetic Engineering" Institute of Science in Society. *i-sis.org.uk*, 19 Aug. 2000. Web. Nov. 2015. <http://www.i-sis.org.uk/horizontalGeneTransfer.php>

72. "Health risks of genetically modified foods." National Center for Biotechnology Information, National Library of Medicine, National Institutes of Health, PubMed. *Ncbi.nlm.nih.gov*, (2010). Web. Nov. 2015. <http://www.ncbi.nlm.nih.gov/pubmed/18989835>

73. Latham, Jonathan and Allison Wilson. "Regulators Discover a Hidden Viral Gene in Commercial GMO Crops." Independent Science News. *Independentsciencenews.org*, 21 Jan. 2013. Web. Nov. 2015. <http://www.independentsciencenews.org/health/regulators-discover-a-hidden-viral-gene-in-commercial-gmo-crops/>

Chapter 3 Principles of Poison

1. "Pesticides 101." Pesticide Action Network (PAN).

2. *panna.org*, n.d. Online. Dec. 2015. <http://www.panna.org/pesticides-big-picture/pesticides-101>

3. Morris, Jeff. "Health/Nutrition Effects of Genetically Engineered Crops." E-journal of Age Management Medicine. *Agemed.org*, July 2012. Online. Dec. 2015. <https://www.agemed.org/AMMGejournal/July2012/Morris-HealthandGMOFoodsJuly2012.aspx>

4. Grieve, Carol. Dr. Robert Kremer: GMOs, Glyphosate and Soil Biology, Interview. Food Integrity Now. *foodintegritynow.org*, 15 April. 2015. Online. Dec. 2015. <http://foodintegritynow.org/2015/04/15/dr-robert-kremer-gmos-glyphosate-and-soil-biology/>

5. "10 Reasons to Avoid GMOs." Institute for Responsible Technology. *Responsibletechnology.org*, n.d. Online. Dec. 2015. <http://responsibletechnology.org/10-reasons-to-avoid-gmos/>

6. "Analysis: Super weeds pose growing threat to U.S. crops." Reuters. *Reuters.com*. 19 Sept. 2011. Web. Dec. 2015. <http://www.reuters.com/article/2011/09/19/us-monsanto-superweeds-idUSTRE78I4BA20110919>

7. "Glyphosate Formulations and their use for the inhibition of 5-enolpy-ruvylshikimate-3-phosphate synthase. US7771736 B2. Grant." Google Patents. Filing Date: 29 Aug. 2003. *google.com*, Publication Date: 10 Aug. 2010. Online. Dec. 2015. <http://www.google.com/patents/US7771736>

8. Hyman, Mark. "How Good Gut Health Can Boost Your Immune System." EcoWatch. *Ecowatch.com*, 26 Feb. 2015. Web. Dec. 2015. <http://ecowatch.com/2015/02/26/gut-health-boost-immune-system/>

9. "Bought, The Truth Behind Big Pharma, Vaccines and your Food." Dir. Bobby Shehan. *Boughtmovie.com*. Capstone Entertainment, 2014. Film. July. 2015. <http://www.boughtmovie.com/ >

10. Cassidy, Emily. "Monsanto's GMO Herbicide Doubles Cancer Risk." Environmental Working Group, AgMag. *Ewg.org*. 6 Oct. 2015. Web. Dec. 2015. <http://www.ewg.org/agmag/2015/10/monsanto-s-gmo-herbicide-doubles-cancer-risk>

11. Cassidy, Emily. "California Moves To Protect Citizens From Monsanto's GMO Weed Killer." Environmental Working Group. AgMag. *Ewg.org*, 10 Sept. 2015. Web. Dec. 2015. <http://www.ewg.org/agmag/2015/09/california-moves-protect-citizens-monsanto-s-gmo-weed-killer>

12. Cassidy, Emily. ""Extreme Levels" of Herbicide Found In Food." Environmental Working Group AgMag. *Ewg.org*, 18 Apr. 2014. Web. Dec. 2015. <http://www.ewg.org/agmag/2014/04/extreme-levels-herbicide-roundup-found-food>

13. Kruger, Monika, Phillipp Schledorn and et al. "Detection of Glyphosate Levels in Animals and Humans." Journal of Environmental and Analytical Toxicology. *Omicsonline.org*, 31 Jan. 2014. 4:210. doi: 10.4172/2161-0525.1000210. Web. Dec. 2015. <http://www.omicsonline.org/open-access/detection-of-<glyphosate-residues-in-animals-and-humans-2161-0525.1000210.php?aid=23853>

14. Bohn, Thomas and Marek Cuhra. "How "Extreme Levels" of Roundup in Food Became the Industry Norm." Independent Science News Food Health and Agriculture Bioscience News. *IndependentScienceNews.org*, 24 Mar. 2014. Web. Dec. 2015. <https://www.independentsciencenews.org/news/how-extreme-levels-of-roundup-in-food-became-the-industry-norm/>

15. Benachour, Nora and Gilles-Eric Séralini. "Glyphosate Formulations Induce Apoptosis and Necrosis in Human Umbilical, Embryonic, and Placental Cells." Chemical Research in Toxicology. pp 97–105. DOI: 10.1021/tx800218n. *Pubs.acs.org*, 23 Dec. 2008. Web. Dec. 2015. < http://pubs.acs.org/doi/abs/10.1021/tx800218n>

16. Thongprakaisang, S., Apinya Thiantanawat and et al. "Glyphosate induces human breast cancer cells growth via estrogen receptors." Food and Chemical Toxicology. ResearchGate. *Researchgate.net*, June 2013. Web. Dec. 2015. <https://www.researchgate.net/publication/237146763_Glyphosate_induces_human_breast_cancer_cells_growth_via_estrogen_receptorsGlyphosate induces human breast cancer cells growth via estrogen receptors>

17. Thongprakaisang, S., Apinya Thiantanawat and et al. "Glyphosate induces human breast cancer cells growth via estrogen receptors." Food

and Chemical Toxicology. *ncbi.nlm.nih.gov*. U.S. Library of Medicine, National Institutes of Health. *ncbi.nlm.nih.gov*, June 2013. Web. Dec. 2015. <http://www.ncbi.nlm.nih.gov/pubmed/23756170>

18. Cressey, Daniel. "Widely Used Herbicide Linked to Cancer." Scientific American- Nature. *scientificamerican.com*, 25 March. 2015. Web. Dec. 2015. <http://www.scientificamerican.com/article/widely-used-herbicide-linked-to-cancer/>

19. "Monsanto's Roundup (Glyphosate) Damages DNA, Says World Health Organization Expert." GM Watch. *Gmwatch.org*. 15 July 2015. Web. Dec. 2015. <http://www.gmwatch.org/news/latest-news/16302-glyphosate-damages-dna-says-world-health-organisation-expert>

20. "Soil Association calls for ban on Glyphosate: the world's most widely sold weedkiller." Soil Association of Scotland, *Soilassociationsscotland.org*, 2015. Web. Jan. 2016. <https://www.soilassociationscotland.org/resource-centre/press-releases/soil-association-calls-for-ban-on-glyphosate-the-world-s-most-widely-sold-weedkiller/>

21. Jahnke, G.D., C.W. Jameson and et al. "Carcinogenicity of tetrachlorvinphos, parathion, malathion, diazinon, and glyphosate." The Lancet Oncology, DOI: 10.1016/S1470-2045(15)70134-816 (5), pp. 490-491. *thelancet.com*, May 2015. Web. Dec. 2015. <http://www.thelancet.com/journals/lanonc/article/PIIS1470-2045(15)70134-8/abstract>

22. Colborn, Theo, Dianne Dumanoski and John Peterson Myers. "Does "the Dose Make the Poison?"" Our Stolen Future. *ourstolenfuture.org*, n.d. Web. Dec. 2015. <http://www.ourstolenfuture.org/NewScience/lowdose/lowdoseeffects.htm>

23. Wiley, Ion. "Glyphosate is a 'probably carcinogenic' pesticide. Why do cities still use it?" The Guardian, U.S. Edition. *theguardian.com*, 21 April. 2015. Web. Dec. 2015. <http://www.theguardian.com/cities/2015/apr/21/glyphosate-probably-carcinogenic-pesticide-why-cities-use-it>

24. Ávila-Vázquez, Medardo and Carlos Nota. "Devastating Effects of Glyphosate Use with GMO Seeds in Argentina." Institute of Science in Society. *i-sis.org.uk*, 15 Feb. 2015. Web. Dec. 2015. <http://www.isis.org.uk/Devastating_Impacts_of_Glyphosate_Argentina.php>

25. Ávila-Vázquez, Medardo and Carlos Nota. "Report from the First National Meeting of Physicians in the Crop-Sprayed Towns." La Red Universitaria de Ambiente y Salud (The University Network for Environment and Health). *Reduas.com*, Oct 7/2011. PDF. Dec. 2015. <http://www.reduas.com.ar/wp-content/uploads/downloads/2011/10/INGLES-Report-from-the-1st-National-Meeting-Of-Physicians-In-The-Crop-Sprayed-Towns.pdf>

26. "Argentina, Santa Fe: Estudio vincula fumigaciones con enfermedades en los pueblos." Argenpress. *Argenpress.info*, May 2013. Web. Nov. 2015. <http://www.argenpress.info/2013/08/argentina-santa-fe-estudio-vincula.html>

27. Cáncer en Córdoba: en el este provincial, la mortalidad más alta. La Voz del Interiror. Lavoz.com, 29 May. 2014. Web. Nov. 2015. <http://www.lavoz.com.ar/interactivo/el-mapa-del-cancer-en-cordoba>

28. Chow, Lorraine. "85% of Tampons Contain Monsanto's 'Cancer Causing' Glyphosate." EcoWatch. *ecowatch.com*, 26 Oct. 2015. Web. Dec. 2015 <http://ecowatch.com/2015/10/26/cotton-glyphosate-cancer/>

29. "Tampons, sterile cotton, sanitary pads contaminated with glyphosate—study." RT News. *Rt.com*, 23 Oct. 2013. Web. Dec. 2015. <https://www.rt.com/usa/319524-tampons-cotton-glyphosate-monsanto/#.VirHea3uV8g>

30. "Researchers Discover that 85% of Tampons are contaminated with Cancer Causing Herbicide." Daily Health Post. *Dailyhealthpost.com*, 27 Oct. 2015. Web. Dec. 2015. <http://dailyhealthpost.com/researchers-discover-that-85-of-tampons-are-contaminated-with-cancer-causing-herbicide/>

31. "Possible developmental early effects of endocrine disrupters on child health." World Health Organization. Geneva, Switzerland. ISBN 978 92 4 150376 1. *apps.who.int*, 2012. PDF. Dec. 2015. <http://apps.who.int/iris/bitstream/10665/75342/1/9789241503761_eng.pdf>

32. "List of Potential Endocrine Disruptors." TedX—The Endocrine Disruption Exchange. *endocrinedisruption.org*, n.d. Web. Dec. 2015. <http://endocrinedisruption.org/endocrine-disruption/tedx-list-of-potential-endocrine-disruptors/overview>

33. "Hormone Hacking." The Detox Project. *detoxproject.org*, n.d. Web. Dec. 2015. <http://detoxproject.org/glyphosate/hormone-hacking/>

34. "Monsanto's Minions: US EPA Hikes Glyphosate Limits in Food and Feed Once Again." Monsanto's Minions: US EPA Hikes Glyphosate Limits in Food and Feed Once Again. Organic Consumers Assoc. *organicconsumers.org*, n.d. Web. Dec. 2015. <https://www.organicconsumers.org/news/monsantos-minions-us-epa-hikes-glyphosate-limits-food-and-feed-once-again>

35. "Pesticide Tolerances: Glyphosate." Final Rule, ID: EPA-HQ-OPP-2012-0132-0009. (Your voice in federal decision making ;). Environmental Protection Agency. *Regulations.gov*, 1 July 2013. Online. Mar. 2016. <https://www.regulations.gov/#%21documentDetail;D=EPA-HQ-OPP-2012-0132-0009>

36. Swanson, Dr. Nancy. "It's time to declare a truce in the chemical war on weeds." Seattle Examiner. *Gmofreewashington.com*, 8 June 2015. Dec. 2015. < http://gmofreewashington.com/our-experts/nancy-swanson/ >

37. State Indiana Crop Weather. IN-CW042511. USDA. *usda.gov*, 24 April. 2011. Web. Dec. 2015. <http://www.nass.usda.gov/Statistics_by_State/Indiana/Publications/Crop_Progress_&_Condition/2011/wc042511.txt>

38. Seralini, GE and et al. "New Analysis of a rat feeding study with a

genetically modified maize reveals signs of hepatorenal toxicity."
National Center for Biotechnology Information (NCBI), National
Library of Medicine (NLM), National Institutes of Health (NIH).
Pubmed.gov, May 2007. Web. Dec. 2015. <http://www.ncbi.nlm.nih.gov/
pubmed/17356802>

39. de Vendômois JS, F. Roullier , D. Cellier D and GE. Séralini GE. A
Comparison of the Effects of Three GM Corn Varieties on Mammalian
Health. Int J Biol Sci 2009; 5(7):706-726. doi:10.7150/ijbs.5.706. Dec.
2015. <http://www.ijbs.com/v05p0706.htm>

40. Huguley, Charles M., Jr. *Clinical Methods: The History, Physical, and
Laboratory Examinations*, 3rd edition. Chapter 145, An overview of the
Hematopoietic System. Atlanta: Emory U School of Medicine, 1990.
Book. <http://www.ncbi.nlm.nih.gov/books/NBK252/>

41. Charles, Dan. "Insects Find Crack in Biotech Corn's Armor."
The Salt, What's on your plate. Oregon Public Broadcasting, *Npr.org*, 5 Dec. 2011. Web. Jan. 2016. <http://
www.npr.org/sections/thesalt/2011/12/05/143141300/
insects-find-crack-in-biotech-corns-armor>

42. Scott, April. Jeffrey Smith Phone Interview, 19 June. 2015.

43. "The Precautionary Principle." World Commission on Ethics of Scientific
Knowledge and Technology (COMEST). United Nations Educational,
Scientific and Cultural Organization (UNESCO). Paris., Mar. 2005.
PDF. Jan. 2016. Courtesy of gmofreeusa.org <http://www.gmofreeusa.
org/wpcontent/uploads/2014/11/ThePrecautionaryPrinciple_UNESCO_
COMEST_Report_2005.pdf>

44. Heuer, Sarah. "Monsanto vs. Schmeiser Case Study." Iowa State University Bioethics Program. *Public.iastate.edu*, n.d. PDF. Jan. 2016. <http://
www.public.iastate.edu/~ethics/SCHMEISERCASESTUDY.pdf>

45. Leonard, Christopher "Monsanto's practices weed out competition."
AP Investigation. Associated Press, via Capital Press. *captialpress.com*, 23
Dec. 2009. Print. Jan. 2016. <http://www.capitalpress.com/apps/pbcs.
dll/article?avis=CP&date=20091223&category=ARTICLE&lopen-
r=312239999&Ref=AR&profile=1020&template=printart> Grunwald,
Michael. "Monsanto Hid Decades of Pollution—PCBs Drenched Ala.
Town, But No One Was Ever Told." The Washington Post, via Common-
Dreams. *Commondreams.org*, 1 Jan. 2002. Web. Jan. 2016. <http://www.
commondreams.org/headlines02/0101-02.htm>

46. U.S. Lawsuits build against Monsanto over alleged Roundup Cancer
Link. Reuters. *Reuters.com*, 15 Oct. 2015. Web. Dec. 2015. <http://www.
reuters.com/article/usa-monsanto-lawsuits-idUSL1N12E18J20151015>

47. Burd, Lori Ann. "Lawsuit Targets EPAs Failure to Release Public Records
on Toxic Herbicide." Center for Biological Diversity. *Biologicaldiversity.org*,
16 Feb. 2016. PDF. Feb. 2016. <https://www.biologicaldiversity.org/news/
press_releases/2016/enlist-duo-02-03-2016.html> and <https://www.

biologicaldiversity.org/campaigns/pesticides_reduction/pdfs/2016-02-03_Dkt_1_16-175_Complaint.pdf>

48. "Glyphosate – Unsafe On Any Plate," Food Democracy Now! and the Detox Project. Fooddemocracynow.org, Nov. 2016. PDF. Nov. 2016 <https://s3.amazonaws.com/media.fooddemocracynow.org/images/FDN_Glyphosate_FoodTesting_Report_p2016.pdf>

Chapter 4 The GMO Gut-Brain Connection & the Big Fail

1. "Gut Microbiota Information—Everything You Ever Wanted to Know about Gut Microbiota." Gut Microbiota for Health Public Information Service from European Society of Neurogastroenterology and Mobility. *Gutmicrobiotawatch.org*, n.d. Web. Dec. 2015. <http://www.gutmicrobiotawatch.org/en/gut-microbiota-info/>

2. Dinan, Timothy G, Roman M. Stilling and et al. "Collective Unconscious: How gut microbes shape human behavior." Journal of Psychiatric research, Vol. 63 1-9. *Journalofpsychiatricresearch.com*, 17 Feb. 2015. Print. Dec. 2015. <http://www.journalofpsychiatricresearch.com/article/S0022-3956(15)00065-5/abstract?cc=y>

3. Stein, Rob. "Finally a map of all the microbes in your body." All things Considered. National Public Radio. *npr.org*, 13 June 2012. Radio broadcast. Dec. 2015. <http://www.npr.org/sections/health-shots/2012/06/13/154913334/finally-a-map-of-all-the-microbes-on-your-body>

4. "The Human Microbiome." Human Microbiome RSS. Human Microbiome Project. Data Analysis and Coordination Center. *hmpdacc.org*, n.d. Web. Dec. 2015. <http://hmpdacc.org/overview/about.php>

5. Qin, Junjie, and Li Ruiqiang and et.al. "A Human Gut Microbial Gene Catalogue Established by Metagenomics Sequencing." *Nature* 464, (2010): 59-65. Nature Publishing Group, *Nature.com*, 4 Mar. 2010. Web. Dec. 2015. <http://www.nature.com/nature/journal/v464/n7285/full/nature08821.html>

6. "Half of All Children Will Be Autistic by 2025, Warns Senior Research Scientist at MIT." Alliance for Natural Health. *anh-usa.org*. n.d. Web. Jan. 2016. <http://www.anh-usa.org/half-of-all-children-will-be-autistic-by-2025-warns-senior-research-scientist-at-mit/>

7. "Aromatic Aminoacid Biosynthesis Inhibitors." Purdue Agriculture. *purdue.edu*, n.d. Web. Jan. 2016. <https://www.btny.purdue.edu/Weed-Science/MOA/Aromatic_amino_acid_inhibitors/text.html>

8. Annigan, Jan. "How Many Amino Acids Does the Body Require."

SFGate. *sfgate.com* n.d. Web. Jan. 2016. <http://healthyeating.sfgate.com/many-amino-acids-body-require-6412.html>

9. Samsel, Anthony, and Stephanie Seneff. "Glyphosate, Pathways to Modern Diseases II: Celiac Sprue and Gluten Intolerance." Interdisciplinary Toxicology. Slovak Toxicology Society SETOX, Dec. 2013. Web. Jan. 2016. <http://www.ncbi.nlm.nih.gov/pmc/articles/ PMC3945755/>

10. Bassler, Bonnie. "How Bacteria Talk." Ted Talks, *ted.com*, Feb. 2009. Online Video. Aug. 2016. <**https://www.ted.com/talks/bonnie_bassler_on_how_bacteria_communicate?language=en#t-73788** >

11. Obrien, Robyn. "A Former GMO Scientist Sends an Open Letter to Canada's Minister of Health." Robyn Obrien, *robynobrien.com*, 2 Nov. 2014. Web. Dec. 2015. <http://robynobrien.com/a-former-gmo-scientist-sends-an-open-letter-to-canadas-minister-of-health/>

12. "Bought, The Truth Behind Big Pharma, Vaccines and your Food." Dir. Bobby Shehan. Capstone Entertainment, *Boughtmovie.com* (2014). Film. July. 2015. <http://www.boughtmovie.com/>

13. Vrain, Thierry. Organic Growers Video. "Engineered food and your health: the nutritional status of GMOs." Online video. YouTube. *YouTube.com*, 16 Nov. 2014. Web. Dec. 2015. <https://www.youtube.com/watch?v=yiU3Ndi6itk>

14. Bock, Kenneth. *Healing the New Childhood Epidemics: Autism, ADHD, Asthma, and Allergies: The Groundbreaking Program for the 4-A Disorders.* New York: Ballantine, 2008. Print. <http://www.amazon.com/Healing-New-Childhood-Epidemics-Groundbreaking/dp/0345494512>

15. Profet, Margie. The Function of Allergy: Immunological Defense Against Toxins." The Quarterly Review of Biology. DOI: 10.1086/417049 66(1):23-62, (1991): *Researchgate.com*. Web. Jan. 2016. <https://www.researchgate.net/publication/21102700_The_Function_of_Allergy_Immunological_Defense_Against_Toxins>

16. Branum, Amy M and et al. "Food Allergy Among U.S Children: Trends in Prevalence and Hospitalizations." Center for Disease Control and Prevention. (CDC), National Center for Health Statistics. *Cdc.gov*, Oct. 2008. Web. Jan. 2016. <http://www.cdc.gov/nchs/data/databriefs/db10.htm>

17. "Autism Prevalence Rise to 1 in 88." Autism Speaks, *Autismspeaks.org*, n.d. Web. Jan. 2016. <https://www.autismspeaks.org/science/science-news/autism-prevalence-rises-1-88>

18. "The Autism and Allergy Overlap." The Autism File. *autismfile.com*, 5 Mar. 2015. Web. Feb. 2016. <http://www.autismfile.com/science-research/the-autism-and-allergy-overlap>

19. "Study May Help ADHD Kids." All Things Considered. NPR News. *Npr.org*, 12 Mar. 2011. Web. Feb.

2016. http://www.npr.org/2011/03/12/134456594/study-diet-may-help-adhd-kids-more-than-drugs>

20. Blakeslee, Sandra. "Complex Hidden Brain in Gut Makes Stomach-aches and Butterflies." The New York Times. Ny*times.com*, 23 January. 1996. Print. Jan. 2016. <http://www.nytimes.com/1996/01/23/science/complex-and-hidden-brain-in-gut-makes-stomachaches-and-butterflies.html?pagewanted=all>

21. Stephens, Krysteena. "Food Inflammation and Autism: Is There a Link?" Psychology Today. *Psychologytoday.com*. 13 July 2013. Web. Jan. 2016. <https://www.psychologytoday.com/blog/mental-wealth/201307/food-inflammation-and-autism-is-there-link>

22. Gray, John. "How to Stay Focused in a Hyper World." Video Interview by Zen Honeycutt, Moms Across America. YouTube. *Youtube.com*, 15 Sept. 2015. <https://www.youtube.com/watch?v=oD7B4_Nsw4k>

23. Cromie, William J. "Study points to more targeted use of Ritalin—Drug not effective for all." Harvard University Gazette. *Harvard.edu*, 18 May. 2000. Web. March 2016. <http://news.harvard.edu/gazette/2000/05.18/adhd.htm>

24. Gray, John. "Natural Solutions for treating Autism." YouTube. *Youtube.com*, 8 March. 2012. Video. Dec. 2016. <https://www.youtube.com/watch?v=Ivduj7-ZPIM>

25. Gray, John. "Understanding. ADHD—ADD—Attention Deficit Disorder—Attention Hyperactivity Disorder." YouTube. *Youtube.com*, 23 Feb. 2012. Video, Dec. 2016. <https://www.youtube.com/watch?v=SVeKZRVkIY4>

26. "The Gluten Free/Casein Free (GF/CF) Diet." Autism Hope and Healing. *Autismhopeandhealing*, n.d. Web. Mar. 2016. <http://www.autismhopeand-healing.com/GFCF.html>

27. "What are Neurotransmitters?" Neurogistics—The Brain Wellness Program, *neurogistics.com*. n.d. Web. Mar. 2016. <https://www.neurogistics.com/TheScience/WhatareNeurotransmi09CE.asp>

28. Deans, Emily. "Dopamine Primer." *Psychologytoday.com*. Psychology Today, 13 May 2011. Web. Mar. 2016. <https://www.psychologytoday.com/blog/evolutionary-psychiatry/201105/dopamine-primer >

29. Bennington, Vanessa. "Understanding our Adrenal System: Dopamine." Breaking Muscle, *Breakingmuscle.com*. n.d. Web. Mar. 2016 <http://breakingmuscle.com/health-medicine/understanding-our-adrenal-system-dopamine >

30. Spector, Michael. "Germs are US." New Yorker Magazine. *Newyorker.com*, 22 Oct. 2012. Web. Mar. 2016. <http://www.newyorker.com/magazine/2012/10/22/germs-are-us >

31. Wenner, Melinda. "Gut Bacteria May Play a Role in Autism." Scientific American. *Scientificamerican.com*, 1 Sept. 2014.

Web. Dec. 2015. <http://www.scientificamerican.com/article/gut-bacteria-may-play-a-role-in-autism/>

32. Pollan, Michael. "Some of My Best Friends are Germs." The New York Times Magazine. *nytimes.com*, 15 May 2013. Web. Dec. 2015. http://www.nytimes.com/2013/05/19/magazine/say-hello-to-the-100-trillion-bacteria-that-make-up-your-microbiome.html?pagewanted=all&_r=1>

33. Molloy, Aimee. "Mothers facing C-section look to vaginal 'seeding' to boost their babies health." The Guardian. *theguardian.com*, 17 Aug. 2015. Web. Dec. 2015. <http://www.theguardian.com/lifeandstyle/2015/aug/17/vaginal-seeding-c-section-babies-microbiome >

34. Seneff, Stephanie, and Wendya Morley. "Diminished Brain Resilience Syndrome: A Modern Day Neurological Pathology of Increased Susceptibility to Mild Brain Trauma, Concussion, and Downstream Neurodegeneration." Surgical Neurology International Surg Neurol Int 5.1. *Sni.wpengine.com*, (2014): 97. PDF. Jan. 2016. <http://sni.wpengine.com/wp-content/uploads/2015/05/3992/SNI-5-97.pdf>

Chapter 5 GMO-Free Testimony

1. Scott, April. Phone Interview—Jennifer Lawrenson, 22 July. 2015.

2. Scott, April. Phone Interview—Julianna Denney Sauber, 21 July. 2015. <https://www.facebook.com/The-Whole-Body-Renewal-Center-LLC-290882387622804/?pnref=lhc>

3. Scott, April Phone Interview—Diana Reeves, 4 Aug. 2015. GMO FREE USA <https://www.facebook.com/search/top/?q=gmo%20free%20usa>

4. Scott, April. Phone Interview—Amanyah Gustovson, 15 Aug. 2015.

5. Scott, April. Phone Interview—Maureen Wheeler, 2015. 15 Aug. 2015.

6. Scott, April. Phone Interview—Amber King, 13 Dec. 2015. <www.gofundme.com/2016amberking907>

7. Scott, April. Phone Interview—Sophiah Pickel, 24 July 2015.

Chapter 6 GMO-Free Doctors

1. "Snapshots: Health Care Spending in the United States & Selected OECD Countries." The Henry J. Kaiser Family Foundation. Kff.org. 12 April. 2011. Web. Jan. 2016. <http://www.healthsystemtracker.org/interactive/health-spending-explorer >

2. American Academy of Environmental Medicine (AAEM), *aaemonline.org*. n.d. Web. Jan. 2016. <https://www.aaemonline.org/gmo.php>

3. Smith, Jeffrey M. "Dramatic Health Recoveries Reported." GMO Food and Issues. Vitality Magazine, *vitalitymagazine.com*, n.d. Web. Jan. 2016.

<http://vitalitymagazine.com/article/dramatic-health-recoveries-reported/#sthash.3X7FYTV5.dpuf) >

4. "Genetic Roulette: The Gamble of Our Lives." Dir. Jeffrey M. Smith. The Institute for Responsible Technology. *geneticroulettemovie.com*, 1 Jan. 2012. Web. July 2015 <http://rapeutation.com/geneticroulettescreenplay.pdf>

5. Andersen, Arden "Real Medicine, Real Health." Bionutrient Food Assoc. bionutrient.org, n.d. Web. <http://bionutrient.org/library/reviews/real-medicine-real-health>

6. Edwards, Joel. "Doctors Against GMOs—Hear From Those Who Have Done The Research." Organic Lifestyle Magazine. *Organiclifestylemagazine.com*, 2 Aug. 2015. Web. Jan. 2016. <http://www.organiclifestylemagazine.com/doctorsagainst-gmos-hear-from-those-who-have-done-the-research>

7. Weiss, Ron. Ethos health. Primary Care Practice. Long Valley, New Jersey. *myethoshealth.com*, n.d. Web. Jan. 2016. <http://www.myethoshealth.com/>

8. Wolfe, David. "This Doctor Sold His New York Practice To Start A 348-Acre Organic Farm To Treat Patients" David Wolfe. *DavidWolfe.com*, 06 Oct. 2015. Web. Jan. 2016. <http://www.davidwolfe.com/this-doctor-sold-his-new-york-practice-to-start-a-348-acre-organic-farm-to-treat-patients/>

9. "Medical Doctor Sells Practice, Opens Up." Cornucopia Institute. *Cornucopia.org*, 05 Nov. 2015. Web. Jan. 2016. <http://www.cornucopia.org/2015/11/medical-doctor-sells-practice-opens-up-farmacy-using-food-as-medicine/>

10. Perro, Michelle. "Dr. Michelle Perro paediatrician talks leaky gut, NCGS, toxicity & children." YouTube. *Youtube.com*, 17 May. 2015. <https://www.youtube.com/watch?v=PbhnIVcKLQ8&feature=youtu.be>

11. Perro, Michelle. "GMOs in baby formula? A paediatrician provides answers." Moms Advocating Sustainability. *momsadvocatingsustainability.org*, 4 June 2013. Web. Jan. 2016. <http://www.momsadvocatingsustainability.org/gmos-in-baby-formula-what/>

12. "So What is a GMO?" Bayshore Pediatric Assoc. *bayshorepediatric.com*, 29 April. 2014. Web. Jan. 2016. <http://www.bayshorepediatric.com/blog/gmo/>

13. Pala, Christopher. "Pesticides in Paradise: Hawaii spike in birth defects puts focus on GM crops." The Guardian, *Theguardian.com*, 23 August. 2015. Web. Jan. 2016. <http://www.theguardian.com/us-news/2015/aug/23/hawaii-birth-defects-pesticides-gmo>

14. Bethell, CD and et al. "A national and state profile of leading health problems and health care quality for U.S Children: key insurance disparities and across state variations." Acad. Pediatr. 2011 May-Jun;11 (3

Suppl):S22-33. doi: 10.1016/j.acap.2010.08.011. *ncbi.nlm.nih.gov*. Print. Jan. 2016. <http://www.ncbi.nlm.nih.gov/pubmed/21570014>

15. Boyles, Salynn. "CDC: Autism Rates Higher Than Thought- But More Aggressive Diagnosis May Explain Increase in Cases." WebMD - Mental Health Center. *webmd.com*, 31 Dec. 2002. Web. Nov. 2016. <http://www.webmd.com/mental-health/news/20021231/cdc-autism-rates-higher-than-thought>

16. "Autism Spectrum Disorder – Data and Statistics." Centers for Disease Control and Prevention. *cdc.gov*, 2012. Web. Nov. 2016. <http://www.cdc.gov/ncbddd/autism/data.html>

17. Wing L, Potter D. "The epidemiology of autistic spectrum disorders: is the prevalence rising?" Ment Retard Dev Disabil Res Rev. 2002;8(3):151–61.doi:10.1002/mrdd.10029. PMID 12216059. Print. Mar. 2016.

18. MacDorman, Marian F and et al. International Comparisons of Infant Mortality and Related Factors: United States and Europe, 2010. Volume 63, Number 5. National Vital Statistics Report. *cdc.gov*, 24 Sept. 2014. PDF. Jan. 2016. <http://www.cdc.gov/nchs/data/nvsr/nvsr63/nvsr63_05.pdf>

19. "Infant Mortality and Life Expectancy for Selected Countries" CIA, World Factbook. Infoplease.© 2000–2015 Sandbox Networks, Inc., publishing as Infoplease. CIA, World Factbook, 2014 <http://www.infoplease.com/world/statistics/infant-mortality-life-expectancy.html >

20. "Infant Mortality Rate (Deaths per 1000 live births)." Kaiser Family Foundation. Kff.org. 2014 < http://kff.org/other/state-indicator/infant-death-rate/>

21. "State-Of-The-Science on the Health Risks of GM Foods." Institute for Responsible Technology. *Responsibletechnology.org*, 15 Feb. 2010. Print. Jan. 2016. <http://responsibletechnology.org/docs/145.pdf >

Chapter 7 GMO-Free Tips, Tricks & Tools

1. Mercola, Joseph. A Special Interview with Joey Jones, "What You Need to Know About Grass-Fed Beef." Courtesy of *Grassfedexchange.com* and *Mercola.com*, 21 Dec. 2014. Video Transcript. Feb. 2016. <http://articles.mercola.com/sites/articles/archive/2014/12/21/grass-fed-beef-production.aspx> **Secondary source**: "Scientific Literature that Supports the Health Benefits of Grass Fed Beef." Access to compiled evidence proving health benefits of Grass Fed vs. Grain Fed beef. Mercola.com, n.d. Apr. 2016. <http://www.mercola.com/beef/references.htm>

2. Gunnars, Kris. "How to Optimize Your Omega-6 to Omega-3 Ratio." Authority Nutrition, *authoritynutrition.com*, Nov. 2013. Web. Feb. 2016. <http://authoritynutrition.com/optimize-omega-6-omega-3-ratio/>

3. Van Elswyk, Mary E. and Shalene H. McNeill. "Impact on grass forage feeding versus grain finishing on beef nutrients and sensory quality: The US Experience." Meat Science, Volume 96, Issue 1, Pages 535–540. *Sciencedirect.com,* Jan. 2014. PDF. Apr. 2016. <http://www.sciencedirect.com/science/article/pii/S0309174013004944>

4. Clancy, Kate. "Greener Pastures—How grass-fed beef and milk contribute to healthy eating." Union of Concerned Scientists, UCS Publications, Cambridge, MA. *ucsusa.org,* 2006. PDF. Apr. 2016. <http://www.ucsusa.org/sites/default/files/legacy/assets/documents/food_and_agriculture/greener-pastures.pdf>

5. Daley, Cynthia A., Amber Abbott and et al. "A review of fatty acid profiles and antioxidant content in grass-fed and grain-fed beef." BioMed Central Ltd. Nutrition Journal, 9:10. DOI: 10.1186/1475-2891-9-10. *Nutritionj.biomedcentral.com,* 10 Mar. 2010. PDF. Apr. 2016. <http://nutritionj.biomedcentral.com/articles/10.1186/1475-2891-9-10>

6. Organic Store Locator—All Natural and Organic Food Directory with state-by- state search option for stores and restaurants, n.d. Web. Apr. 2016. <http://www.organicstorelocator.com/organic.org/storefinder>

7. *Eatwild.com*—Getting Wild Nutrition from Modern Food. Directory of U.S., Canadian and International Farms & Ranches. Contains over 1400 pasture-based farms. By Jo Robinson. 2002-2016. Web. Apr. 2016. <http://Eatwild.com>

8. *Localharvest.com*—'Grassroots' directory of over 30,000 family farms and farmers markets, along with restaurants and grocery stores that feature local food. Founded by Guillermon Payet and Erin Barnett, n.d. Web. Apr. 2016 <http://www.localharvest.org/>

9. *Ams.usda.gov*—Farmer's Market—National directory for local and regional. United States Department of Agriculture (USDA),16 April, 2016. Web. Apr. 2016. <**https://www.ams.usda.gov/local-food-directories/onfarm**>

10. *Eatwellguide.org*—Curated Directory of over 25,000 hand-picked restaurants, farms markets and other sources of local, sustainable food throughout the U.S. 2016. Web. Apr 2016. <**http://www.eatwellguide.org/info**>

11. *Grassfedexchange.com*—Producers directory and coordinated effort of producers and buyers of grassfed genetics forming the Grassfed Exchange Committee. n.d. Web. Apr. 2016. <**http://www.grassfedexchange.com/about/**>

12. *Greepeople.org*—Organic Consumers Association/Green People Directory. State-by-State search of U.S Based Green Businesses, n.d. Web. Apr. 2016. <http://www.greenpeople.org/btc/BuyingGuide.cfm>

13. *Foodroutes.org*—provides communications tools, technical support, networking and information resources to organizations nationwide that are

working to rebuild local, community-based food systems, n.d. Web. Apr. 2016. <http://foodroutes.org/5>

14. Coopdirectory.org—Co-op Listing Directory Service. 1999-2013. Web. Apr. 2016. <http://www.coopdirectory.org/directory.htm>

15. *ams.usda.gov* —Community—Supported Agriculture (CSA) Directory. United States Department of Agriculture (USDA). 19 Apr. 2016. Web. April. 2016. <http://www.ams.usda.gov/local-food-directories/csas>

16. *Wewantorganicfood.com* –Information about organic food and related topics. Cofounded by George Vigil. 2007-2016. Web. Apr. 2016. <http://wewantorganicfood.com/directory/>

17. *Whatonmyfood.org*—Pesticide Action Network (PAN) compiled database of cross-referenced information from the USDA's Pesticide Data Program and toxicological data from the EPA and other authoritative listings. 2011-2014. Web. Apr. 2016. <http://www.whatsonmyfood.org/level.jsp?food=BN&pesticide=160>

18. Katie. "What are the safest cookware options?" Wellness Mama. *well-nessmama.com*, n.d. Web. Feb. 2016. <http://wellnessmama.com/5148/safest-cookware- options/>

19. "Adverse Health Effects of Plastics." Ecology Center. *ecologycenter.org*, n.d. Web. Feb. 2016. <http://ecologycenter.org/factsheets/adverse-health-effects-of-plastics/>

20. Our Stolen Future. Current Scientific Literature and News Updates re: the chemical Bisphenol a (BPA). *ourstolenfuture.org*, n.d. Online Database. Dec. 2015. <http://www.ourstolenfuture.org/newscience/oncompounds/bisphenola/bpauses.htm>

21. Webber, Valerie. Health Risks of Cooking in Aluminum. Livestrong.com. *Livestrong.com*, 6 May 2015. Web. Feb. 2016. <http://www.livestrong.com/article/475155-health-risks-of-cooking-in-aluminum/>

22. "Healthy Home Tips: Tip 6—SKIP THE NON-STICK TO AVOID THE DANGERS OF TEFLON." Environmental Working Group, *ewg.org*, n.d. Feb. 2016. <http://www.ewg.org/research/healthy-home-tips/tip-6-skip-non-stick-avoid-dangers-teflon>

23. Wayne, Anthony and Lawrence Newell. "The Hidden Hazards of Micro-wave Cooking." Health-Science, *Health-science.com*, n.d. Web. Apr. 2016. <https://www.health-science.com/microwave_ hazards.html>

24. Lipman, Frank "What do those codes on stickers of fruits and some veggies mean." Dr. Frank Lipman, *drfranklipman.com*, 2 Nov. Web. Apr. 2016. <http://www.drfranklipman.com/what-do-those-codes-on-stickers-of-fruits-and-some-veggies-mean/>

Chapter 8 GMO Detoxification

1. Issels, Ilse Marie. "Information on Detoxification." Issels Immuno-Oncology. *issels.com*, 2001. Web. Apr. 2016. <http://www.issels.com/newissels/publication-library/information-on-detoxification/>

2. "Detoxification." Texas A&M University, *peer.tamu.edu*, n.d. Web. Apr. 2016. <http://peer.tamu.edu/curriculum_modules/organsystems/Module_3/index.htm

3. Cabot, Sandra. "The Liver and Detoxification." Liver Doctor. *Liverdoctor.com*, n.d. Web. May 2016. <https://www.liverdoctor.com/liver/the-liver-and-detoxification/>

4. Axe, Josh. "The Lymphatic System: How to Make It Strong & Effective." Dr. Axe. n.d. Web. May 2016. <http://draxe.com/lymphatic-system/>

5. Toledo, Chelsea and Katie Saltsman. "Genetics by the Numbers." Inside Life Science. National Institute of General Medical Sciences, 11 July. *nih.gov*, 2012. Web. Feb. 2016. <http://publications.nigms.nih.gov/insidelifescience/genetics-numbers.html>

6. "The Meaning of Methylation." Genetics Based Integrative Medicine. *Autismnti.com*, 13 Jan. 2012. PDF. Feb. 2016. <http://www.autismnti.com/images/The_Meaning_of_Methylation_1-13-12.pdf>

7. Douillard, John. "Remove Toxins from your fat cells." John Douillard's LifeSpa. Lifespa.com, 15 Oct. 2015. Web. April 2016 <http://lifespa.com/remove-toxins-from-your-fat-cells/>

8. "All 48 Fruits and Vegetables with Pesticide Residue Data." Environmental Working Group. *ewg.org*, n.d. Web. Apr. 2016. <http://www.ewg.org/foodnews/clean_fifteen_list._php>

9. Dunn, Jon. "Methylation and Mystery Disease." Naturopathic Healthcare, Inc. *Drjondunn.com*, Sept. 2013. Web. Feb. 2016. <http://www.drjondunn.com/Newsletters/2013-09Methylation.html>

10. Kresser, Chris. "9 Steps to Perfect Health—#5: Heal Your Gut." Chris Kresser. *chriskresser.com*, 24 Feb. 2011. Web. Feb. 2016. <https://chriskresser.com/9-steps-to-perfect-health-5-heal-your-gut/>

11. Gunnars, Kris. "10 Proven Health Benefits of Coconut Oil." Authority Nutrition. *authoritynutrition.com*, Apr. 2016. Web. Feb. 2016. <http://authoritynutrition.com/top-10-evidence-based-health-benefits-of-coconut-oil/>

12. "Oil Pulling: Safe, Simple and Effective!" EarthClinic. *Earthclinic.com*, 5 Feb. 2016. Web. Mar. 2016. <http://www.earthclinic.com/remedies/oil_pulling._html>

13. Scott, April. "Bisphenol A—Political Hell Freezes Over." *salem-news.com*, 27 Jan. 2010. Web. 27 Jan. 2010. <http://www.salem-news.com/articles/january272010/bisphenol_as.php> Also check out all the current

scientific literature and news updates re: the chemical Bisphenol-a (BPA). *ourstolenfuture.org*, n.d. Web. Jan. 2010.

14. Hearn, Nancy. "Drinking Spring Water Health Pros and Cons." Water Benefits Health. *waterbenefitshealth.com*, n.d. Web. Feb. 2016. <http://www.waterbenefitshealth.com/drinking-spring-water.html>

15. "Benefits of Apple Cider Vinegar." The Healthy Eating Site. *Thehealthyeatingsite.com*, n.d. Web. Feb. 2016. <http://thehealthyeatingsite.com/benefits-of-apple-cider-vinegar/>

16. "Glutathione Foods." Immune Health Science. *Immunehealthscience.com*, n.d. Web. Mar. 2016. <http://www.immunehealthscience.com/glutathione-foods.html>

17. "How to Raise Glutathione." Immune Health Science, *Immunehealthscience.com*, n.d. Web. Mar. 2016. <http://www.immunehealthscience.com/how-to-raise-glutathione.html>

18. Demova, S, PH Hoet and et al. "Acetaminophen decreases intracellular glutathione levels and modulates cytokine production in human alveolar macrophages and type II pneumocytes in vitro." Volume 37, Issue 8, Aug. 2005. Vol. 37, Issue 8. <http://www.sciencedirect.com/science/article/pii/S1357272505001159>

19. "Don't Suppress that fever! (and why I don't like Tylenol)" *Naturopathicpediatrics.com*, 30 Dec. 2012. Web. Mar. 2016. <http://naturopathicpediatrics.com/2012/12/30/dont-suppress-that-fever/>

20. "Glutathione Foods." *Immunehealthscience.com*, n.d. Web. Apr. 2016. <http://www.immunehealthscience.com/glutathione-foods.html >

21. "The Six Thousand Hidden Dangers of Processed Foods (and What to Choose Instead)." Body Ecology. *Bodyecology.com*. 18 Oct. 2007. Web. 28 Jan. 2016. <http://bodyecology.com/articles/hidden_dangers_of_processed_foods.php>

22. "EWG's Shopper's Guide to Pesticides in Produce." Environmental Working Group, *Ewg.com*. 2016. Web. Jan. 2016. <http://www.ewg.org/foodnews/summary.php>

23. Guthrie, Catherine. "Glutathione: The Great Protector." Experience Life. Life Time Fitness. *experiencelife.com*, 01 Apr. 2011. Web. Jan. 2016. <https://experiencelife.com/article/glutathione-the-great-protector/>

24. "14 Healthy Tips to Detox Your Kids." Wellness Achiever. *Wellnessachiever.net*, 26 Sept. 2013. Web. Jan. 2016. <http://wellnessachiever.net/14-healthy-tips-detox-kids/>

25. Cordain, Loren. "What to Eat on The Paleo Diet" The Paleo Diet, thepaleodiet.com, n.d. Web. Jan. 2016. <http://thepaleodiet.com/what-to-eat-on-the-paleo-diet/#.Vu9TbeIrLIU>

26. "ABC's of Nutrition—Weston A Price." The Weston A. Price Foundation for Wise Traditions in Food, Farming, and the Healing Arts. Dr. Weston

A. Price, *westonaprice.org*. n.d. Web. 28 Dec. 2015. <http://www.westona-price.org/abcs-of-nutrition/>

27. Wilson, Lawrence. "POSSIBLE SYMPTOMS WITH TOXIC METAL REMOVAL." TOXIC METALS. The Center for Development. *drlwilson. com*, June 2015. Web. 28 Apr. 2016. < http://drlwilson.com/articles/ TOXIC%20METALS.htm>

28. "Toxic Load Reduction Quiz." Created by April Scott, Oct. 19. 2015.

29. Campbell-McBride, Natasha. "About." International Nutrition, Inc. GAPS Diet, *gapsdiet.com*, n.d. Web. May 2016. <http://www.gapsdiet. com/about.html>

30. Campbell-McBride, Natasha. "GAPS Introduction Diet." International Nutrition, Inc. GAPS Diet, *gapsdiet.com*, n.d. Web. May 2016. <http:// www.gapsdiet.com/gaps-introduction-diet.html>

31. Campbell-McBride, Natasha. "GAPS Protocol Outline." International Nutrition, Inc. GAPS Diet, *gapsdiet.com*, n.d. Web. May 2016. <http:// www.gapsdiet.com/gaps-outline.html>

32. Walsh, Bryan. "Food Sensitivities and Intolerances: How and Why to Do an Elimination Diet | Precision Nutrition." Precision Nutrition. *Precisionnutrtion.com*, 11 May 2011. Web. May 2016. <http://www.preci-sionnutrition.com/elimination-diet>

33. Foucher, Ray. "Lactic Acid Bacteria Benefit Digestion and Produce B Vitamins, Even B12." Natural Pain Relief .*Natural-pain-relief-guide.com*. n.d. Web. Jan. 2016. <http://www.natural-pain-relief-guide.com/lactic-ac-id-bacteria.html>

34. "Cultured Vegetable, Fruit, and Condiment Recipes." Cultured Vegetable, Fruit and Condiment Recipes. Cultures for Health. *cultures-forhealth.com*, n.d. Web. Mar. 2016. <http://www.culturesforhealth.com/ cultured-vegetable-fruit-condiment-recipes#salsa>

35. Zurich, Linda. "7 Ways to Avoid Detox Symptoms on a Cleanse." The Healthy Home Economist. *Healthyhomeeconomist.com*, 16 May 2013. Web. Feb. 2016. <http://www.thehealthyhomeeconomist. com/7-ways-to-avoid-detox-symptoms-on-a-cleanse/>

36. "Top 7 Fermented Foods to Add to Your Diet." *Superfoods-for-superhealth. com*, n.d. Online Database. Mar. 2016. <http://www.superfoods-for-super-health.com/fermented-foods.html>

Chapter 9 GMO-Free Recipes

All chapter 9 sources cited in the body of the recipes.

Chapter 10 The GMO-Free Movement

1. "Jeffrey M. Smith Biography." Institute for Responsible Technology. *responsibletechnology.org*, n.d. Web. Nov. 2015. <http://responsibletechnology.org/jeffrey-m-smith-biography/>

2. "Andrew Kimbrell, CFS Executive Director." Center for Food Safety. *centerforfoodsafety.org*, n.d. Web. Nov. 2015. <http://www.centerforfoodsafety.org/andrew-kimbrell/>

3. "Ronnie Cummins—International Director." Organic Consumers Assoc. *Organicconsumers.org*, n.d. Web. Nov. 2015. <https://www.organicconsumers.org/staff>

4. "About Us." AllergyKids. Robyn Obrien, n.d. Web. Nov. 2015. <http://www.allergykids.com/about-us/about-us/>

5. "For the Freedom to Choose Our Families Food." Zen Honeycutt. Moms Across America. momsacrossamerica.com, n.d. Web. Nov. 2015. <http://www.momsacrossamerica.com/about> <https://www.facebook.com/MomsAcrossAmerica/?fref=ts>

6. "Navdanya." Dr. Vandana Shiva. *Navdanya.org*, n.d. Web. Nov. 2015. <http://www.navdanya.org/>

7. "Dr Vandana Shiva." Dr Vandana Shiva. *vandanashiva.com*, n.d. Web. Nov. 2015. <http://vandanashiva.com/?page_id=2>

8. "Global Food, Farming and Environmental Justice Groups to Put Monsanto on Trial for Crimes Against Human Health and the Environment in the International People's Court in The Hague." Organic Consumers Assoc. *Organicconsumers.org*, 03 Dec. 2015. Web. Nov. 2016. <https://www.organicconsumers.org/press/global-food-farming-and-environmental-justice-groups-put-monsanto-trial-crimes-against-human>

9. "Monsanto Swung to a Loss in the First Fiscal Quarter Announces a 1,000 More Job Cuts." U.S News and World Report. *usnews.com*, 06 Jan. 2016. Web. Jan. 2016. <http://www.usnews.com/news/business/articles/2016-01-06/monsanto-swings-to-1q-loss-amid-lower-seed-sales>

10. "Monsanto Cuts 16% of Work Force as Sales in Roundup Herbicide Fall 34%—Sustainable Pulse." Sustainable Pulse. *Sustainablepulse.com*, 07 Jan. 2016. Web. Jan. 2016. <http://sustainablepulse.com/2016/01/07/monsanto-cuts-16-of-work-force-as-sales-in-roundup-herbicide-fall-34/#.Vqmq5_krLIU>

11. "GMO Facts, Frequently Asked Questions." The NonGMO Project RSS. *Nongmoproject.org*, n.d. Web. Nov. 2015. <http://www.nongmoproject.org/learn-more/>

12. Bonar, Samantha, "Hungary Destroys Genetically Modified Corn Crops." LA Weekly. *laweekly.com*, 28 July 2011. Web. Dec.

2015. <http://www.worldculturepictorial.com/blog/content/ hungary-destroys-gm-corn-africa-no-place-for-gmo-eu-bans>

13. "Majority of EU Nations Seek Opt-out from Growing GM Crops." Reuters. Thomson Reuters, 04 Oct. 2015. Web. Dec. 2015. <http://www. reuters.com/article/eu-gmo-opt-out-idUSL6N0M01F620151004>

14. "Taiwan Bans GMOs in School Meals over Health Fears—Sustainable Pulse." Sustainable Pulse. *Sustainablepulse.com*, 14 Dec. 2015. Web. Nov. 2015. <http://sustainablepulse.com/2015/12/14/taiwan-bans-gmos-in-school-meals-over-health-fears/#.VpHbjPkrLIU>

15. Sukhoterina, Yelena. "Sorry, Monsanto: GMO Crops Now Banned in 38 Countries, Grown in Only 28." AltHealthWorks.com RSS2. *Althealthworks.com*, 21 Apr. 2016. Web. Apr. 2016. <http://althealthworks. com/9778/list-of-38-countries-that-banned-gmos-and-28-that-grow-the-myelena/?c=ngr#sthash.rvAvlRYW.dpuf>

16. Lee, Jaeah. "CHARTS: World's GMO Crop Fields Could Cover the US 1.5 Times Over." Mother Jones. *Motherjones.com*, 26 Feb. 2013. Web. July 2016 <http://www.motherjones.com/blue-marble/2013/02/ gmo-farming-crops-more-popular-than-ever-world-charts>

17. Fryar, John. "Boulder County to Phase out GMO Crops on County-owned Lands."—Boulder Daily Camera. *Dailycamera.com*, 17 Mar. 2016. Web. Mar. 2016. <http:// www.dailycamera.com/longmont-local-news/ci_29653129/ boulder-county-phase-out-gmo-crops-county-owned>

18. Prupis, Nadia. "Organic Farmers Win GMO Fight in Jackson County, Oregon." EcoWatch. *Ecowatch.com*, 07 Jan. 2016. Web. May 2016. <http:// ecowatch.com/2016/01/07/jackson-county-gmo-free/>

19. SCHULZ FAMILY FARMS LLC v. JACKSON COUNTY and CHRISTOPHER HARDY, Individual; OSHALA FARM, LLC, an Oregon Limited Liability Company; OUR FAMILY FARMS COALITION. Doc. 96 Case 1:14-cv-01975-CL. UNITED STATES DISTRICT COURT FOR THE DISTRICT OF OREGON MEDFORD DIVISION. 22 Dec. 2015. Print. <http://www.centerforfoodsafety.org/files/2015-12-22-dkt-96—order—granting-mot-stay_14439.pdf>

20. "Europe Rejects GM Crops as New Report Highlights 20 Years of Failures." Greenpeace EU Unit. *Greenpeace.org*, 05 Nov. 2015. Web. Mar. 2016. <http://www.greenpeace.org/eu-unit/en/News/2015/ Europe-rejects-GM-crops-as-new-report-highlights-20-years-of-failures/>

21. "In Twenty Years 89 of the World's Top Chemical Companies Have Asked SD to Design Their Plants. Why?" Chemical & Engineering News Chem. Eng. News 44.27 (1966): n. pag. Green Peace. *Greenpeace.org*, Nov. 2015. PDF. Dec. 2015. <http://www.greenpeace.org/international/Global/ international/publications/agriculture/2015/Twenty%20Years%20of%20 Failure.pdf>

22. Bleakly, Claire. "GE Animals in New Zealand—Genetically Engineered

Animals The First Fifteen Years." GE FREE New Zealand. *Gefree.org*, Sept. 2015. PDF. Mar. 2016. <http://www.gefree.org.nz/assets/pdf/GE-Animals-in-New-Zealand.pdf>

23. "UNDER THE INFLUENCE—THE NATIONAL RESEARCH COUNCIL AND GMOS." ISSUE BRIEF. Food & Water Watch. *Foodandwaterwatch.org*, May 2016. PDF. May 2016. <http://www.foodandwaterwatch.org/sites/default/files/ib_1605_nrcinfluence-final-web_0.pdf>

24. Servick, Kelly. "Once Again, U.S. Expert Panel Says Genetically Engineered Crops Are Safe to Eat." Science. *sciencemagazine.org*, 17 May 2016. Web. May 2016. <http://www.sciencemag.org/news/2016/05/us-panel-releases-consensus-genetically-engineered-crops>

25. Weise, Elizabeth. "Academies of Science Finds GMOs Not Harmful to Human Health." USA Today. Gannett, 17 May 2016. Web. May 2016. <http://www.usatoday.com/story/tech/2016/05/17/gmos-safe-academies-of-science-report-genetically-modified-food/84458872/>

26. National Academies of Sciences, Engineering, and Medicine. *Genetically Engineered Crops: Experiences and Prospects*. Washington, DC: The National Academies Press, 2016.doi:10.17226/23395. <http://www.nap.edu/catalog/23395/genetically-engineered-crops-experiences-and-prospects>

27. "Sanders Celebrates as GMO Labeling Dark Act Is Blocked in US Senate. "Sustainable Pulse. *Sustainablepulse.com*, 16 Mar. 2016. Web. Mar. 2016. <http://sustainablepulse.com/2016/03/16/sanders-celebrates-as-new-gmo-labeling-dark-act-is-blocked-in-us-senate/#.Vuy2deIrLIV>

28. Chow, Lorraine. "Cereal Giant General Mills to Start Labeling GMOs Nationwide as Vermont Law Looms." EcoWatch. *Ecowatch.com*, 19 Mar. 2016. Web. Mar. 2016. <http://ecowatch.com/2016/03/19/general-mills-label-gmos/>

29. "Campbell Soup Switches Sides In The GMO Labeling Fight." NPR. *Npr.org*, 08 Jan. 2016. Web. Feb. 2016. <http://www.npr.org/sections/thesalt/2016/01/08/462422610/campbell-soup-switches-sides-in-the-gmo-labeling-fight>

30. Jackson, Rev. Jesse. Letter to President Obama. Rainbow Push Coalition. *sustainablepulse.com*. 14 July. 2016. PDF. July 2016. <http://sustainablepulse.com/wp-content/uploads/2016/08/jesse-jackson-letter-to-obama_12626.pdf>

31. Bjerga, Alan and Angela Greiling Keane. "Obama Ready to Sign Food-Label Bill Consumer Groups Dislike" Bloomberg Politics. *Bloomberg.com*, 13 July 2016. Web. July 2016. <http://www.bloomberg.com/politics/articles/2016-07-13/obama-ready-to-sign-food-label-bill-consumer-groups-find-suspect>

32. Gillam, Carey. "Consumer Groups Demand GMO Labeling, question food safety." Reuters. Reuters.com, 27 Mar.

2012 Web. Dec. 2015. <http://www.reuters.com/article/
us-usa-food-idUSBRE82Q10820120327>

33. Harwell, Drew. "Bayer agrees to buy Monsanto in $66 billion deal that
could reshape agriculture" The Washington Post. Washingtonpost.com,
September 14, 2016. Web. Oct. 2016 <https://www.washingtonpost.
com/business/economy/bayer-agrees-to-buy-monsanto-in-66-billion-deal-
that-could-reshape-agriculture/2016/09/14/4599de48-7aa6-11e6-ac8e-
cf8e0dd91dc7_story.html>

34. Adams, Mike. "Nazi-founded Bayer chemical company wants to buy
Satan-inspired Monsanto for $42 billion… it's a perfect match made in
chemical Hell" Natural News. naturalnews.com, 20 Mar. 2016. Web. Oct.
2016. <http://www.naturalnews.com/054092_Monsanto_acquisition_
Bayer_Nazi_origins.html#ixzz4MA3pl8YY>

35. "Fritz ter Meer" Wikipedia. wikipedia.org. n.d. Web. Oct. 2016 <https://
en.wikipedia.org/wiki/Fritz_ter_Meer>

36. Edwards, Jim. "Bayer Admits it Paid "Millions" in HIV Infection Cases—Just Not in English." CBS News. cbsnews.com 28
Jan. 2011. Web. Oct. 2016. <http://www.cbsnews.com/news/
bayer-admits-it-paid-millions-in-hiv-infection-cases-just-not-in-english/>

37. "Farmer's vs. Monsanto." Food Democracy Now. Fooddemocracynow.org,
n.d. Web. Mar. 2016. Web. April 2016. <http://www.fooddemocracynow.
org/farmers-vs-monsanto>

38. Philpot, Tom. "No, GMOs Didn't Create India's Farmer Suicide
Problem, But…" Mother Jones. Motherjones.com, Sept. 2013. Web.
Mar. 2016. <http://www.motherjones.com/tom-philpott/2015/09/
no-gmos-didnt-create-indias-farmer-suicide-problem>

39. "Indigenous Mayans Win Stunning Repeal of Hated 'Monsanto Law'" Waking Times. Wakingtimes.com, 19 Oct. 2015.
Web. Mar. 2016. <http://www.wakingtimes.com/2015/10/19/
indigenous-mayans-win-stunning-repeal-of-hated-monsanto-law/>

40. Chopra, Mallika. "The Tragedy of Farmers Suicides in India." The
Huffington Post. TheHuffingtonPost.com, 22 May 2011. Web. Mar. 2016.
<http://www.huffingtonpost.com/mallika-chopra/the-tragedy-of-farmers-
su_b_189843.html>

About the Author

April is The *"Cleanfood Advocate."* She recently married and lives with her new husband, daughter and too many pets. Her passion for children's health issues and the role of GMOs and glyphosate has led to her commitment of out-reach and advocacy for the wellness and safety of our children and the food they eat.

Propelled through rabbit holes of information following the discovery that her four year old had 62 food allergies, April delved into the realities of our GMO food supply and the consequences they appear to deliver.

Questioning the corporate model, patents on life, industry science and back door policies that led to the "GMO Revolution," her edgy nature and cheeky poetic perspectives will fire you up, make you think, change you and make you a better parent.

Her original published works can be viewed at:

<http://www.salem-news.com/by_author.php?reporter=April%Scott>

and <http://www.salem-news.com/by_author.php?reporter=April%20Scott&offset=10>

CPSIA information can be obtained
at www.ICGtesting.com
Printed in the USA
FSOW02n0440140317
31712FS